TUMORS of the ADRENAL

Arnold M. Schwartz
1987

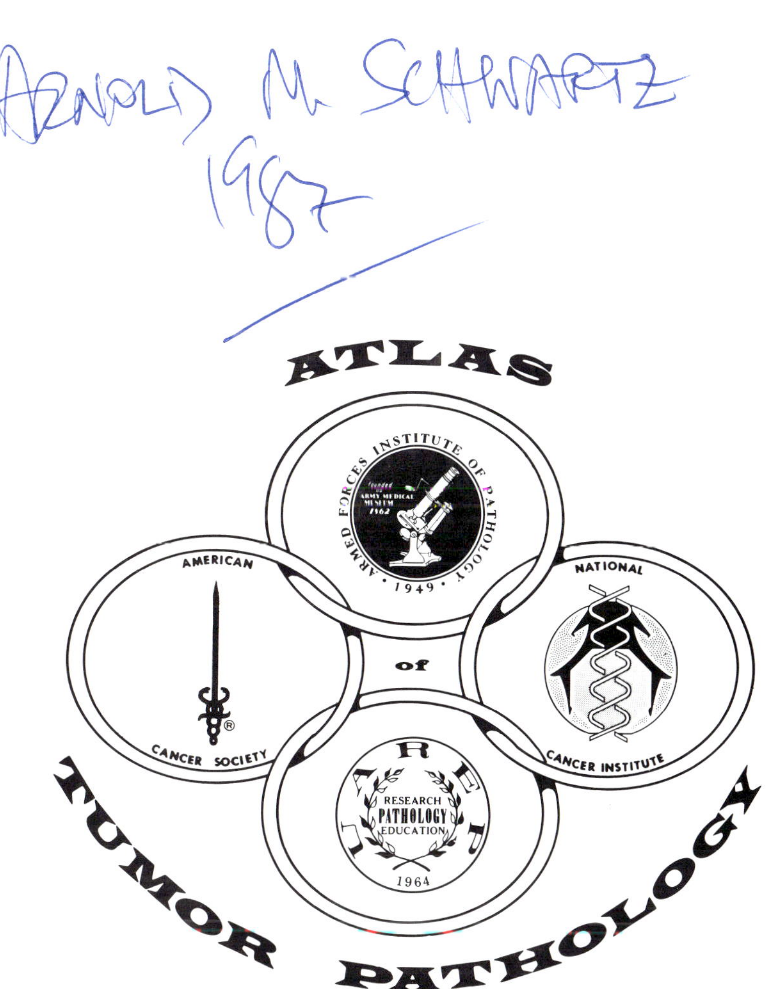

ATLAS OF TUMOR PATHOLOGY

Second Series
Fascicle 23

TUMORS OF THE ADRENAL

by

DAVID L. PAGE, M.D.
Department of Pathology
Vanderbilt University School of Medicine
Nashville, Tennessee 37232

RONALD A. DeLELLIS, M.D.
Department of Pathology
Tufts University School of Medicine
Boston, Massachusetts 02111

and

AUBREY J. HOUGH, Jr., M.D.
Laboratory Services, Veterans Administration Hospital
and
Vanderbilt University School of Medicine
Nashville, Tennessee 37203

Current Address
Professor and Chairman, Department of Pathology
University of Arkansas for Medical Sciences
Little Rock, Arkansas 72205

Published by the
ARMED FORCES INSTITUTE OF PATHOLOGY
Washington, D.C.

Under the Auspices of
UNIVERSITIES ASSOCIATED FOR RESEARCH AND EDUCATION IN PATHOLOGY, INC.
Bethesda, Maryland
1986

Accepted for Publication
1983 — Revised 1985

For sale by the Armed Forces Institute of Pathology
Washington, D.C. 20306-6000
ISSN 0160-6344

ATLAS OF TUMOR PATHOLOGY

Sponsored by

AMERICAN CANCER SOCIETY
ARMED FORCES INSTITUTE OF PATHOLOGY
NATIONAL CANCER INSTITUTE, NATIONAL INSTITUTES OF HEALTH
UNIVERSITIES ASSOCIATED FOR RESEARCH AND EDUCATION IN PATHOLOGY, INC.

EDITOR
WILLIAM H. HARTMANN, M.D.
Professor and Chairman, Department of Pathology
Vanderbilt University School of Medicine
Nashville, Tennessee 37232

COEDITOR
LESLIE H. SOBIN, M.D.
Armed Forces Institute of Pathology
Washington, D.C. 20306-6000

EDITORS' NOTE

The Atlas of Tumor Pathology was originated by the Committee on Pathology of the National Academy of Sciences—National Research Council in 1947. The form of the Atlas became the brainchild of the Subcommittee on Oncology and was shepherded by a succession of editors. It was supported by a long list of agencies; many of the illustrations were made by the Medical Illustration Service of the Armed Forces Institute of Pathology; the type was set by the Government Printing Office; and the final printing was done by the Armed Forces Institute of Pathology. The American Registry of Pathology purchased the Fascicles from the Government Printing Office and sold them at cost, plus a small handling and shipping charge. Over a period of 20 years, 15,000 copies each of 40 Fascicles were produced. They provided a system of nomenclature and set standards for histologic diagnosis which received worldwide acclaim. Private contributions by almost 600 pathologists helped to finance the compilation of an index by The Williams & Wilkins Company to complete the original Atlas.

Following the preparation of the final Fascicle of the first Atlas, the National Academy of Sciences—National Research Council handed over the task of further pursuit of the project to Universities Associated for Research and Education in Pathology, Inc. Grant support for a second series was generously made available by both the National Cancer Institute and the American Cancer Society. The Armed Forces Institute of Pathology has expanded and improved its press facilities to provide for a more rapid and efficient production of the new series. A new Editor and Editorial Advisory Committee were appointed, and the solicitation and preparation of manuscripts continues.

This second series of the Atlas of Tumor Pathology is not intended as a second edition of the first Atlas and, in general, there will be variation in authorship. The basic purpose remains unchanged in providing an Atlas setting standards of diagnosis and terminology. Throughout the rest of this series, the terminology chosen for the World Health Organization's series "International Histological Classification of Tumours" will be used when available. Hematoxylin and eosin stained sections still represent the keystone of histologic diagnosis; therefore, most of the photomicrographs will be of sections stained by this technic, and only sections prepared by other technics will be specifically designated in the legends. It is hoped that in many of the new series a broader perspective of tumors may be offered by the inclusion of special stains, histochemical illustrations, electron micrographs, data on biologic behavior, and other pertinent information when indicated for a better understanding of the disease.

The format of the new series is changed in order to allow better correlation of the illustrations with the text, and a more substantial cover is provided. An index is included in each Fascicle.

It is the hope of the Editors, past and present, the Editorial Advisory Committees, past and present, and the Sponsors that these changes will be welcomed by the readers. Constructive criticisms and suggestions will always be appreciated.

William H. Hartmann, M.D.
Leslie H. Sobin, M.D.

Permission to use copyrighted illustrations has been granted by:

Annual Reviews Inc.:
  Ann. Rev. Pharmacol. 10:199-218, 1970. For figure 29.

Churchill Livingstone:
  Functional Pathology of the Human Adrenal Gland, 1969. For figures 3, 5, 10, and 77.

Gustav Fischer Verlag:
  Beitr. Pathol. 159:371-397, 1976. For figures 78, 80, 81, and 82.

Japan Endocrine Society:
  Endocrinol. Japn. 22:555-560, 1975. For figures 44 and 45.

Lippincott/Harper & Row:
  Am. J. Pathol. 83:177-196, 1976. For figures 4, 199, 200, 201, 202, and 203.
  Am. J. Clin. Pathol. 72:390-399, 1979. For figure 94.
  Am. J. Clin. Pathol. 73:443-447, 1980. For figure 144.

Massachusetts Medical Society:
  N. Engl. J. Med. 300:1322-1328, 1979. For figures 88, 89, and 90.

W. B. Saunders Company:
  Hum. Pathol. 11:205-207, 1980. For figure 186.
  Pediatri. Clin. North Am. 23:161-170, 1976. For figure 225.

PREFACE AND ACKNOWLEDGMENTS

In the three decades since the publication of Tumors of the Adrenal in the first series of Fascicles, our understanding of adrenal disease has been greatly expanded. These changes have come about not so much through elucidation of heretofore undescribed histopathologic entities, but from a greater understanding of pathophysiology and its association with certain recognizable anatomic findings. For these reasons, we have chosen to consider adrenal neoplasms and related conditions from both anatomic and functional standpoints.

This extensive discussion of function as well as anatomy has led to repetition, but, hopefully, also to clarification and increased usefulness of this volume. The anatomic study of the enlarged or neoplastic adrenal is often secondary in importance to the definition of hormonal dysfunction. This is due to the primacy of disease causation by hormonal excess or deficiency and the need to diagnose these conditions by biochemical, physiologic, and pharmacologic means before anatomic correlation is attempted. We hope the usefulness of this volume is enhanced because clinicians may begin with the functional aspects and proceed to histopathology. Conversely, anatomic pathologists will better appreciate the necessity of understanding the functional attributes of an individual case rather than attempting a diagnosis without reference to clinical data. The anatomic approach in each clinical setting is different, as are the questions to ask or to expect to be answered. For example, in most pheochromocytomas, the diagnosis is made by biochemical and pharmacologic means. At the other extreme, the possible adrenal origin of poorly differentiated retroperitoneal neoplasms will often rest solely on anatomic study. The histopathologist can only hope that endocrine evaluation had been or can be done to help in this task. The primary function of surgical pathologists in adrenal disease lies in predicting the likelihood of malignant behavior, recognizing previously unsuspected adrenal origin, and classifying the nature of lesions to predict the status of the contralateral glands.

Although the three authors have collaborated on all portions of this Fascicle, discussions concerning the adrenal medulla are primarily the work of one author (R.D.). The presentations relative to the adrenal cortex are the result of close collaboration between the remaining two authors (D.P. and A.H.) over a considerable number of years.

We wish to thank Dr. James Oertel, Chief of the Endocrinology Branch, Armed Forces Institute of Pathology, and Dr. Elgin Cowart and Dr. William R. Cowan, Directors, Armed Forces Institute of Pathology, for making the facilities of this institute available to us. The aid of Mrs. Audrey Cyr and Mrs. Sherry Kloak of the editorial office was invaluable, as was the expert secretarial support of Annelle Johnson.

The preparation of the section on localization of adrenal disease is largely due to the efforts of Drs. Craig Coulam and A. James Gerlock, Jr., of Vanderbilt University School of Medicine, Nashville, TN. We acknowledge with thanks helpful consultations with the following physicians: Drs. H. William Scott, Jr., Grant W. Liddle, David N. Orth, John Hollifield, Ian Burr, and James Sullivan, all of Vanderbilt University School of Medicine, Nashville, TN;

Richard B. Cohen and James Connolly, Beth Israel Hospital and Harvard University School of Medicine, Boston, MA; Arthur Tischler of Tufts University School of Medicine, Boston, MA; Sir Thomas Symington, University of Edinburgh, Edinburgh, Scotland; and Professor A. Munro Neville, Ludwig Institute for Cancer Research, Royal Marsden Hospital, Sutton, Surrey, England.

We are indebted to the staff of the Medical Illustrations Service of the Nashville Veterans Administration Medical Center, Mr. Ron Gregory of Vanderbilt University School of Medicine, and Mr. Steven Halpern of the Tufts University Medical School for expert preparation of many of the photomicrographs.

Finally, we wish to thank the following physicians for having generously shared their case material with us: Albert Stanek, State University of New York, Downstate Medical Center, NY; Samuel L. Orr, Charlotte Memorial Hospital, Charlotte, NC; G.A.K. Missen, Guy's Hospital, London, England; James Connolly, Harvard University, Boston, MA; Ella H. Oppenheimer, Johns Hopkins School of Medicine, Baltimore, MD; Hideo Hidai, Yokohama City University School of Medicine, Yokohama, Japan; Karin Gorgas, University of Cologne, Cologne, Federal Republic of Germany; Albert E. Kalderon, University of Arkansas for Medical Science, Little Rock, AR; G. Richard Dickersin, Massachusetts General Hospital and Harvard Medical School, Boston, MA; A. Munro Neville, Ludwig Institute for Cancer Research, Royal Marsden Hospital, Sutton, Surrey, England; William A. Gardner, Nashville Veterans Administration Medical Center and Vanderbilt University School of Medicine, Nashville, TN; George F. Gray, Cornell University Medical School, New York, NY; Alan D. Glick, Vanderbilt University School of Medicine, Nashville, TN; Louis S. Graham, Jr., St. Thomas Hospital, Nashville, TN; J.D. Maynard, Gordon Museum, Guy's Hospital, London, England; Clifton K. Meador, St. Thomas Hospital, Nashville, TN; and Barbara Carter, Victor Millan, and John Leonidas, all of New England Medical Center Hospital, Boston, MA. The Departments of Pathology at the following medical centers generously made their museums of specimens available to us: Leeds University, Leeds, England; Radcliffe Infirmary, Oxford University, Oxford, England; Royal Marsden Hospital, London, England; and the Johns Hopkins Hospital, Baltimore, MD.

David L. Page, M.D.
Ronald A. DeLellis, M.D.
Aubrey J. Hough, Jr., M.D.

TUMORS OF THE ADRENAL

Contents

TUMORS OF THE ADRENAL

INTRODUCTION

HISTORICAL ASPECTS

Early Theories and Discoveries
(1563-1856)

One searches in vain among the works of classical Greco-Roman medicine for descriptions of the adrenal glands. The first accurate anatomic description of the adrenal glands (fig. 1) is attributed to Bartholomeaus Eustachius (1563), although his works were not edited and published until 1722 (Eustachius). Some authors (Bachmann) maintain that the adrenals were well known in Biblical times, due to references in Leviticus. However, descriptions of the adrenal glands are conspicuously absent from treatises of anatomy prior to Eustachius and from several subsequent to that time (Biedl).

Erroneous anatomic interpretations during the early seventeenth century fostered misconceptions about adrenal pathophysiology which persisted for over 200 years. Schenk, in 1600, described a central cavity (the dilated central vein) in the adrenal glands (Rolleston). Thomas Bartholinus postulated that this cavity contained black bile which was purified and drained by a vein to the kidney. This view of the adrenals or "capsule atrabilariae," as Bartholinus named them, as detoxifying organs dominated medical thought for over 200 years and persisted as late as 1930 (Sorkin). Although this concept and its many variations may now seem absurd, it was but a

logical outgrowth of the humoral theory of medicine which had led Galen to postulate the pituitary as the secretor of nasal mucus (Rolleston). Riolan, who discounted the central cavity, advocated in 1629 that the adrenals functioned only in fetal life. Erroneous interpretations of the genitourinary vasculature led several authors to postulate nonexistent excretory ducts draining to various organs.

The elaboration of a conceptual theory preceded the period of great discoveries about the adrenal glands. This theory was that of glands of internal secretion as described by DeBordeu (1752) and subsequently popularized by Claude Bernard (1855). Addison (1849, 1855) described the clinical syndrome of adrenal hypofunction, and Brown-Séquard (1856) showed that the adrenals were essential to life in dogs. After these concepts became popular, discoveries about the adrenal glands began to occur rapidly.

Adrenal Medulla

Although identification of a pressor substance contained within the adrenal medulla was not achieved until 1895 (Oliver and Schafer), by the late nineteenth century the functional and embryologic dichotomy between cortex and medulla was becoming apparent. Vulpian (1856) and Henle (1865) demonstrated that the central regions of the gland differed in staining characteristics from the outer portions, and Kölliker (1861)

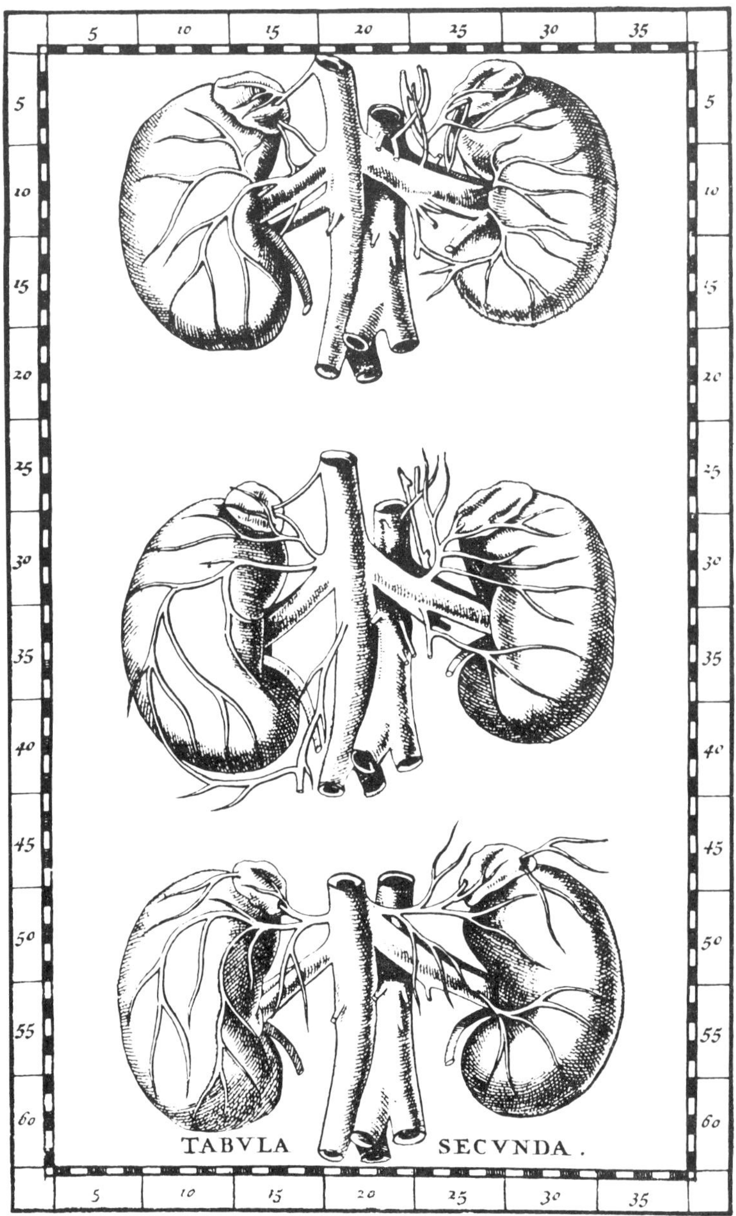

Figure 1
GROSS ANATOMY
Early description of adrenal glands by Eustachius in 1563 was accompanied by this
illustration. (Courtesy of Vanderbilt University History of Medicine Collection.)

showed that the cortex formed first during fetal development and was subsequently invaded by the neural elements of the medulla. Kohn, in 1898, applied the term "chromaffin" to describe these cells, since they selectively darkened after exposure to potassium dichromate. Epinephrine was isolated from the gland by Abel and Crawford in 1897 and Takamine first obtained crystalline preparations of l-epinephrine in 1901. Fränkel (1886) is generally credited with the first description of pheochromocytoma. His patient, an 18 year old woman with a one year history of headache, vomiting, pallor, and recurrent episodes of palpitation, was found to have bilateral adrenal medullary tumors. Manasse, in 1896, was the first to demonstrate that these neoplasms of the adrenal medulla gave a positive chromaffin reaction. In 1908, Alezais and Peyron used the term "paraganglioma" to describe extra-adrenal chromaffin positive neoplasms. A considerable period of time passed, however, before the association between paroxysmal hypertension and adrenal medullary tumors was firmly established (Coller et al., 1934). Both vonEuler and Holtz and his associates demonstrated norepinephrine in the sympathetic nervous system. Holtz and associates later showed that the adrenal medulla contained norepinephrine in addition to epinephrine. In the early 1950's, vonEuler showed that patients with pheochromocytoma excreted increased amounts of epinephrine and norepinephrine in the urine. These workers set the stage for the application of sensitive methods for the detection of catecholamines and their metabolites in the urine of patients with pheochromocytoma and other tumors of the adrenal medulla and associated paraganglia.

Adrenal Cortex

The characteristic histologic zones of the adrenal cortex were described by Arnold in 1866. However, the debate whether cortex or medulla were essential to life continued until 1917 (Wheeler and Vincent). Subsequently, Hartman and associates (1927) proved that relatively pure adrenal cortical extracts free of epinephrine cured the clinical syndrome of adrenal insufficiency. By 1929 (Moehlig), the concept of a pituitary hormone controlling the adrenal cortex was firmly established.

The 75-year period (1855-1930) of landmark studies of adrenal hypofunction was followed by an era of equally important discoveries about the hyperfunctioning adrenal cortex (Albright, 1943). Cushing (1932) described the association of adrenal cortical hyperplasia and small basophilic adenomas of the anterior pituitary. It became apparent to Walters and associates (1934) that a syndrome identical to that described by Cushing occurred in patients without pituitary adenomas. These patients had adenomas and carcinomas of the adrenal cortex instead.

The association between adrenal tumors and virilism had been seen at autopsy in 1811 (Rolleston). Early surgical attempts to remove virilizing adrenal cortical tumors were reported by 1890 (Thornton), with the observation that the virilism recurred in parallel with the growth of the tumor. However, many such tumors were reported as sarcomas (Adams, 1905) or tumors of other organs.

Retrospective analysis of art and literature suggests that virilism and precocious puberty of the type associated with adrenal malignancies were known in the middle ages (Rolleston). However, a general recognition of the adrenogenital syndrome due to either congenital hyperplasia or tumor occurred in the twentieth century (Krabbe).

Although the unique histologic character of the zona glomerulosa was appreciated in the mid-nineteenth century, the specific contribution of the cells to mineral metabolism, aldosterone, was not isolated until 1952 (Simpson et al.) and the clinical syndrome of hyperaldosteronism was not described until 1955 (Conn).

The contributions of physicians and scientists of the past 400 years form an extensive framework on which the clinical and pathologic diagnoses of adrenal tumors and their associated syndromes are based. For more information than that provided in this brief overview, the reader is directed to comprehensive reviews on the subject by Bachmann (1954), Rolleston (1936), Sorkin (1957), and Thorn (1968).

References

Abel, J. J. and Crawford, A. C. On the blood-pressure-raising constitutent of the suprarenal capsule. Bull. Johns Hopkins Hosp. 8:151-156, 1897.

Adams, C. E. A case of precocious development associated with a tumour of the left suprarenal body. Trans. Pathol. Soc. Lond. 56:208-212, 1905.

Addison, T. Anemia — Disease of the Supra-renal Capsules, pp. 517-518. In: The London Medical Gazette. London: Longman, Brown, Green, and Longmans, 1849.

__________. On the Constitutional and Local Effects of Disease of the Supra-renal Capsules. London: S. Highley, 1855.

Albright, F. Cushing's Syndrome. Harvey Lectures 38:123-186, 1943.

Alezais, H. and Peyron, A. Un Groupe Nouveau de Tumeurs Epithéliales: Les Paragangliomes, pp. 745-747. In: Société de Biologie, 2d. Ed. Paris: Masson et Cie, 1908.

Arnold, J. Ein beitrag zu der feineren structur und dem chemismus der nebennieren. Virchows Arch. 35:64-107, 1866.

Bachmann, R. Die nebenniere. I. Die Geschichte der Nebenniereforschung, pp. 1-14. In: Handbuch der Mikroskopischen Anatomie des Menschen Bd. 6, Teil 5. Berlin: Springer-Verlag, 1954.

Bartholinus, T. Anatomica Ex Caspari Bartholini Parentis Institutionibus. Lugdini Batavorum: Apud Franciseum Hackium, 1651. London: John Streater, 1668.

Bernard, Claude. Remarques sur la sécrétion du sucre dans le foie faites à l'occasion de la communication de M. Lehmann. Comptes Rendus 40:589-592, 1855.

Biedl, A. Die geschichtliche entwicklung der kenntnisse ueber die nebenniere bis Addison (1855). Janus 15:192-219, 1910.

Brown-Séquard, E. Recherches expérimentales sur la physiologie et la pathologie des capsules surrénales. Arch. Généales de Médecine 8:385-401, 1856.

Coller, F. A., Field, H., Jr., and Durant, T. M. Chromaffin cell tumor causing paroxysmal hypertension, relieved by operation. Arch. Surg. 28:1136-1148, 1934.

Conn, J. W. Part II. Primary aldosteronism: a new clinical syndrome. J. Lab. Clin. Med. 45:3-17, 1955.

Cushing, H. The basophil adenomas of the pituitary body and their clinical manifestations (pituitary basophilism). Bull. Johns Hopkins Hosp. 50:137-195, 1932.

DeBordeu, T. Recherches Anatomique sur la Position des Blandes et sur Leur Action, p. 227. Paris: 1752.

Eustachius, B. Tabulae Anatomicae. Edited by Lancisius. Amsterdam, 1722.

Fränkel, F. Ein Fall von doppelseitigem, völlig latent verlaufenen Nebennierentumor und gleichzeitiger. Nephritis mit veränderungen am circulations apparat und retinitis. Virchows Arch. Pathol. Anat. 103:244, 1886.

Hartman, F. A., MacArthur, C. G., and Hartman, W. E. A substance which prolongs the life of adrenalectomized cats. Proc. Soc. Exp. Biol. Med. 25:69-70, 1927.

Henle, J. Ueber das Gewebe der Nebenniere und der Hypophyse, pp. 143-152. In: Zeitschrift für Rationalle Medicin. Henle, J. and Pfeufer, C. (Eds.). Leipzig and Heidelberg: C. F. Wintersche Verlagshandlung, 1865.

Holtz, P., Credner, K., and Kroneberg, G. Über das sympathicomimetische pressorische Prinzip des Harns ("Urosympathin"). Arch. Exp. Pathol. Pharmakol. 204:228-243, 1947.

Kohn, A. Das chromaffine Gewebe. Ergeb. Anat. Entwicklungsgesch 12:253-348, 1902.

Kölliker, A. Entwickelungsgeschichte des Menschen und Hoheren Thiere. 1861.

Krabbe, K. H. The relation between the adrenal cortex and sexual development. New York Med. J. 114:4-8, 1921.

Manasse, P. Zur histologie und histogenese der primären Nierengeschwülste. Virchows Arch. 145:113-157, 1896.

Moehlig, R. C. The pituitary gland and the suprarenal cortex. Arch. Int. Med. 44:339-343, 1929.

Oliver, G. and Schäfer, E. A. The physiological effects of extracts of the suprarenal capsules. J. Physiol. 18:230-276, 1894.

Pick, L. Das ganglioma embryonale sympathicum (sympathoma embryonale). Berl. Klin. Wschr. 49:16-22, 1920.

Riolan, J. Les Oeuvres Anatomiques. Paris, 1629.

Rolleston, H. D. The Endocrine Organs in Health and Disease with an Historical Review, pp. 301-384. London: Oxford University Press, 1936.

Simpson, S. A., Tait, J. F., and Bush, I. E. Secretion of a salt-retaining hormone by the mammalian adrenal cortex. Lancet 2:226-228, 1952.

Sorkin, S. Z. The adrenals before Addison. Mt. Sinai Hosp. J. 24:1238-1247, 1957.

Takamine, J. The blood-pressure-raising principle of the suprarenal glands — a preliminary report. Therapeutic Gazette 25:221-224, 1901.

Thorn, G. W. The adrenal cortex. Johns Hopkins Med. J. 123:49-77, 1968.

Thornton, J. K. Abdominal Nephrectomy for Large Sarcoma of the Left Suprarenal Capsule: Recovery, pp. 150-153. In: Transactions of the Clinical Society of London, Vol. 23. London: Longmans, Green, and Co., 1890.

von Euler, U. S. Increased urinary excretion of noradrenaline and adrenaline in cases of pheochromocytoma. Ann. Surg. 134:929-933, 1951.

__________. III. Epinephrine and norepinephrine. Pharmacol. Rev. 6:15-22, 1954.

Vulpian, A. Note sur quelques reactions propres à la substance des capsules surrénales. C. R. Acad. Sci. [D] (Paris) 43:663-665, 1856.

Walters, W., Wilder, R. M., and Kepler, E. J. The suprarenal cortical syndrome with presentation of ten cases. Ann. Surg. 100:670-688, 1934.

Wheeler, T. D. and Vincent, S. The question as to the relative importance to life of cortex and medulla of the adrenal bodies. Trans. Roy. Soc. Canada 11:125-127, 1917.

Wiesel, J. Zur pathologie des chromaffinen systemes. Virchows Arch. 176:103-114, 1904.

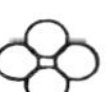

ANATOMY

GROSS ANATOMY

In man, the adrenal glands sit as caps over the medial aspects of the kidneys. The convex surface of the kidney produces a concave inferolateral surface in each adrenal. The right adrenal is roughly triangular in outline, with its anterior surface approaching the posteromedial border of the left kidney and the lateral aspect of the aorta. Usually, the two glands are completely surrounded by perirenal fat. Occasionally, part of the glands, particularly their lateral portions, may lie within the renal capsule. Much more rarely, a portion of the gland may be included within the hepatic capsule (fig. 2).

The adult human adrenal gland may be considered to have a tripartite structure and includes head, body, and tail regions (figs. 3, 4). The head is placed medially in the body. Medullary tissue is not uniformly present throughout the gland, but is concentrated in the head and body regions. The medulla occupies 8 to 10 percent of the volume of the gland. In an autopsy study of adrenal glands of accident victims, Quinan and Berger, after careful dissection of cortical tissue, found mean medullary weights of 0.43 and 0.44 g for the left and right adrenals, respectively. Utilizing a morphometric technic, DeLellis and associates found an estimated average medullary weight of 0.47 ± 0.15 g. In the adult gland, the average cortico:medullary ratios are 5:1 and 14.7:1 in the head and body regions, respectively (fig. 4). Medullary tissue is absent from the tail region of the gland. The medullary tissue is light gray and is

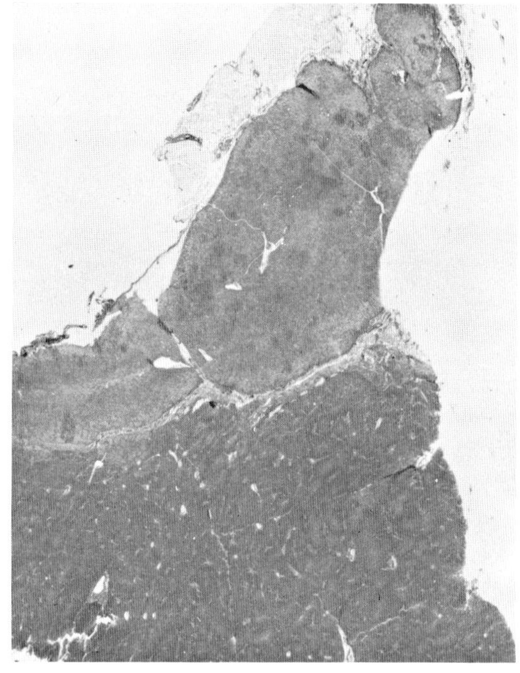

Figure 2
GROSS ANATOMY
Fusion of adrenal gland (upper) and liver (lower) is seen as an incidental finding at autopsy. Hematoxylin and eosin stain.* X5.

immediately surrounded by an inner portion of the cortical tissue, which is brown (pl. I-A). The outer cortex is yellow because of lipid content, although this lipid is often reduced at autopsy.

The weight of the normal adult adrenal gland varies, but tends to be about 4 g each in cases of sudden, unexpected death, as well as in glands removed surgically for disease in the kidney (Symington). Combined weights of about 12 g for both adrenals may be expected at autopsy following an extended illness. Therefore, a surgically excised adrenal weighing over 6 g after careful removal of surrounding fat is

---

*Throughout the Fascicle where the stain is not designated, hematoxylin and eosin stain has been used.

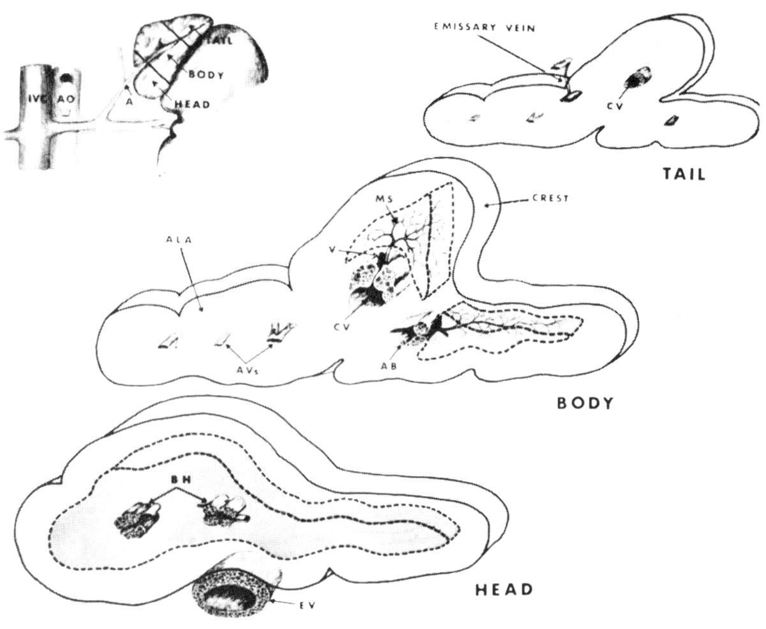

Figure 3
GROSS ANATOMY
Schematic representation of left adrenal gland showing head, body, and tail with distribution of venous drainage and illustrating discontinuous nature of central adrenal vein musculature. AO = aorta; IVC = inferior vena cava; EV = external vein; BH = branches to head; AVs = alar veins; CV = central vein; V = venule; MS = medullary sinuses; AB = alar branch; A = adrenal vein. (From Symington, T. In: Functional Pathology of the Human Adrenal Gland. Edinburgh: Churchill Livingstone, 1969).

probably enlarged (Bloodworth). There is no difference in adrenal weight between the sexes.

The adrenal glands have an abundant arterial supply from branches of the inferior phrenic artery superiorly, the aorta and the renal artery inferiorly (fig. 5). In addition, branches from the ovarian and internal spermatic artery on the left side and branches from the intercostal arteries on either side are often present. Sixty or more small arterial branches pass from these sources to the anterior and posterior surfaces of the gland, where they form an extensive subcapsular plexus. On the right, the short adrenal vein drains directly into the vena cava, while the left adrenal vein drains either into the left renal vein or the vena cava. A small vein on each side courses along with the inferior phrenic vessels and other small veins may be present. It is evident that many arteries reach the adrenal, piercing the cortex, and that one major vein drains each gland.

MICROSTRUCTURE, CORTEX

The classical division of the adrenal cortex into three histologic layers is useful (Bachmann), although the functional relationship(s) are not completely clarified (Neville and Davidson). The **zona glomer ulosa** lies immediately beneath the thick

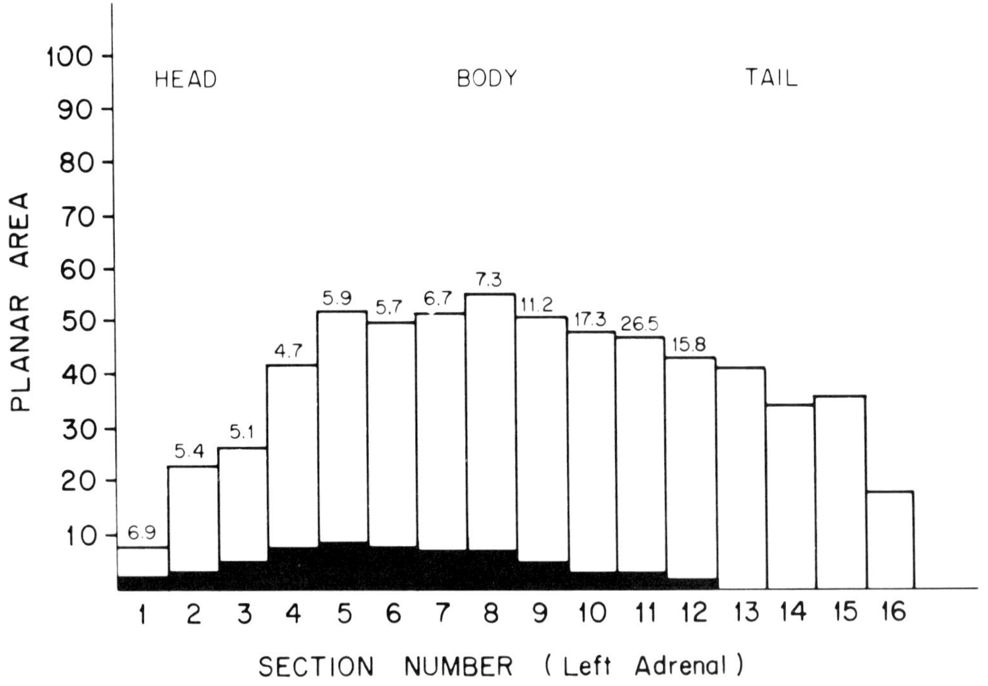

Figure 4
GROSS ANATOMY
This histogram illustrates the ratios of cortical and medullary areas in a normal human adrenal gland. The x-axis represents the section number proceeding from the head of the gland (1) to the tail (16). The y-axis represents the planar area in square millimeters. The medulla is indicated by the closed columns, while opened columns represent cortical areas (From DeLellis, R.A., Wolfe, H.J., Gagel, R.F., et al. Adrenal medullary hyperplasia. Am. J. Pathol. 83:177-196, 1976.)

fibrous capsule and is made up of rounded collections of several cells in thickness, bordered by delicate connective tissue and capillaries. The nuclei are smaller and darker than in other layers, centrally placed in a relatively clear cytoplasm with lipid content intermediate between that of the other two layers (fig. 6). This layer is not clearly demarcated from inner zones and precise identification is further hampered by the discontinuity of this layer, as the fasciculate zone (zona fasciculata) often extends to the capsule.

The **zona fasciculata** is the thickest of the three layers, with cells present in long regular columns between the other two layers (pl. I-B). The columns are roughly radially symmetrical about the central vein, although later in life nodular irregularities in this arrangement are relatively common. In the unstressed patient, the cells have a large amount of clear cytoplasm (fig. 6), representing lipid storage (clear cells). In situations of stress or ACTH administration, the cells of this zone, focally and later diffusely, lose cytoplasmic lipid and come to resemble the compact cells of the reticular zone (fig. 7).

The innermost zone of the cortex, **zona reticularis,** is usually well demarcated from

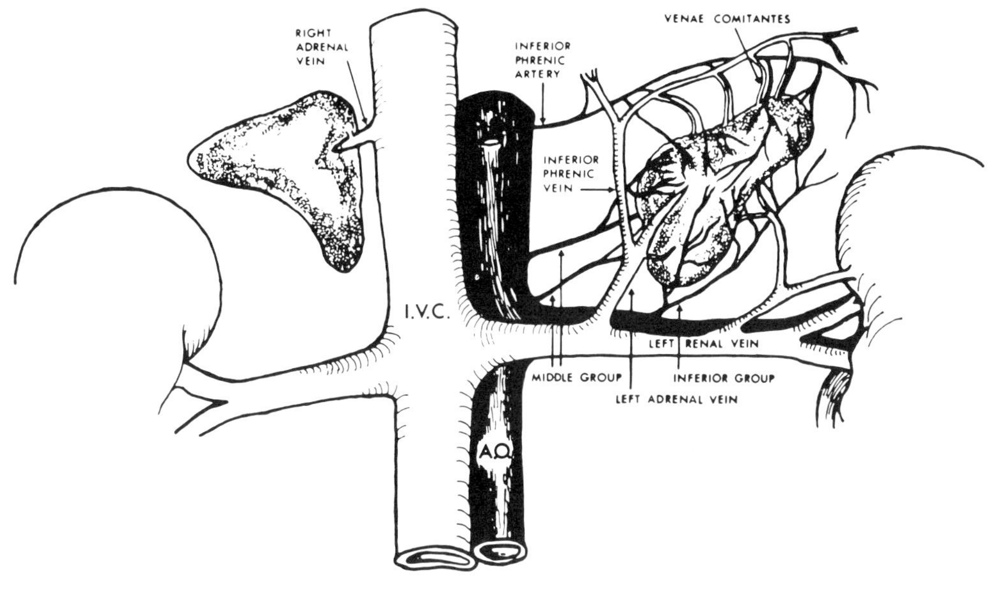

Figure 5
GROSS ANATOMY
Schematic demonstrates arterial supply to and venous drainage from the left adrenal gland. IVC = inferior vena cava; AO = aorta. (From Symington, T. In: Functional Pathology of the Human Adrenal Gland. Edinburgh: Churchill Livingstone, 1969.)

the medulla internally (fig. 8) and in the unstressed state is abruptly separated from the fasciculate zone. The cells of this reticular zone are arranged in slightly irregular columns or cords, somewhat larger than those of the zona glomerulosa. There is a tendency for these cords to be arranged with a long axis parallel to those of the overlying fasciculate zone. The cytoplasm is eosinophilic, as opposed to clear. Little lipid is present and there is a prominent reticulin framework. In adults, lipofuscin is often seen within this layer (pl. I-C, D).

The biochemical-physiologic definition of three adrenal steroid types (glucocorticoids, mineralocorticoids, and sex steroids), coupled with the histologic definition of three layers in the adrenal cortex, made the assumption of a 1·1 relationship inevitable. This assumption has been termed the zonation theory, ascribing one hormone type to each histologic region. A seemingly opposed notion was termed the migration theory, maintaining that the varied appearances of the cortex were related to migration of cells centripetally from the subcapsular region where cell division took place. Currently, it appears that each theory holds partial truth. It is certain that in the intact adrenal, aldosterone is released from cells of the zona glomerulosa and that the glomerulosa does not atrophy in the absence of ACTH. The remainder of the adrenal cortex appears to have no definite regional variation as to steroid type released, although the quantity released and responsiveness to ACTH probably varies between the two inner zones. ACTH administration causes the clear cells at the interface of the zona fasciculata and zona reticularis to change to compact cells, losing their lipid. This change extends

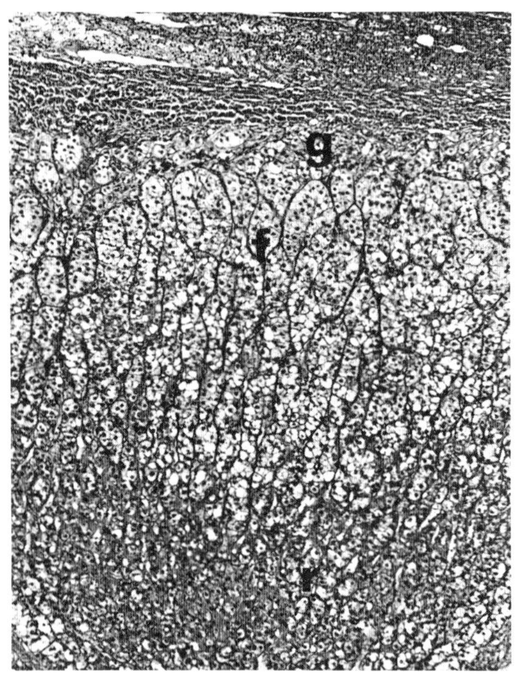

Figure 6
MICROSTRUCTURE, CORTEX
Normal unstressed adrenal gland of patient dying acutely of gunshot wound demonstrates prominent lipid filled fasciculate (f) zone. The small band of zona glomerulosa (g) lies immediately beneath the capsule. This photograph demonstrates the full cortical thickness, with dark compact cells of the zona reticularis (r) inferiorly. X40.

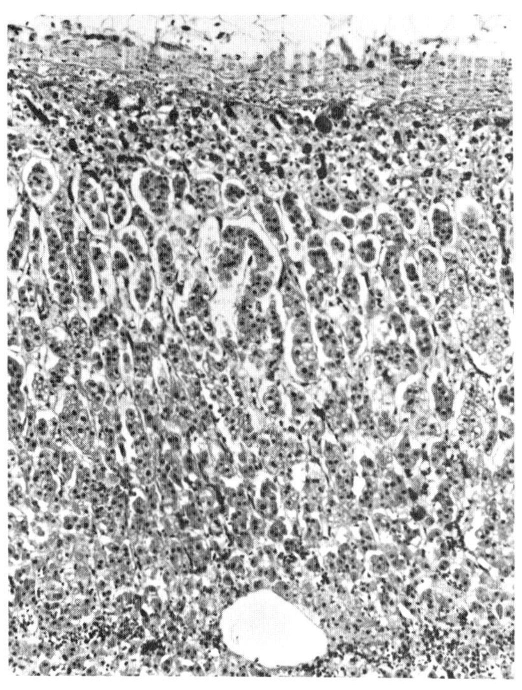

Figure 7
MICROSTRUCTURE, CORTEX
Stressed adrenal gland from patient dying from debilitating carcinomatosis demonstrates lipid depletion of fasciculate zone. X75.

centrifugally toward the capsule, resulting in alteration of all zona fasciculata cells into compact cells under the prolonged influence of ACTH. The stimuli causing increase in cell numbers are not understood.

Cells removed from their in situ framework do not remain functionally fixed. Specifically, after a short time in culture, cells from any part of the adrenal cortex are capable of responding to ACTH primarily by release of glucocorticoids (O'Hare et al.). Cultured glomerulosa cells tend to lose their ability to assemble aldosterone with time; however, evidence of local increase of steroids in culture medium will allow maintenance of differentiated zona glomerulosa function (Crivello et al.). Thus, the relationship of cells to each other, the influences of vascular pattern, or microenvironment must be determinants of activity and biosynthetic pathways in situ (Bertholet; Dickerman et al.). Therefore, the zones are not closed compartments with defined function and, thus, the zonation theory is not completely explanatory. It has been demonstrated in rats, and is likely true in man, that patterns of adrenal cortical cell renewal involve most cell division occurring in the zona glomerulosa with few mitoses in other layers (Wright and Voncina). Cell migration occurs into the inner zones and most cell death occurs in the adrenal cortex

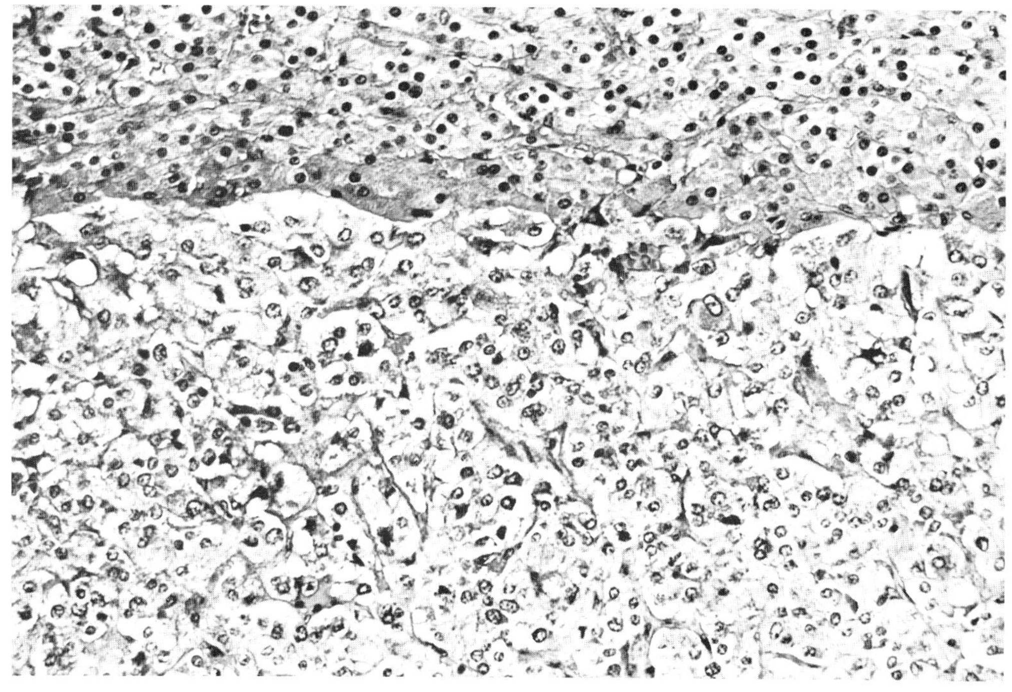

Figure 8
MICROSTRUCTURE, CORTEX
Sharp demarcation between inner zone of cortex (above) and medulla (below) is usually apparent. X100.

adjacent to the adrenal medulla (Wyllie et al.) Therefore, some combination of the migration and zonation theories appears to explain the cell renewal and functional patterns in the adrenal cortex.

The practical significance of zonation in the anatomic evaluation of adrenals in man relates primarily to changes which occur during heightened ACTH stimulation. Particularly, the work of Symington, in Glasgow, showed that the alteration of lipid filled cells to compact cells under the extreme influence of ACTH is followed by the peculiar "reversion pattern" which tends to occur when the ACTH stimulus is lessened. This produces a very odd histologic appearance in the adrenal because the return of a clear cell status proceeds, as does the change to compact cells, from central region toward the capsule. Thus, an increased number of compact cells may be seen in the outer portion of the zona fasciculata adjacent to the zona glomerulosa. These cells mimic zona glomerulosa in appearance and may lead to the false impression that the zona glomerulosa is increased in cell number.

Cortical cells are characteristically present in discontinuous foci adjacent to the central veins (fig. 9). These seemingly displaced cells are thus separated from the reticulate zone by cells of the medulla in areas where medullary tissue is present and may be intermixed with cells of the medulla. This perivenous zone of cortical cells resembles glomerulosa adjacent to the vein and fasciculata in the outer portions, although precise identification is usually impossible.

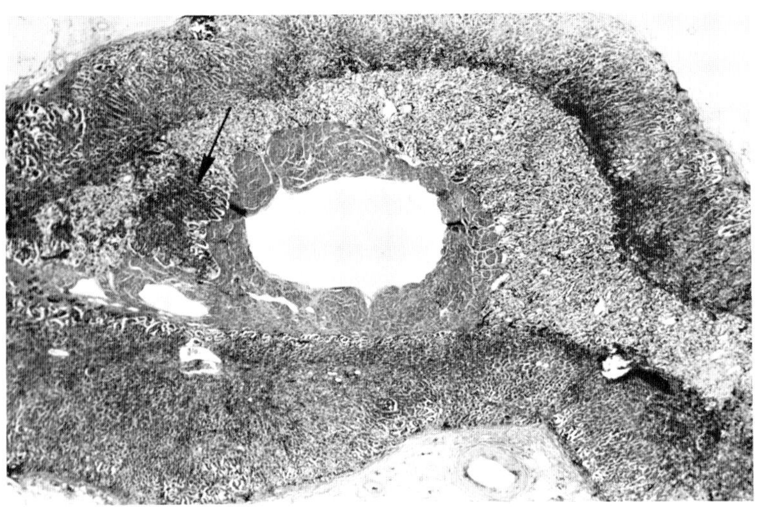

Figure 9
MICROSTRUCTURE, CORTEX
Foci of cortex are often present in the medulla adjacent to the central vein as noted
(arrow) in this case at the left of the discontinuous muscle bundles of central vein.
These cortical cells are surrounded by lighter cells of the medulla. X12.

The arrangement of microvasculature follows from the gross arrangement (fig. 10). A great number of small arteries and arterioles ramify over the capsule and divide to form a subcapsular plexus of arterioles. Some of these arterioles traverse the cortex and supply the medulla directly. Most arterioles of the subcapsular area branch into the rich mass of anastomosing capillaries (Motta et al.) around the columns of the cells of the reticulate zone to a rich plexus in the zona reticularis. From the region of the cortico-medullary junction, blood drains into branches of the central vein which has prominent longitudinal muscle bundles, often varying in thickness. This characteristic is a regular feature of the central vein and its tributaries (Dobbie and Symington).

Histochemical procedures in the adrenal cortex have been developed (Arvy), but have not yet realized general diagnostic usefulness. Demonstration of steroid specific enzymes, particularly steroid 3-B -ol dehydrogenase, may be useful in establishing adrenal origin for metastatic neoplasm (Idelman; Dawson et al.). Despite this promise, we are not aware that they have been used for this purpose. Immunohistochemical localization of specific steroid hormones has been used to aid in the understanding of function in testicular and ovarian tumors (Taylor et al.; Kurman et al.). The usefulness of this technic in the identification of functional correlates in adrenal tissue is evident and is currently being developed (Okano et al).

Some generally available special stains are useful in specific situations. Stains for fat, such as oil red O (pl. I-E), are useful for the demonstration of variations in cytoplasmic lipid content associated with nodular adrenal glands and the characteristic "Maltese cross" appearance of cholesterol may be seen when fresh frozen sections of adrenal cortex are viewed in polarized light. The PAS stain gives remarkably good

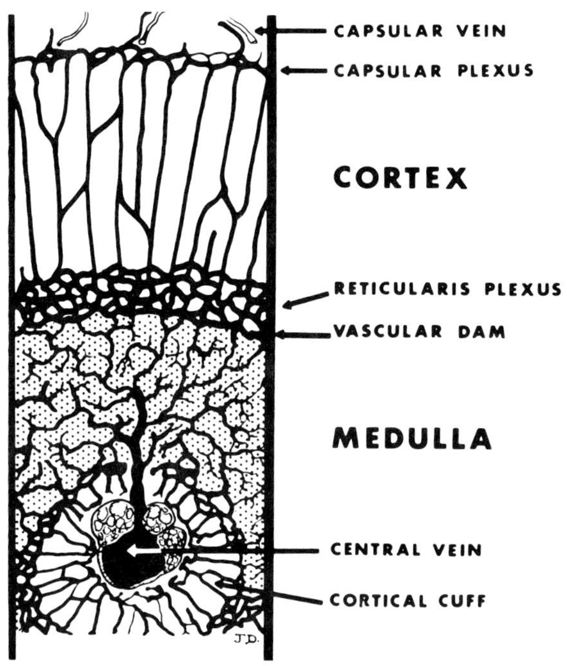

Figure 10
MICROSTRUCTURE, CORTEX
Diagrammatic representation of intraglandular venous drainage of adrenal demonstrates rich capillary plexuses of head and body regions. (From Symington, T. In: Functional Pathology of the Human Adrenal Gland. Edinburgh: Churchill Livingstone, 1969.)

visualization of the excessive lipofuscin pigment associated with several forms of adrenal cortical disease (pl. I-D). The luxol fast blue technic is a method for differentiating medullary tissue (normal, hyperplastic, or neoplastic) from adrenal cortex. This stain demonstrates nerves present between groups of medullary cells.

Adrenal cortical cells possess ultrastructural characteristics typical of cells adapted for synthesis of steroid hormones (Mackay; Fawcett et al.). Therefore, the ultrastructural appearance of adrenal cortical cells is not dissimilar from that of the steroid producing cells of the ovary or testis. Features common to these cells include numerous liposomes, extensive smooth endoplasmic reticulum (SER), a prominent Golgi apparatus, parallel arrays of rough endoplasmic reticulum, and numerous specialized mitochondria (Mackay). In the absence of ACTH, adrenal cortical cells lose their specialized features both in vivo and in vitro.

The distribution and types of cellular organelles vary from zone to zone within the adrenal cortex (Table 1). However, the relatively sharp transitions between the zones noted with light microscopy are less apparent at the ultrastructural level, since transition zones are noted between both zona glomerulosa and fasciculata and between zona fasciculata and reticularis (Mackay; Tannenbaum, 1973; Bloodworth; Neville and O'Hare).

The zona glomerulosa (ZG) is characterized by relatively scanty SER, lipid and lysosomes, and many elongated mitochondria containing small lamellar cristae. Stimulation of this region by angiotensin II produces lipid depletion, cytoplasmic volume increase, and hypertrophy of mitochondria as well as smooth endoplasmic reticulum (Mazzocchi et al.). The Golgi apparatus is

Table 1

ULTRASTRUCTURE OF HUMAN ADRENOCORTICAL CELLS

Parameter	Zona Glomerulosa	Zona Fasciculata		Zona Reticularis
		Outer	Inner	
Cytoplasmic volume	Small	Very large	Large	Intermediate
Smooth endoplasmic reticulum (SER)	Scanty	Scanty	Prominent	Densely packed
Mitochondria	Elongated, small, lamellar cristae	Ovoid, small, few internal short tubules and vesicles	Spherical, variable size, many internal vesicles	Ovoid, medium sized tubulovesicular cristae
Lipid content	Scanty, free, osmiophilic	Many osmiophilic free droplets or empty vacuoles	Many osmiophilic free droplets or empty vacuoles	Very few vacuoles or osmiophilic droplets
Lysosomes and lipofuscin granules	Few	Few	Intermediate	Many
Microvilli	Occasional	Occasional	Prominent	Numerous

Modified from Mackay (1969); Neville and Mackay (1972); and Neville and O'Hare (1979).

more prominent in the zona glomerulosa than in the inner zones of the cortex.

The zona fasciculata (ZF) is characterized by prominent ovoid or spherical (fig. 11) mitochondria with tubular cristae and many osmiophilic lipid droplets or empty vacuoles (fig. 12) which presumably once contained lipid. Stimulation by ACTH leads to an extensive development of surface filopodia and enlarged intercellular spaces (Pudney et al.). Many authors consider the inner or transition zone of the ZF a distinct entity (Mackay; Neville and O'Hare) populated by cells possessing characteristics of both zona fasciculata and reticularis.

The zona reticularis (ZR) is composed of cells containing numerous large ovoid tubulovesicular mitochondria, many lysosomes (fig. 13), and lipofuscin pigment granules (fig. 14). Although parallel rows (stacks) of rough (granular) endoplasmic reticulum may be seen in any of the zones of the cortex, they are most commonly found in the compact cells of the zona reticularis.

There is abundant work supporting the concept that the cells of the zona fasciculata are converted to those of the zona reticularis under the aegis of ACTH (Symington; Neville and O'Hare). This concept is underscored by the inability of most authors (Neville and O'Hare) to identify ultrastructural differences between androgen- and cortisol-secreting tumor cells. Thus, ultrastructure, although valuable in establishing the identity of adrenal cells, is of limited usefulness in relating production of specific steroids to a specific cell type (Symington; Neville and O'Hare).

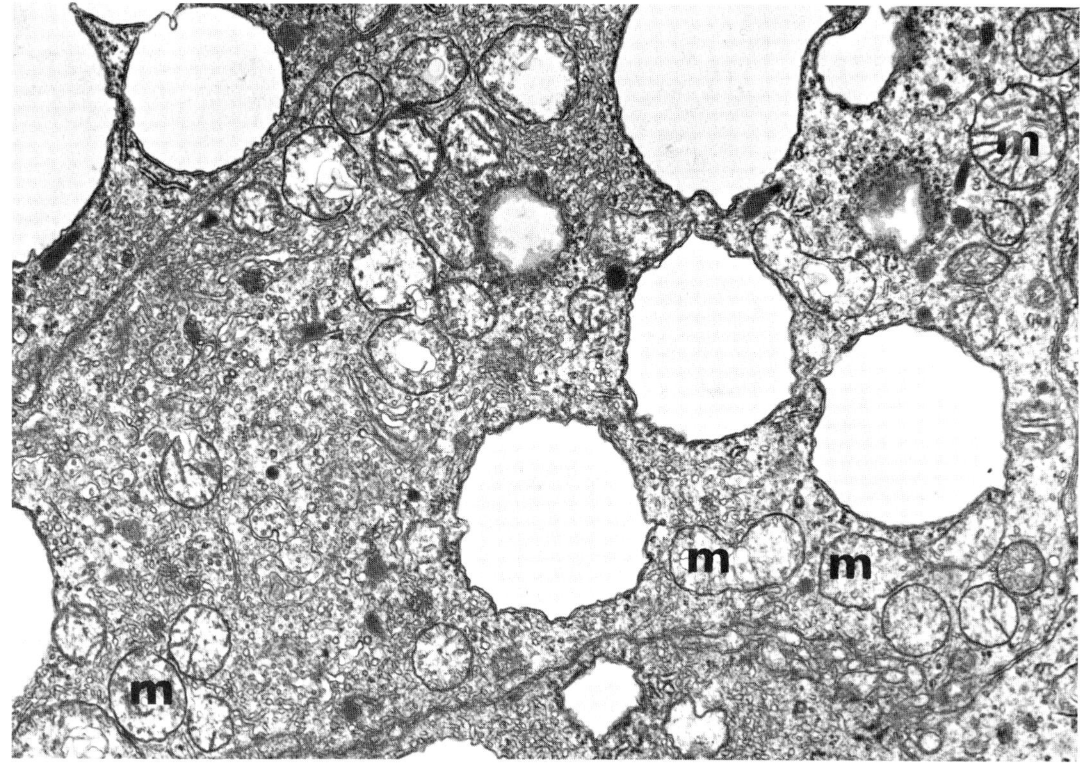

Figure 11
MICROSTRUCTURE, CORTEX
Ovoid tubulovesicular mitochondria (m) from fasciculate zone demonstrate characteristic arrangement seen in steroid secreting cells. Lipid vacuoles are present. Uranyl acetate-lead citrate. X12,000.

Although some authors have described cells at the boundary of the cortex and medulla with characteristics of each (Hashida and Yunis), others have discounted this concept (Neville and O'Hare) and we are in agreement with the latter.

The ultrastructure of the fetal (provisional) adrenal cortical cells reveals light and dark variants, with the former being distinctive due to their abundant cytoplasm, lipid content, and giant mitochondria (Tannenbaum, 1973). Although neither type of fetal cortical cell resembles those seen in the adult cortex, there is substantial evidence that these fasciculata-like cells are capable of responding to both ACTH and to HCG.

MICROSTRUCTURE, MEDULLA

Although the boundaries between the cells of the zona reticularis and the medulla are often sharply defined, occasional human adrenals may show an irregular interface between these anatomic compartments of the glands. In addition to the cortical cuff which surrounds the central vein, occasional groups of apparently isolated cortical cells may be found within the substance of the medulla (fig. 9). The medulla is characteristically chromaffin positive following fixation in Zenker's or Orth's solution. A more detailed review of the histochcmistry of the medulla is presented in the section on Pheochromo-

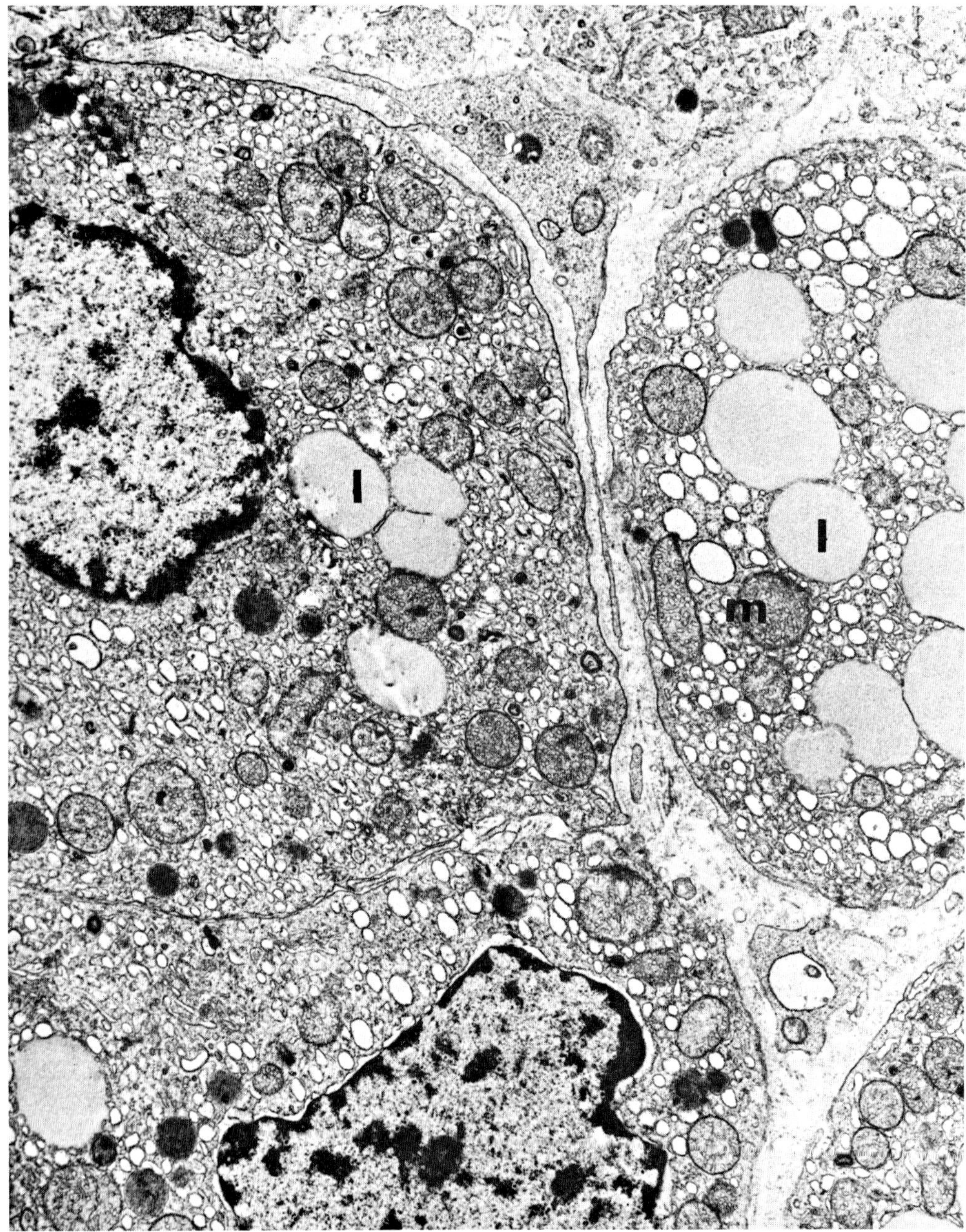

Figure 12
MICROSTRUCTURE, CORTEX
Inner zona fasciculata of normal adrenal reveals cells containing lipid droplets (l) and numerous ovoid mito-chondria (m). Smooth endoplasmic reticulum forms fill the cytoplasm. Uranyl acetate-lead citrate. X10,500.

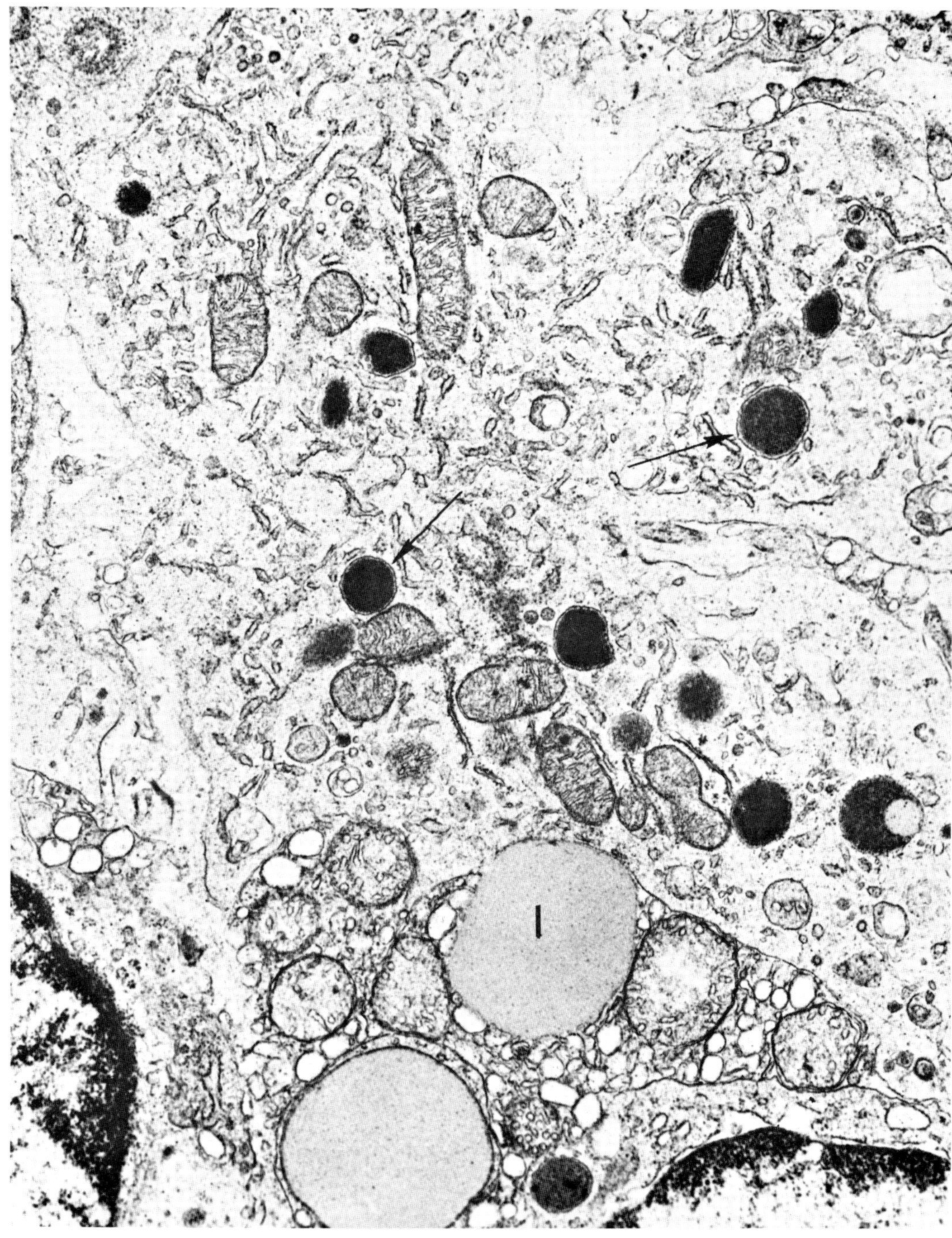

Figure 13
MICROSTRUCTURE, CORTEX
Cell of zona reticularis demonstrates sparse lipid (l), elongate mitochondria, and numerous lysosomes (arrows). Lipofuscin pigment is present in several lysosomes. Uranyl acetate-lead citrate. X21,000.

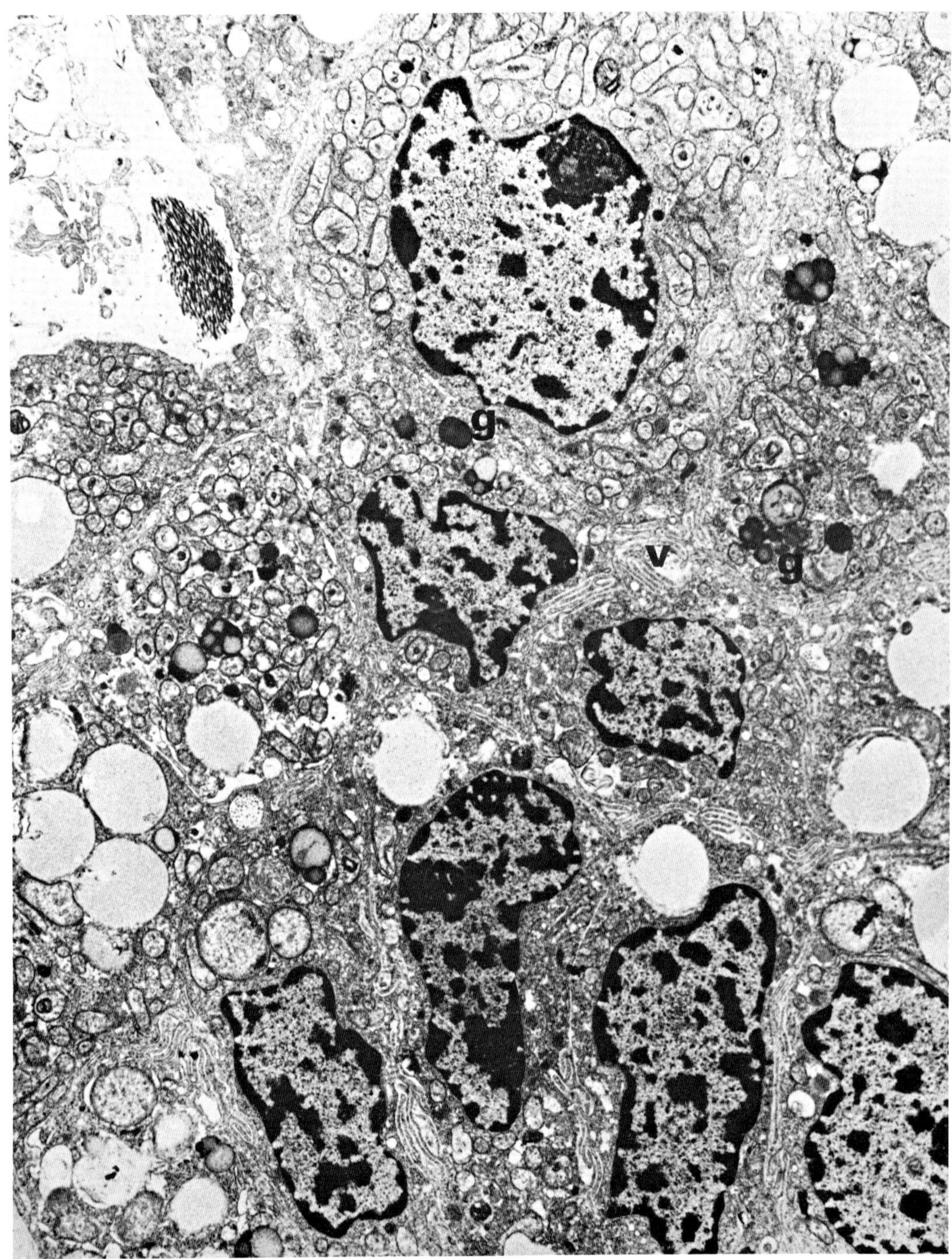

Figure 14
MICROSTRUCTURE, CORTEX
Cells of zona reticularis show numerous lysosomes and lipofuscin granules (g) and many microvilli (v). Note the elongate mitochondria as compared to the spherical ones seen in figure 12. Uranyl acetate-lead citrate. X8500.

cytoma. Medullary (chromaffin) cells are arranged in small nests or short cords and are separated by a rich capillary network. Individual medullary cells are round to polyhedral in shape and often have a finely granular basophilic cytoplasm (fig. 8). In some specimens, the cytoplasm may appear extensively vacuolated. Nuclei are round to ovoid and often occupy a slightly eccentric position within the cytoplasm. Chromatin is coarsely clumped and a single distinct nucleolus is often apparent. Nuclei of medullary cells often show variation in size and shape with occasional giant hyperchromatic forms, particularly in juxtacortical regions. Rare eosinophilic intranuclear "inclusions" may be found in some medullary cells. At the ultrastructural level, these "inclusions" represent cytoplasmic-nuclear invaginations which are similar to those described in other normal and neoplastic tissues. Sympathetic ganglion cells are present, both singly and as small groups, particularly in the walls of central veins. Groups of small cells with round hyperchromatic nuclei and scanty cytoplasm are found commonly in the medulla of adults. These cells, originally thought to represent primitive sympathetic cells, probably represent mature lymphocytes. True primitive sympathetic cells, however, may be found in the adrenal medulla in newborns and children up to the age of three years (see section on Embryology and Postnatal Development).

Although they are difficult to recognize in routinely stained sections, sustentacular (satellite) cells, similar to those present in extra-adrenal paraganglia, are present at the peripheries of the medullary cell cords. The sustentacular cells may be stained selectively with antibodies to S-100 protein (Nakajima et al.; Blaivas et al.). Chromogranin proteins, on the other hand, are present within the adrenal medullary cells, but are absent from the sustentacular elements (Lloyd and Wilson; O'Connor et al.). Medullary cells contain neurofilament-rich intermediate (10 nm) filaments, while the cortical cells contain cytokeratin proteins (Miettinen et al.).

Cytoplasmic hyaline inclusions occurring singly or in small groups have been described both in normal and in neoplastic adrenal medullary cells. These inclusions, which are eosinophilic in hematoxylin and eosin stained sections, measure 1 to 25 μm in diameter. They are PAS positive, variably acid fast, and are autofluorescent. Hyaline inclusions may be found in up to 79 percent of unselected autopsies, but are numerous in only 3 percent of cases. They are most commonly located in the juxtacortical medullary cells. At the ultrastructural level, the hyaline inclusions are membrane bound and have a finely granular to amorphous matrix in which are embedded degenerated secretory granule-like structures. The inclusions are thought to represent residual type bodies. Although some authors have suggested that their presence reflects intense cellular secretory activity, the significance of these inclusions remains unknown. Studies of Dekker and Oehrle have indicated that the presence of these inclusions is unrelated to age, sex, race, or any specific disease process.

The ultrastructural characteristics of adrenal medullary cells of various species have been studied extensively. The most striking feature of these cells is the presence of membrane bound, dense core secretory granules within the cytoplasm (fig. 15). In addition to the granules, adrenal medullary cells have well developed Golgi regions and prominent stacks of

PLATE I
ANATOMY

(Plate I-A and B from same patient)

A. Cross section of normal adrenal glands removed from a 23 year old man dying acutely of trauma. Combined weight was 8 g. Dark inner ring of tissue is normal zona reticularis. A small amount of medulla is present (arrows). X2.

B. Histology of normal adrenal gland reveals thin zona glomerulosa (arrow) immediately under the capsule seen at upper left and prominent fascicular (f) and reticular (r) zones. X75.

(Plate I-C and D from same patient)

C. Nodular adrenal removed from a patient dying of chronic disease. Pigmented (black) nodule is seen. Pigment results from accentuation of lipofuscin normally present in zona reticularis. X2. (Courtesy of Dr. W.A. Gardner, Jr., Nashville, TN.)

D. Lipofuscin pigment stains positively by the PAS reaction. PAS-hematoxylin. X400.

E. Variation in lipid content among adrenal nodules is commonly seen at necropsy. Oil red O-hematoxylin. X160.

PLATE I

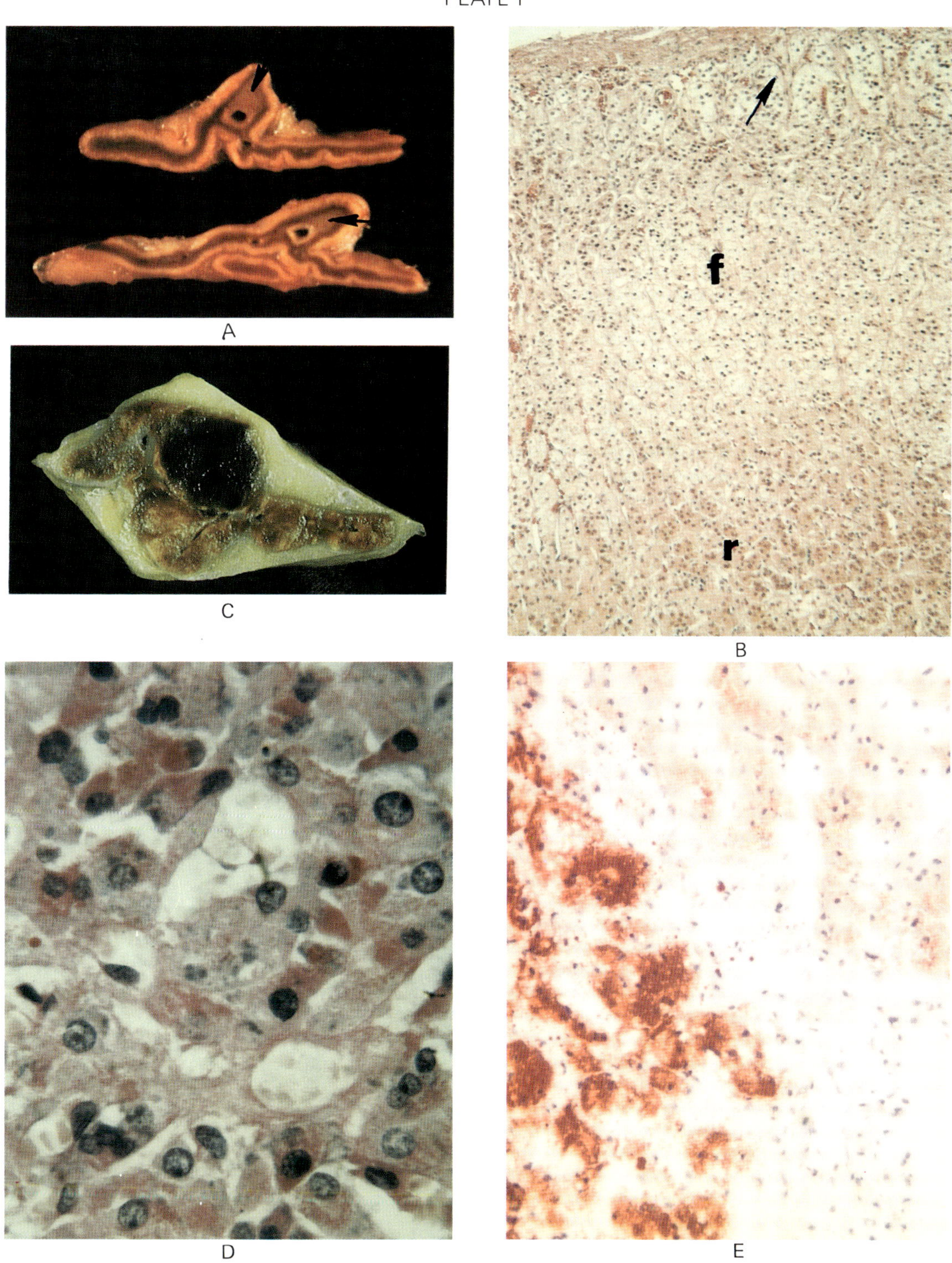

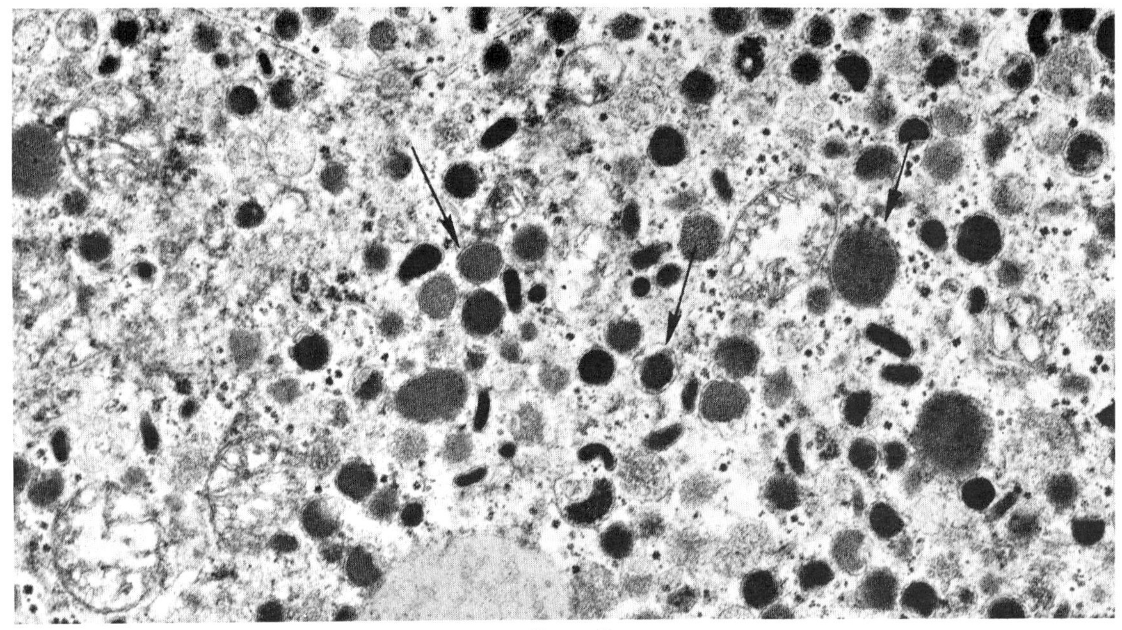

Figure 15
MICROSTRUCTURE, MEDULLA
This normal adrenal medullary cell contains numerous membrane bound granules (arrows). The granules have moderately electron dense matrices and show variation in size and shape. These ultrastructural features are characteristic of the predominant storage of epinephrine in the human adrenal medulla. X24,000.

granular endoplasmic reticulum. The appearance of the granules is dependent upon the type of initial tissue fixation. In species such as the rat, correlative histochemical and ultrastructural studies of glutaraldehyde fixed tissue have revealed two distinctive cell types. Norepinephrine containing cells are characterized by granules with markedly electron dense cores which are separated from the limiting membranes by a prominent electronlucent halo. Epinephrine containing cells, on the other hand, have moderately electron dense finely granular contents which are closely applied to the limiting membranes (fig. 15). Although some studies have revealed both granule types in single cells of human medullary tissue, more recent studies suggest that there may be separate epinephrine and norepinephrine storing cells. In glutaraldehyde and osmium fixed human tissues, the intramembranous diameter of epinephrine granules is 190 nm, while that of norepinephrine granules is 250 nm. The diameter of the dense core of norepinephrine granules, however, is less than that of the epinephrine containing granules.

A third chromaffin cell type, originally described in the bird, has also been identified in most other species, including mammals. This cell type has been referred to as the SGC (small granule chromaffin) or SIF (small intensely fluorescent) cell. This cell type contains membrane bound secretory granules smaller than those of epinephrine or norepinephrine cells and synaptic type vesicles measuring 40-70 nm in diameter. These cells, which have prominent processes, may function as interneurons (Kobayashi and Coupland; Serizawa and Kobayashi).

References

Alexander, D. P., Britton, H. G., Nixon, D. A., Ratcliffe, J. G., and Redstone, D. Corticotrophin and cortisol concentrations in the plasma of the chronically catheterised sheep fetus. Biol. Neonate 23:184-192, 1973.

Arvy, L. Histoenzymology of the Adrenal Glands. Oxford: Pergamon Press, 1971.

Bachmann, R. Die Nebenniere I. Die Geschichte der Nebennierenforschung. In: Handbuch der Mikroskopischen Anatomie des Menschen Bd. 6, Teil 5. Berlin: Springer-Verlag, 1954.

Bertholet, J. Y. Proliferative activity and cell migration in the adrenal cortex of fetal and neonatal rats: an autoradiographic study. J. Endocrinol. 87:1-9, 1980.

Blaivas, M., Lloyd, R. V., and Wilson, B. Distribution of chromogranin and S-100 protein in normal and abnormal adrenal medullary tissue. Lab. Invest. 52:8A, 1985.

Bloodworth, J. M. B., Jr. The Adrenal, pp. 172-192. In: Pathology Annual. Sommers, S. C. (Ed.). New York: Appleton-Century-Crofts, 1965.

Coupland, R. E. Electron microscopic observations on the structure of the rat adrenal medulla. J. Anat. 99:231-254, 1965.

Crivello, J. F., Hornsby, P. J., and Gill, G. N. Metyrapone and antioxidants are required to maintain aldosterone synthesis by cultured bovine adrenocortical zona glomerulosa cells. Endocrinology 3:469-478, 1982.

Dawson, I.M.P., Pryse-Davies, J., and Snape, I. M. The distribution of six enzyme systems and of lipid in the human and rat adrenal cortex before and after administration of steroid and ACTH, with comments on the distribution in human foetuses and in some natural disease conditions. J. Pathol. Bacteriol. 81:181-195, 1961.

Dekker, A. and Oehrle, J. S. Hyaline globules of the adrenal medulla of man. Arch. Pathol. 91:353-364, 1971.

DeLellis, R. A., Wolfe, H. J., Gagel, R. F., Feldman, Z. T., Miller, H. H., Gang, D. L., and Reichlin, S. Adrenal medullary hyperplasia. Am. J. Pathol. 83:177-196, 1976.

Dickerman, A., Grant, D. R., Faiman, C., and Winter, J. S. D. Intraadrenal steroid concentrations in man: Zonal differences and developmental changes. J. Clin. Endocrinol. Metab. 59:1031-1036, 1984.

Dobbie, J. W. and Symington, T. The human adrenal gland with special reference to the vasculature. J. Endocrinol. 34:479-489, 1966.

Fawcett, D. W., Long, J. A., and Jones, A. L. The ultrastructure of endocrine glands. Recent Prog. Horm. Res. 25:315-368, 1969.

Grynszpan-Winograd, O. Ultrastructure of the Chromaffin Cell, pp. 295-308. In: Handbook of Physiology, Section 7, Vol. 6. Greep, R. O. and Astwood, E. B. (Eds.). Washington: American Physiological Society, 1975.

Hashida, Y. and Yunis, E. J. Ultrastructure of the adrenal zona glomerulosa in children with renovascular hypertension. Hum. Pathol. 3:301-315, 1972.

Idelman, S. The Structure of the Mammalian Adrenal Cortex, pp. 1-109. In: General, Comparative and Clinical Endocrinology of the Adrenal Cortex, Vol. 2. Jones, I. C. and Henderson, I. W. (Eds.). London: Academic Press, 1976.

Kobayashi, S. and Coupland, R. E. Two populations of microvesicles in the SGC (small granule chromaffin) cells of the mouse adrenal medulla. Arch. Histol. Jpn. 40:251-259, 1977.

Kurman, R. J., Andrade, D., Goebelsmann, U., and Taylor, C. R. An immunohistological study of steroid localization in Sertoli-Leydig tumors of the ovary and testis. Cancer 42:1772-1783, 1978.

Lloyd, R. V. and Wilson, B. S. Specific endocrine tissue marker defined by a monoclonal antibody. Science 222:628-630, 1983.

Long, J. A. and Jones, A. L. Observations of the fine structure of the adrenal cortex of man. Lab. Invest. 17:355-370, 1967.

Mackay, A. Atlas of Human Adrenal Cortex Ultrastructure, pp. 346-489. In: Functional Pathology of the Human Adrenal Gland. Symington, T. (Ed.). Baltimore: The Williams & Wilkins Co., 1969.

Mazzocchi, G., Meneghelli, V., and Nussdorfer, G. G. Effects of antiotensin II on the zona glomerulosa of sodium-loaded dexamethasone treated rats administered or not with maintenance doses of ACTH: stereology and plasma hormone concentrations. Acta Endocrinol. 102:129-135, 1983.

Miettinen, M., Lehtho, V-P., and Virtanen, I. Immunofluorescence microscopic evaluation of the intermediate filament expression of the adrenal cortex and medulla and their tumors. Am. J. Pathol. 118:360-366, 1985.

Motta, P., Muto, M., and Fujita, T. Three dimensional organization of mammalian adrenal cortex. Cell Tissue Res. 196:23-38, 1979.

Nakajima, T., Kameya, T., Watanabe, S., Hirota, T., et al. S-100 Protein Distribution in Normal and Neoplastic Tissues, pp. 141-158. In: Advances in Immunohistochemistry. DeLellis, R.A. (Ed.). New York: Masson Publishing USA, Inc. 1984.

Neville, A. M. and Davidson, I. K. Diseases of the Adrenal Gland, pp. 261-307. In: Applied Surgical Pathology. Stuart, A. E., Smith, A. N., and Samuel, E. (Eds.). Oxford: Blackwell, 1975.

Neville, A. M. and Mackay, A. M. The Structure of the Human Adrenal Cortex in Health and Disease, pp. 361-395. In: Clinics in Endocrinology and Metabolism, Vol. 1, No. 2. London, Philadelphia, Toronto: W. B. Saunders Company, 1972.

__________ and O'Hare, M. J. Aspects of Structure, Function, and Pathology, pp. 1-65. In: The Adrenal Gland. James, V. H. T. (Ed.). New York: Raven Press, 1979.

O'Connor, D. T., Burton, D., and Deftos, L. J. Chromogranin A: Immunohistology reveals its universal occurrence in normal polypeptide hormone producing endocrine glands. Life Sci. 33:1657-1663, 1983.

O'Hare, M. J., Monaghan, P., and Neville, A. M. The pathology of adrenocortical neoplasia: a correlated structural and functional approach to the diagnosis of malignant disease. Hum. Pathol. 10:137-154, 1979.

Okano, T., Kawaoi, A., and Shikata, T. Immunohisto- and cytochemical demonstration of corticosteroids in the adrenocortical cells. Cancer Treatment Reports 63: 1145, 1979.

Pudney, J., Sweet, P. R., Vinson, G. P., and Whitehouse, B. J. Morphological correlates of hormone secretion in the rat adrenal cortex and the role of filopodia. Anat. Rec. 201:537-551, 1981.

Quinan, C. and Berger, A. A. Observations on human adrenals with especial reference to the relative weight of the normal medulla. Ann. Int. Med. 6:1180-1192, 1933.

Serizawa, Y. and Kobayashi, S. SGC cell of the adrenal medulla. A transient form between neurons and paraneurons. Biomed. Res. (Suppl.) 107:111, 1980.

Stark, E., Gyévai, A., Bukulya, B., Szabó, D., Szalay, K. S., and Mihály, K. Interrelationship between corticosteroid production and fine structure in the fetal adrenal cortex. Gen. Comp. Endocrinol. 25:472-486, 1975.

Symington, T. Functional Pathology of the Human Adrenal Gland. Edinburgh: Churchill Livingstone, 1969.

Tannenbaum, M. Ultrastructural pathology of the adrenal cortex. Pathol. Annu. 8:109-156, 1973.

__________ . Ultrastructural Pathology of Adrenal Medullary Tumors, pp. 145-171. In: Pathology Annual. Sommers, S. C. (Ed.). New York: Appleton-Century-Crofts, 1970.

Taylor, C. R., Kurman, R. J., and Warner, N. E. The potential value of immunohistologic techniques in the classification of ovarian and testicular tumors. Hum. Pathol. 9:417-427, 1978.

Winkler, H. and Smith, A. D. The Chromaffin Granule and the Storage of Catecholamines, pp. 321-339. In: Handbook of Physiology. Endocrinology, Section 7, Vol. 6. Greep, R. O. and Astwood, E. B. (Eds.). Washington: American Physiological Society, 1975.

Wright, N. and Voncina, D. Studies on the postnatal growth of the rat adrenal cortex. J. Anat. 123:147-156, 1977.

Wyllie, A. H., Kerr, J. F. R., and Currie, A. R. Cell death in the normal neonatal rat adrenal cortex. J. Pathol. 111:255-261, 1973.

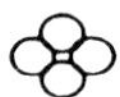

EMBRYOLOGY AND POSTNATAL DEVELOPMENT

Each adrenal gland is composed of two fundamentally distinct endocrine systems enclosed within a single capsule. The cortex develops from mesenchyme adjacent to the urogenital ridge, while the medulla originates in cells derived from the neuroectoderm.

CORTEX

The cells destined to form the primordial adrenal cortex are first seen as plates of mesenchyme connected to the mesothelial lining of the coelomic cavity between the midsagittal mesentery and the mesonephric buds (England). These plates grow in size, bulge from the dorsal coelom, and become highly vascularized (fig. 16). These masses continue to grow throughout fetal life and each is approximately one-third the size of the kidney at birth. This is relatively larger than the normal adult adrenal:kidney ratio (Kissane).

The relatively homogeneous mass of primitive adrenocortical cells is invaded by cells of the mesonephric Bowman's capsule at about the 10 mm stage. These cells form the internal connective tissue framework of the gland. At about the same period, neural elements begin to migrate into the gland, first entering the caudal portions (fig. 17). The cells of the cortex continue to proliferate and become separated from the dorsal coelomic epithelium at the 16 mm stage (Crowder).

By late embryonic life (40 mm stage), an outer glomerular zone has formed, in which cortical cells are rapidly produced. The gland continues to proliferate, and by the 50 mm stage (second trimester) a broad inner

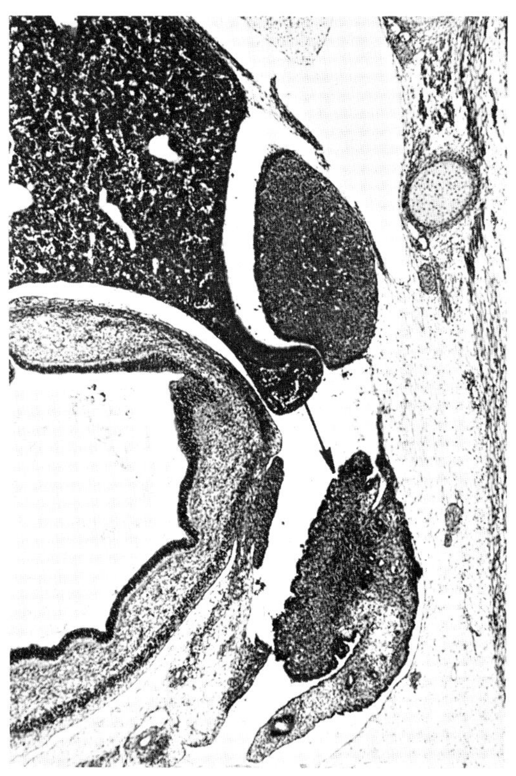

Figure 16
EMBRYOLOGY AND POSTNATAL DEVELOPMENT
Developing gonadal ridge at lower right, with adrenal appearing in an indentation of the liver at upper right. Tubular structure is developing gut. Note developing metanephros (arrow). X30.

zone of large polyhedral eosinophilic cells, termed the fetal cortex, has formed surrounding the central adrenal vein. A separate, outer rim of cells is destined to become the permanent adult cortex. These cells of the definitive cortex remain smaller and more basophilic than cells of the fetal or provisional cortex until birth. Zonation similar to that seen in the adult is not seen, nor is a discrete medulla present (fig. 17). The fetal adrenal cortex is responsive to ACTH (Challis et al.) and its size may be

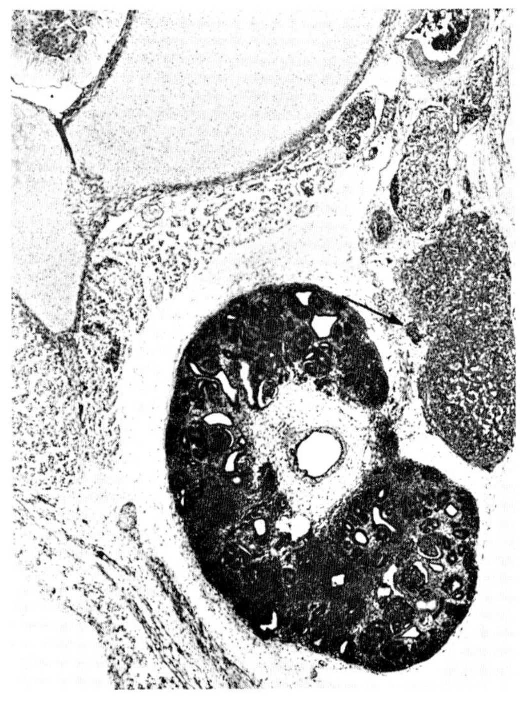

Figure 17
(Figures 17 and 19 from same patient)
EMBRYOLOGY AND POSTNATAL DEVELOPMENT
Human embryo at later stage of development (40 mm) showing well developed metanephros adjacent to adrenal gland. Collection of primitive sympathetic cells is at edge of adrenal (arrow). X30.

reduced experimentally by exogenous corticosteroids (Milkovic and Domac). Although the cells of the fetal cortex do not closely resemble definitive adult adrenal cortical cells ultrastructurally (Fujita and Ihara), they are capable of synthesizing steroid hormones (Stark et al.) and their function may be important to the timing of birth (Serón-Ferré and Jaffe).

At birth, the fetal component occupies 75 percent of the adrenal cortex (Bech et al.). The fetal cortex immediately becomes hypervascular as the cells swell and disintegrate (Crowder; pl. II-D). The fetal cortex continues to degenerate, occupying 58 percent and 23 percent of the cortex at 2 and 12 weeks, respectively (Bech et al). Although the definitive cortex continues to proliferate during this period, the combined weight of the adrenals continues to fall until 2-3 months postdelivery, after which there is a gradual increase in weight concomitant with somatic growth (Tähkä). A separate zona glomerulosa is detectable at birth, with no definable zona reticularis. This latter zone is formed during the first year of life.

MEDULLA

The intra- and extra-adrenal paraganglia and the sympathetic nervous system are intimately associated during embryonic development and arise from the primitive sympathetic cells (small intensely basophilic cells, sympathogonia) of the neural crest. In the course of development of paraganglia, three distinctive cell types have been recognized on the basis of light microscopic and histochemical analysis (Hervonen; Coupland). These include the primitive sympathetic cells, pheochromoblasts, and pheochromocytes. The primitive sympathetic cells have small hyperchromatic nuclei, which measure 4 to 6 μm in diameter, and small amounts of cytoplasm. At the ultrastructural level, the cytoplasm contains dispersed free ribosomes, few polyribosomes, and occasional mitochondria (fig. 18). By approximately seven weeks of development, these cells contain well formed Golgi zones, occasional microtubules, and sparse glycogen rosettes. With further development, empty vesicles appear within the cytoplasm. Despite the negative chromaffin reaction, the primitive sympathetic cells have been shown to contain low levels of norepinephrine by the formaldehyde induced fluorescence technic.

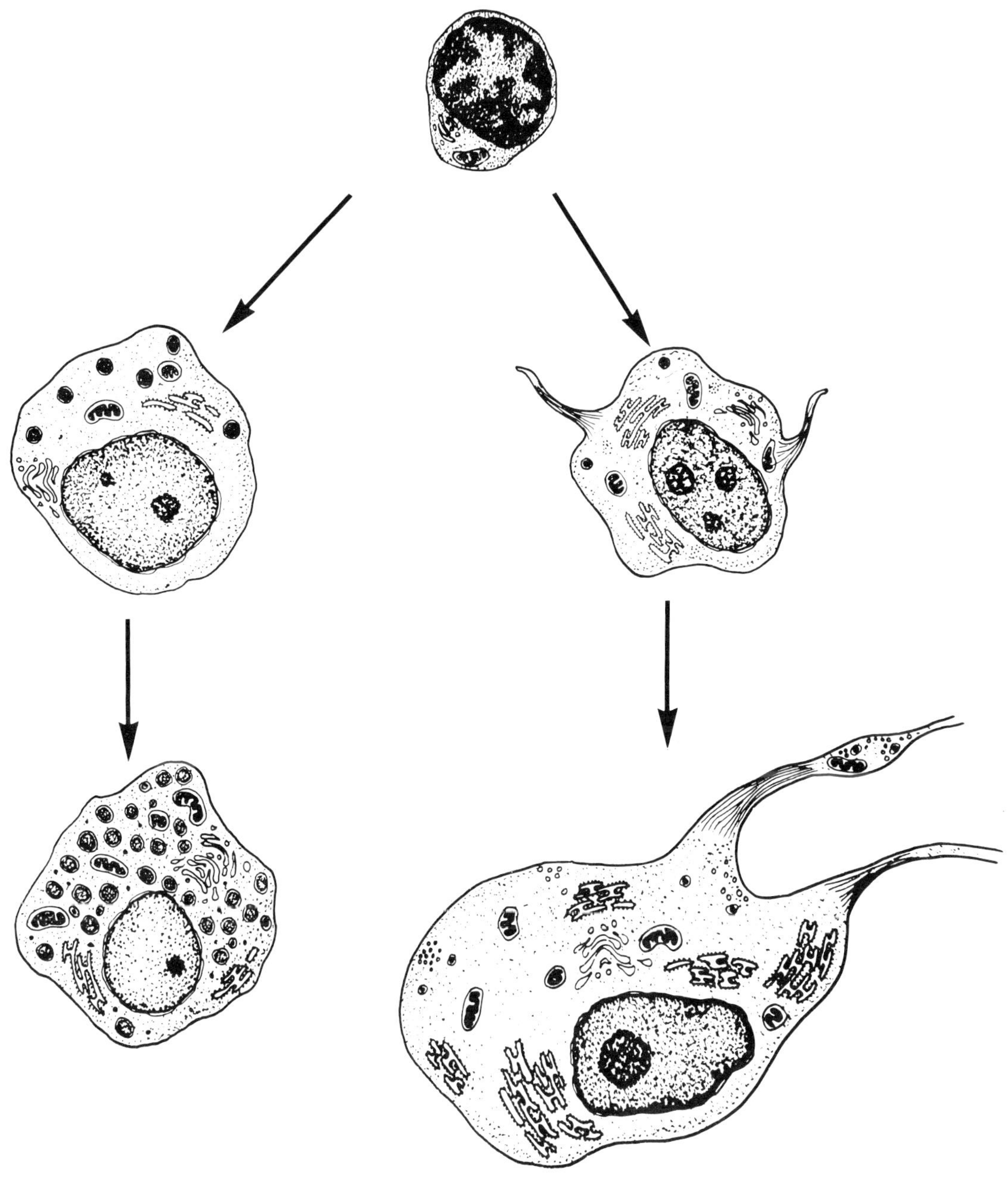

Figure 18
EMBRYOLOGY AND POSTNATAL DEVELOPMENT
This diagram summarizes the stages in the development of primitive sympathetic cells into pheochromocytes or adrenal medullary chromaffin cells (left) and sympathetic ganglion cells (right). The primitive sympathetic cell has a small amount of cytoplasm containing dispersed ribosomes, a few polyribosomes, and occasional mitochondria. Differentiation into pheochromocyte line is characterized by the gradual appearance of chromaffin granules. The mature sympathetic ganglion cells are characterized by the development of neuritic processes containing microtubules, microfilaments, dense core neurosecretory granules, and small clear (synaptic type) vesicles.

PLATE II
EMBRYOLOGY AND POSTNATAL DEVELOPMENT

A. Fusion of adrenal gland with kidney (as in this child) could provide setting for a future ectopic adrenal tumor. X2.5. (Courtesy of Dr. W.A. Gardner, Jr., Nashville, TN.)

B. Anomalous location of adrenal cortical tissue in the spermatic cord is a recognized occurrence. X1.5. (Courtesy of Dr. G. Gray, New York, NY.)

C. These adrenal glands from an infant demonstrate an extreme example of the most common form of adrenal ectopia, capsular extrusions. X.8. (Courtesy of University of Arkansas For Medical Sciences, Little Rock, AR.)

D. Involuting provisional cortex in a 4 month old infant reveals typical ballooning degeneration and interspersed hemorrhage. X125.

PLATE II

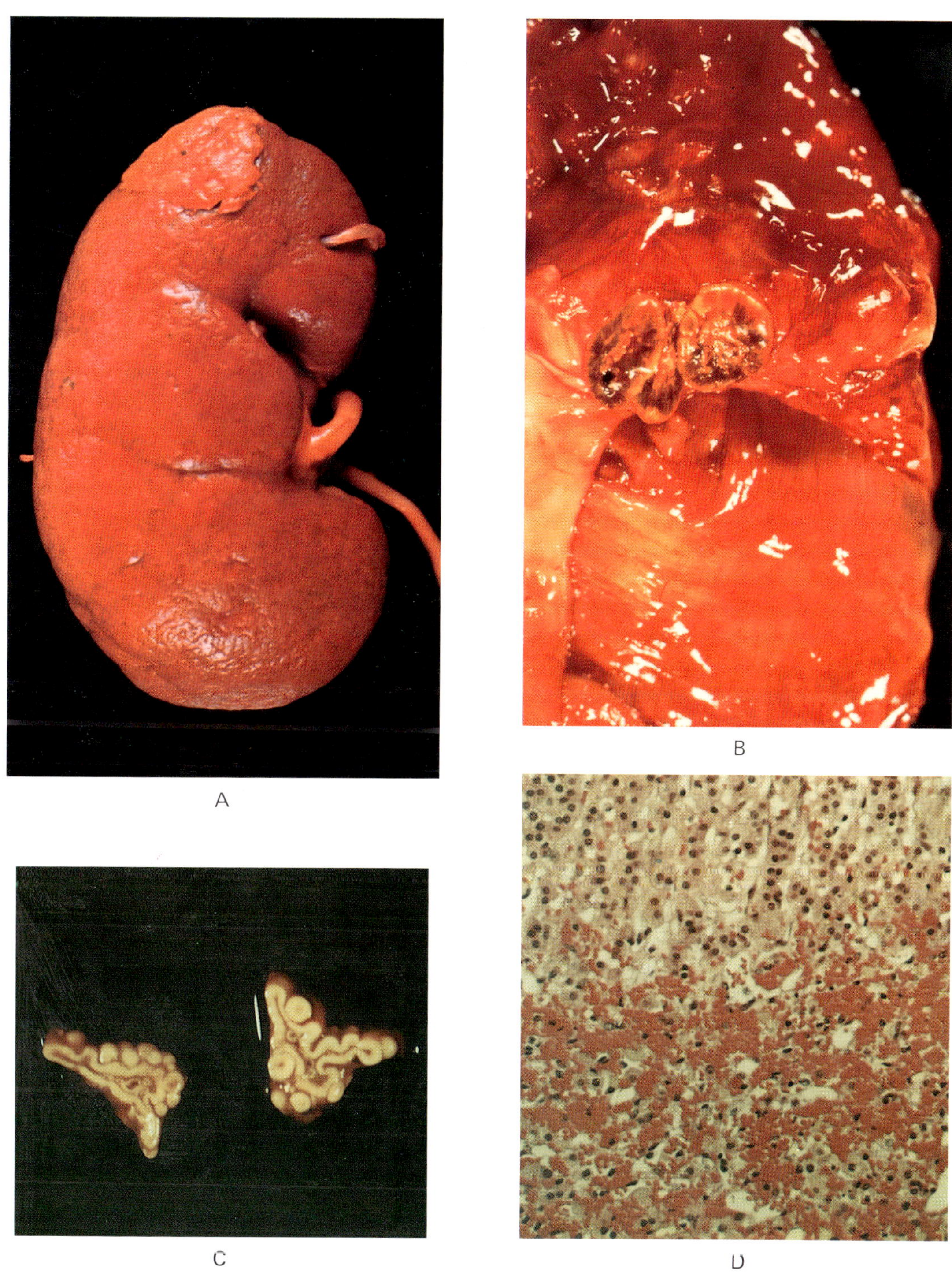

A

B

C

D

In 8 mm embryos, primitive sympathetic cells are found singly or in small groups in paravertebral and in pre- and para-aortic regions. At 10 to 14 mm, these cells become more numerous, particularly at the sites of future paravertebral sympathetic chains. The adrenal cortical anlage forms a well defined group of cells in the medial part of the intermediate cell mass in 10 mm embryos. By the 14 mm stage of development, groups of primitive sympathetic cells begin to invade the cortical anlage (fig. 19). In the 16 mm embryo, a different cell type may be recognized in the para-aortic regions. These cells have nuclei which measure 8 to 10 μm in diameter, with usually two prominent nucleoli and more abundant cytoplasm than the primitive sympathetic cells. These cells represent the pheochromoblasts (fig. 20). Although the chromaffin reaction is generally negative in these cells, norepinephrine may be demonstrated by the formaldehyde induced fluorescence reaction. Ultrastructurally, the Golgi region, particularly the vesicular component, becomes prominent. Cytoplasmic vesicles become more apparent and some of them contain an electron dense secretory material. With further development, the dense core vesicles increase both in number and in size. The pheochromoblasts are largely arranged in a whorl-like pattern which changes to a pattern of anastomosing cell cords as the definitive pheochromocytes or chromaffin cells appear. These cells have nuclei which measure 6 to 8 μm in diameter, with usually a single nucleolus. A definitive positive chromaffin reaction, however, is not observed until the 55 mm stage.

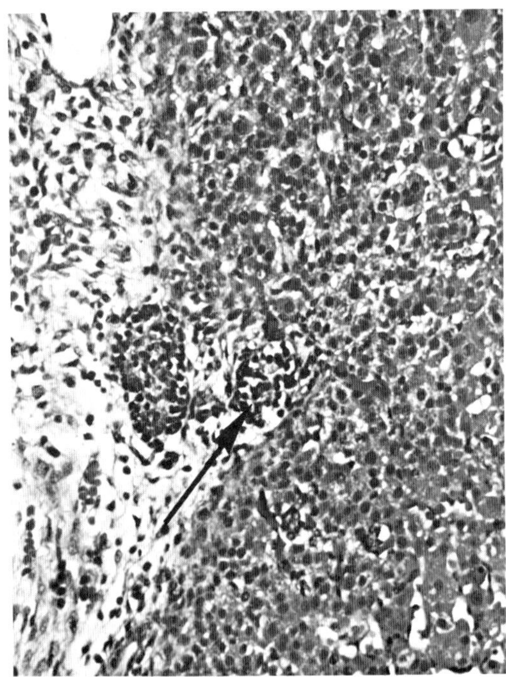

Figure 19
EMBRYOLOGY AND POSTNATAL DEVELOPMENT
High power of figure 17 showing invasion of adrenal cortex by primitive sympathetic cells (arrow). X120.

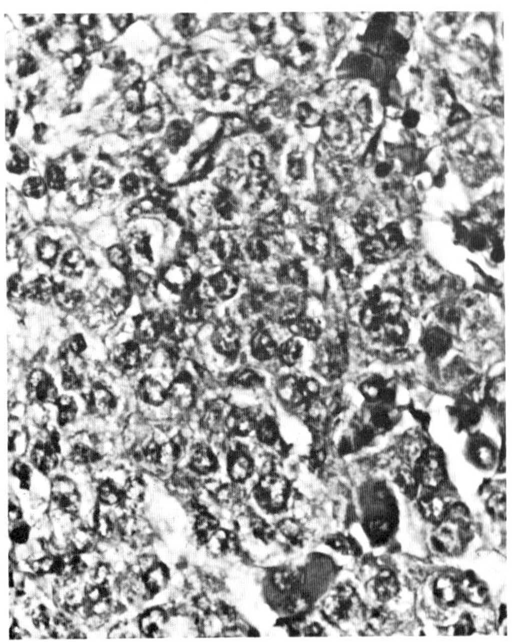

Figure 20
EMBRYOLOGY AND POSTNATAL DEVELOPMENT
Pheochromoblasts (cells with dark cytoplasm) intermixed with fetal cortex. X480.

In the 19.5 mm embryo, definite invasion of the adrenal cortical anlage has occurred. While some primitive sympathetic cells penetrate the anlage with nerve fibers, some invading pheochromoblasts pass directly in from the adjacent cell whorls. Following the invasion of the cortical anlage, intra-adrenal chromaffin cells develop independently of, and more slowly than, those in extra-adrenal sites. In 270 mm specimens, primitive sympathetic cells persist in the adrenal, but are absent from the extra-adrenal paraganglia. In addition to the chromaffin cells and their precursors, neuroblasts and developing sympathetic ganglion cells are found within the medulla. Primitive sympathetic cells persist in the adrenal in the newborn. Most of these cells are associated with nerve fibers or are adjacent to the walls of vascular sinuses. Occasional groups of primitive sympathetic cells may be arranged in rosettes. The medulla undergoes its major development during the first three years of life. Chromaffin cells progressively increase in number as the population of primitive sympathetic cells decreases. Mitotic activity during this time may be striking. Concurrent with this development of the adrenal medulla, the extra-adrenal chromaffin tissue undergoes progressive atrophy.

Recent studies have established that the chromaffin cell and neuronal lineages are neither as divergent nor as irrevocably committed as traditionally believed and that the phenotype of individual cells can be altered by microenvironmental influences. In the presence of nerve growth factor (NGF), for example, cultured normal human adrenal medullary cells show a series of changes which are indicative of neuronal differentiation and which include the extension of neurite-like processes, redistribution of cytoplasmic granules and amine stores, and the formation of synaptic-like vesicles (Tischler et al.).

ECTOPIC SITES

The many cellular contributions to the development of the adrenals and the relatively diffuse nature of the primordium contribute to the frequency with which adrenal tissue is found in ectopic sites. More commonly, this accessory adrenal tissue contains adrenal cortical cells only and, less commonly, both endocrine systems. The latter are found only medial to the adrenal glands at their level (Graham).

Ectopic adrenal cortical tissue is most commonly detected retroperitoneally in the coeliac plexus; kidney (pl. II-A); genitalia (fig. 21); broad ligaments (Falls), epididymis; and spermatic cord (Neville; pl. II-B; fig. 22). More rarely, accessory cortical tissue may occur beneath the capsule of the liver (Dolan and Janovski; figs. 2, 23). Of extreme rarity is the fusion of each adrenal in the midline (fig. 24). Other rare sites which have been reported to contain adrenal cortical cells are the gallbladder wall (Busuttil) and ovary (Symonds and Driscoll). An apparently unique case describes a complete adrenal presenting adjacent to the brain (Wiener and Dallgaard).

ANATOMIC VARIANTS
Capsular Extrusion

Many adrenals present small, rounded collections of cortical cells just outside the glandular capsule (fig. 25). Occasionally these may be striking (pl. II-C). These extrusions usually rest upon the capsule and may contain cells of each histologic zone or appear as zona fasciculata cells only. Diffuse adrenal hyperplasia, particularly pitu-

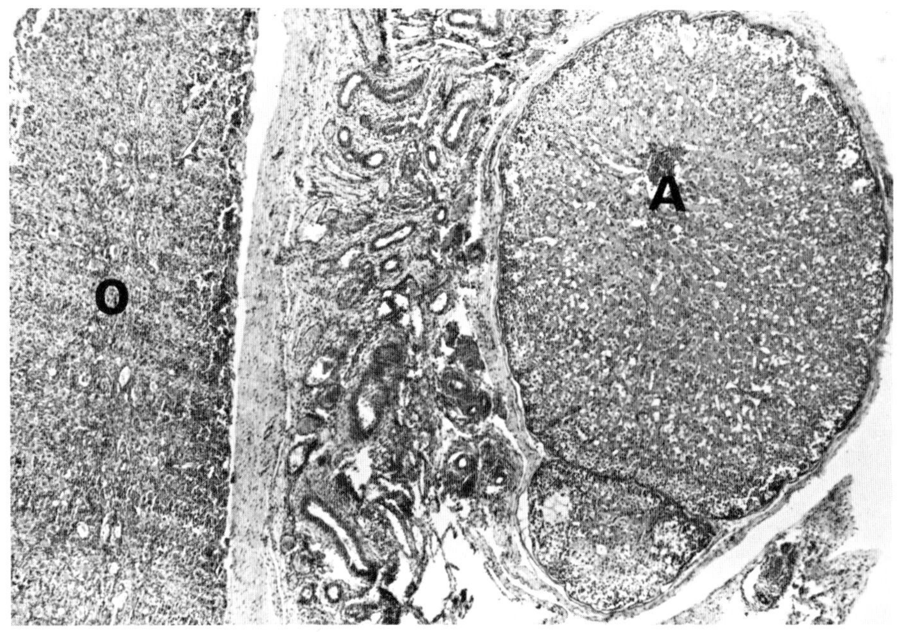

Figure 21
EMBRYOLOGY AND POSTNATAL DEVELOPMENT
Ectopic adrenal (A) adjacent to ovary (O) in a neonate. Intervening structure is vascular plexus. X40.

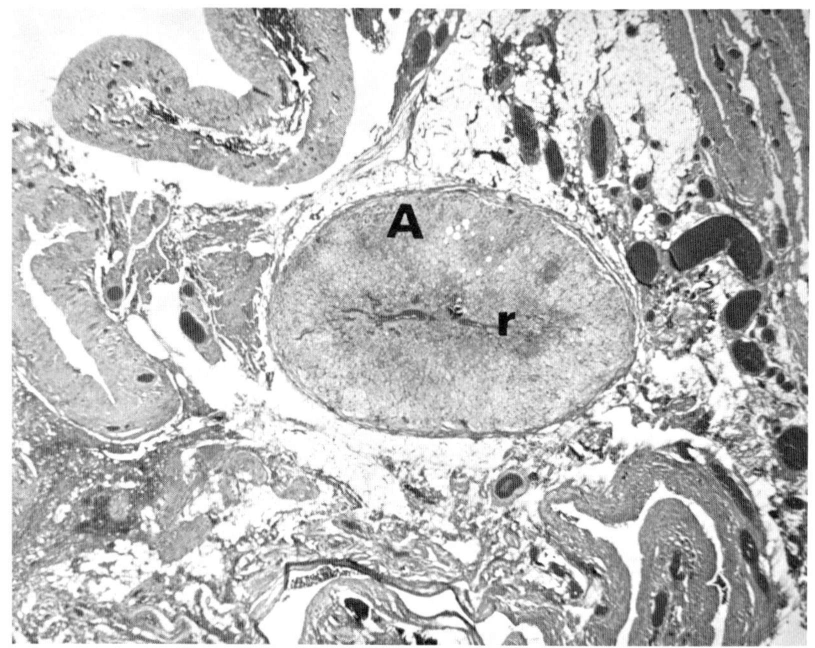

Figure 22
EMBRYOLOGY AND POSTNATAL DEVELOPMENT
Accessory adrenal cortex (A) in a surgically excised inguinal hernia sac. Note darker
reticularis cells (r) present centrally and absence of medulla. X10.

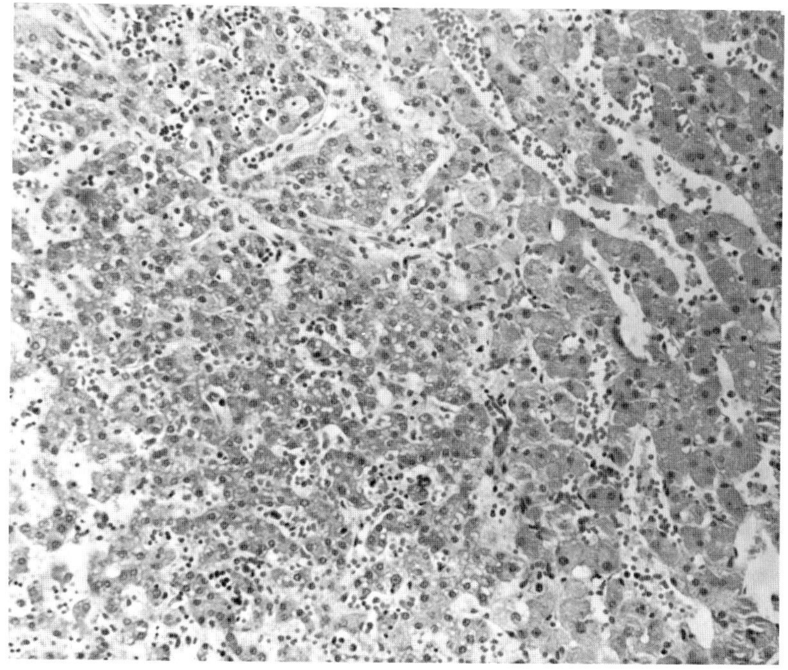

Figure 23
EMBRYOLOGY AND POSTNATAL DEVELOPMENT
Adrenal hepatic fusion. Hepatic cells at right are arranged in plates, sharply sepa-
rated from smaller adrenal cells along a vertical line roughly bisecting the picture.
X75.

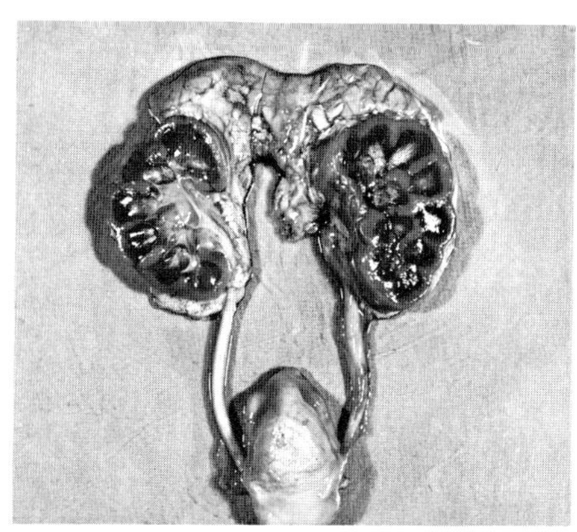

Figure 24
EMBRYOLOGY AND POSTNATAL DEVELOPMENT
Fusion of adrenal across the midline in a newborn baby.
Reduced to 40 percent of actual size.

itary-based hypercortisolism, will demonstrate many of these capsular extrusions.
They are rarely larger than 1-2 mm in
diameter and should not be termed "nodules," as they are clearly separable from the
other conditions for which this term is
used. (See discussion of nodules, p. 73).

Adrenal Cytomegaly

Cells of the fetal cortex may demonstrate
bizarre nuclear features and abundant,
brightly eosinophilic cytoplasm (fig. 26). As
many as 3 percent of newborn infants may
have these cells in the adrenals. They may
also be seen in premature infants or stillborn fetuses. The alteration is common in
Beckwith's syndrome (Borit and Kosek).
The cells are up to 100 μm in diameter, with
densely staining cytoplasm which may be

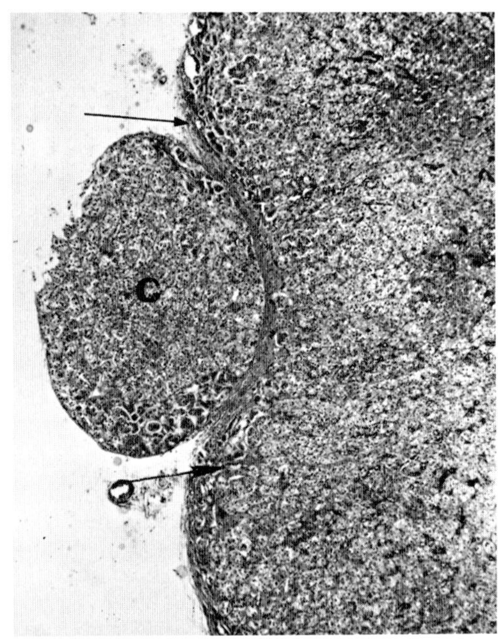

Figure 25
ANATOMIC VARIANTS
Nodular capsular extrusion (c) at left is seen indenting
adrenal capsule. A few zona glomerulosa cells (arrows) are
present in outer portion of extruded adrenal gland. X30.

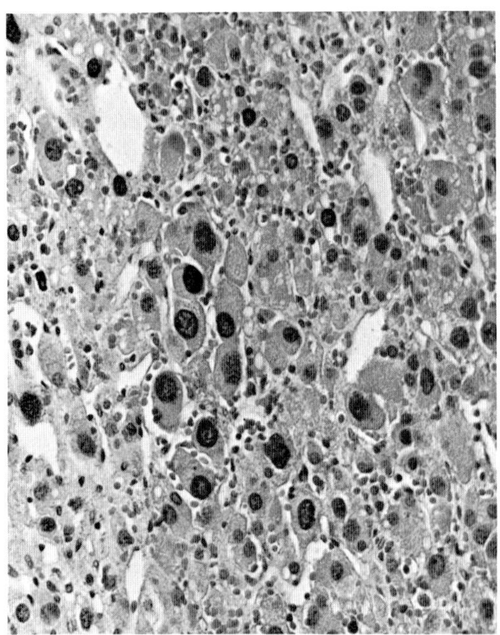

Figure 26
(Figures 26 and 28 from same patient)
ANATOMIC VARIANTS
Neonatal cytomegalic hypoplasia demonstrates extreme
enlargement and variation in nuclear shape. X200.

vacuolated. Nuclei are greatly enlarged with hyperchromasia, irregular margins, and often have rounded cytoplasmic invaginations (Oppenheimer; fig. 27).

Adrenal cytomegaly is of unknown significance, but must not be confused with cytomegalic inclusion disease or neoplasia (Kissane). These adrenals are usually less than 1 g in weight. When the change is diffuse, it may be associated with a clinical picture of Addison's disease (Lindgren). Cytomegaly is usually a focal change, but may involve much of the provisional zone. These changes may be seen in ectopic adrenal cells (fig. 28).

References

Bech, K., Tygstrup, I., and Nerup, J. The involution of the foetal adrenal cortex. Acta Pathol. Microbiol. Scand. 76:391-400, 1969.

Borit, A. and Kosek, J. Cytomegaly of the adrenal cortex. Arch. Pathol. 88:58-64, 1969.

Busuttil, A. Ectopic adrenal within the gall-bladder wall. J. Pathol. 113:231-233, 1974.

Challis, J. R. G., Mitchell, B. F., and Lye, S. J. Activation of fetal adrenal function. J. Dev. Physiology 6:93-105, 1984.

Coupland, R. E. The Natural History of the Chromaffin Cell. London: Longmans, 1965.

Crowder, R. E. Development of the adrenal gland in man with special reference to origin and ultimate locations of cell types and evidence in favor of cell migration theory. Contrib. to Embryol. 36:193-210, 1975.

Dolan, M. F. and Janovski, N. A. Adreno-hepatic union. Arch. Pathol. 86:22-24, 1968.

England, M. A. Color Atlas of Life Before Birth. Normal Fetal Development, p. 152. New York: Year Book Medical, 1983.

Falls, J. L. Accessory adrenal cortex in the broad ligament. Cancer 8:143-150, 1955.

Fujita, H. and Ihara, T. Electron-microscopic observations on the cytodifferentiation of adrenocortical cells of human embryo. Z. Anat. Entwicklungsgesch 142:267-281, 1973.

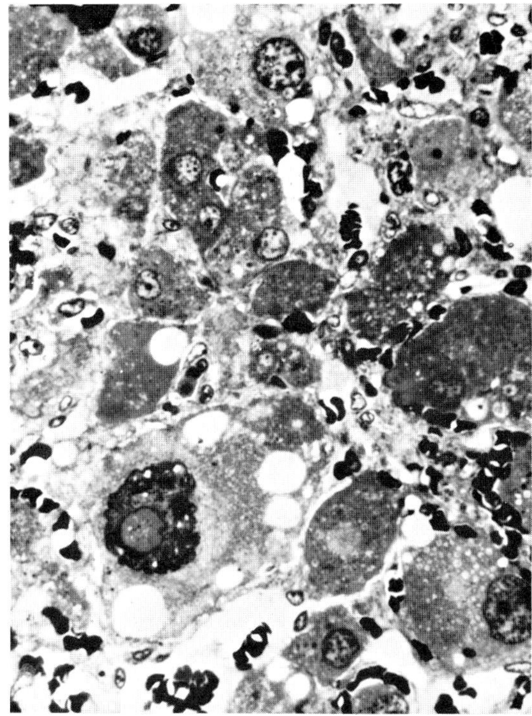

Figure 27
ANATOMIC VARIANTS
Focus of cytomegaly in a premature infant who died six hours after birth. Distinct membrane is seen around the cytoplasmic extrusion into the nucleus in largest cell at lower left. Epoxy embedded, methylene blue, azure II, basic fuchsin stain. X490. (Courtesy of the late Dr. E.H. Oppenheimer, Baltimore, MD.)

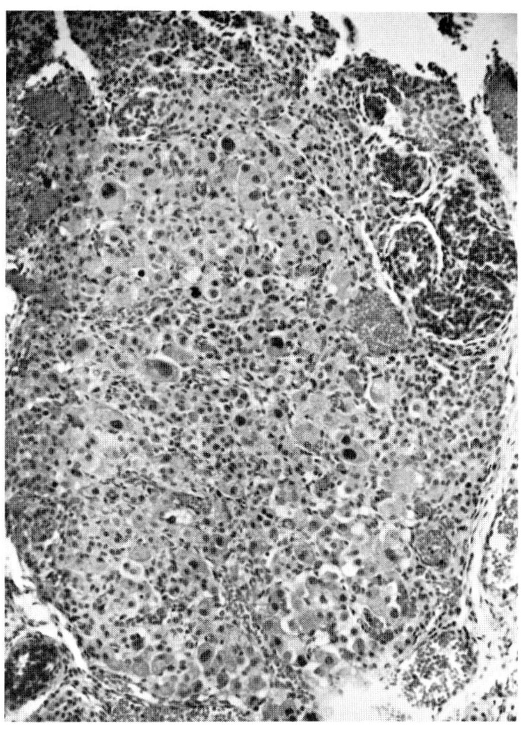

Figure 28
ANATOMIC VARIANTS
Cytomegaly of adrenal rest in testis. X75.

Graham, L. S. Celiac accessory adrenal glands. Cancer 6:149-152, 1953.

Hervonen, A. Development of catecholamine-storing cells in human fetal paraganglia and adrenal medulla. Acta Physiol. Scand. (Suppl.) 368:1-94, 1971.

Kissane, J. M. Pathology of Infancy and Childhood, pp. 746-783. St. Louis: The C. V. Mosby Company, 1975.

Lindgren, S. Congenital primary adrenal hypoplasia. Acta Pathol. Microbiol. Scand. 70:541-548, 1967.

Milkovic, K. and Domac, B. The effect of fetal pituitary ACTH and maternal corticosteroid on the development of fetal rat adrenal cortex. Endokrinologie (Leipzig) 62:17-18, 1973.

Neville, A. M. Disease of the Adrenal Gland, pp. 261-307. In: Applied Surgical Pathology. Stuart, A. E., Smith, A. N,, and Samuel, E. (Eds.). Oxford: Blackwell Scientific Publications, 1975.

Oppenheimer, E. H. Adrenal cytomegaly: Studies by light and electron microscopy. Arch. Pathol. 90:57-64, 1970.

Serón-Ferré, M. and Jaffe, R. B. The fetal adrenal gland. Ann. Rev. Physiol. 43:141-162, 1981.

Stark, E., Gyévai, A., Bukulya, B., Szabó, D., Szalay, K. S., and Mihály, K. Interrelationship between corticosteroid production and fine structure in the fetal adrenal cortex. Gen. Comp. Endocrinol. 25:472-486, 1975.

Symonds, D. A. and Driscoll, S. G. An adrenal cortical rest within the fetal ovary. Am. J. Clin. Pathol. 60:562-564, 1973.

Tähkä, H. On the weight and structure of the adrenal glands and the factors affecting them, in children of 0-2 years. Acta Paediatr. Scand. 40(81):1-95, 1951.

Tischler, A. S., DeLellis, R. A., Biales, B., Nunnemacher, G., Carabba, V., and Wolfe, H. J. Nerve growth factor-induced neurite outgrowth from normal human chromaffin cells. Lab. Invest. 43:399-409, 1980.

Wiener, M. F. and Dallgaard, S. A. Intracranial adrenal gland. Arch. Pathol. 67:228-233, 1959.

ENDOCRINOLOGY AND BIOCHEMISTRY

CORTEX

Normally, a sequence of enzymatic steps governed by enzymatic transformations produce the major corticosteroid hormones from the parent compound cholesterol (Wurtman and Axelrod). The first and rate limiting step in the biosynthesis of steroids is the conversion of cholesterol to pregnenolone. All steroid hormones are derived from this compound by subsequent modifications of the common skeleton (fig. 29). The essential corticosteroids have 21 carbon atoms (C-21 steroids), with cortisol, corticosterone, and aldosterone representing the major products of the adrenal cortex, both physiologically and quantitatively (fig. 30).

The **glucocorticoid** hormones are so termed because of effects on carbohydrate metabolism. They are C-21 steroids which are formed in the reticular and fasciculate zones. The production of cortisol, the most active of the naturally occurring glucocorticoids, and the most abundant one as well, is formed from a series of modifications proceeding from cholesterol which is converted by the 20-22 desmolase system to pregnenolone and by the 3 β (ol) dehydrogenase to progesterone (figs. 29, 30). The 17 hydroxylase enzyme produces 17 hydroxy-progesterone, which is then converted by 21-hydroxylase to form 17, 21-dihydroxyprogesterone or 11-deoxycortisol. Finally, hydroxylation at the 11 position produces cortisol. A small amount of corticosterone, a much less potent glucocorticoid, is produced when the hydroxylation at position 17 is not accomplished. Thus, corticosterone is produced by hydroxylation of progesterone at positions 21 and 11. Adrenocorticotrophic hormone (ACTH) from the anterior pituitary acts at the site of plasma membrane receptor in the adrenal cortex to initiate the synthesis and secretion of cortisol. A feedback control system involves the ability of cortisol to effect the decrease of ACTH release from pituitary either directly or by reducing secretion of corticotrophic releasing factor(s) (CRF) from the hypothalamus (Martin et al.).

The **mineralocorticoids** are also C-21 steroids and affect ion transport, resulting in sodium conservation, particularly in the kidney. Absence of mineralocorticoid activity may result in lethal wastage of sodium and retention of potassium. Many of the naturally occurring steroid hormones have this activity, but aldosterone is the most important and potent. Aldosterone is produced in the zona glomerulosa consequent to the unique presence there of the 18-hydroxylase enzyme and the absence there of a 17-hydroxylase. Thus, after its formation from progesterone, corticosterone is hydroxylated at C-18 to form 18 hydroxycorticosterone, which is converted to aldosterone by the 18-dehydrogenase. Regulation of aldosterone production is largely accomplished by the renin-angiotensin system. Renin is released into the blood by the juxtaglomerular apparatus in the kidney and enzymatically cleaves a plasma globulin, "renin substrate," to release a decapeptide, angiotensin I. This substance is further hydrolyzed to angiotensin II, which stimulates the formation and release of aldosterone (Nussdorfer). A feedback system is

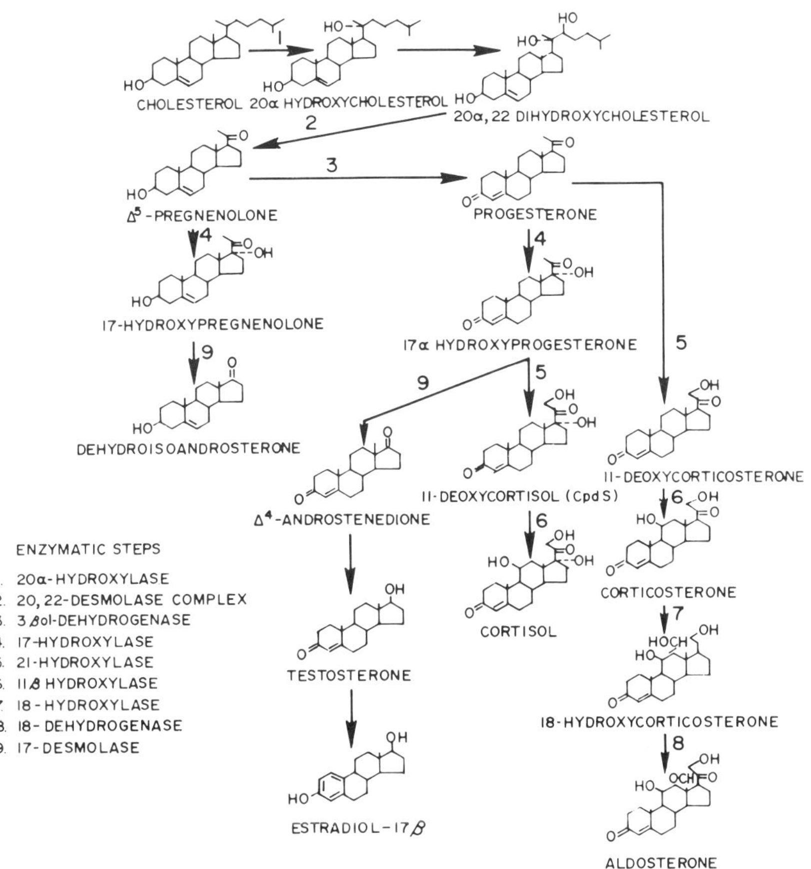

Figure 29
BIOCHEMISTRY
Major biosynthetic pathways for adrenal steroids. (From Temple, T.E. and Liddle, G.W. Inhibitors of adrenal steroid bio-synthesis. Ann. Rev. Pharmacol. 10:199-218, 1970).

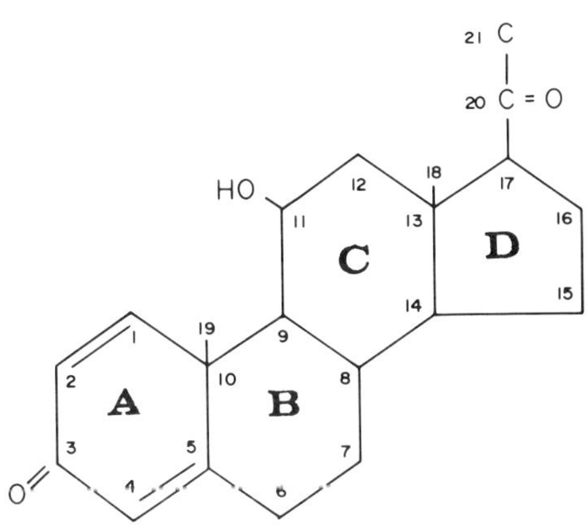

Figure 30
BIOCHEMISTRY
The steroid nucleus is shown with the elements common to all steroids known to have glucocorticoid activity in man. (Adapted from Liddle, G.W., 1974)

also involved in the normal control of this system, as high levels of aldosterone will result in low levels of renin. Despite the apparent preeminence of the renin-angiotensin system in aldosterone control mechanisms, ACTH is involved in the control of cell growth in the zona glomerulosa as well as in the maintenance of enzymatic integrity (Mazzocchi et al.; Hinson et al.).

Androgens contain 19 carbon atoms, and the relatively weak androgen, dehydroisoandrosterone (also known as dehydroepiandrosterone), is the most plentiful steroid produced by the adrenal cortex other than the corticosteroids. A small amount of testosterone, a potent virilizing agent, may also be produced. **Estrogenic steroids** contain 18 carbon atoms with a hydroxy group at position 3. Normally, only very small amounts of estrogenic compounds are produced by the adrenal. Androgens and estrogens are formed by cells of the zona fasciculata and zona reticularis.

Metabolism of the Corticosteroids

Small amounts of intact corticosteroids are excreted. However, most of the corticosteroids undergo inactivation by enzymes which introduce oxygen or hydrogen atoms at one or more positions. These inactive compounds are then conjugated to form water soluble derivatives which are excreted in the urine.

The liver inactivates the corticosteroids by enzymatic reduction of the 4-5 double bond in the A ring to form the dihydrosteroid derivative. This is converted to a tetrahydro derivative by the reduction of the 3-oxo group to a hydroxyl group. Conjugation with glucuronic acid produces the water soluble end product which is, then,

tetrahydrocortisol glucuronide in the case of cortisol and tetrahydroaldosterone glucuronide in the case of aldosterone. Similar compounds are produced from desoxycorticosterone and 11 deoxycortisol.

The major C-19 product of the adrenal, dehydroepiandrosterone (DHEA) is primarily conjugated to form dehydroepiandrosterone sulfate which is bound to plasma protein and is thus not readily excreted. As a result, it circulates in high concentration in the plasma. DHEA is the principal precursor of the urinary 17-ketosteroids. Although DHEA has little androgenic activity, alteration of some of it to testosterone gives it importance as an androgenic substance when it is present in elevated amounts.

MEDULLA

The biologically important catecholamines produced by the adrenal medulla in mammals include dopamine, norepinephrine, and epinephrine. Epinephrine, which is synthesized and stored primarily in the adrenal medulla, is secreted into the peripheral circulation where it exerts its effects on a variety of tissues. Norepinephrine, on the other hand, is synthesized and stored primarily by the peripheral sympathetic nerve endings, where it functions as the principal adrenergic neurotransmitter. In the human adrenal medulla, norepinephrine represents only 15 percent of the total catecholamine content. Both in the sympathetic nervous system and in the adrenal medulla, the catecholamines are stored in characteristic membrane bound secretory granules, which have been referred to as chromaffin or neurosecretory type granules. In addition to the catecholamines, which represent approximately 20 percent of the dry weight of the granules, a variety of other substances are found in the chromaffin granule fraction. These include ATP, dopamine β-hyroxylase, lysolecithin, chromogranins, and chromomembrins. The chromogranins represent a class of highly acidic water soluble proteins which are discharged concurrently with amine release. Although it has been suggested that the chromogranins may be important in the binding of catecholamines, the exact functional significance of these proteins remains obscure (Lloyd and Wilson). The high net negative charge of the chromogranins is largely responsible for the characteristic basophilia of adrenal medullary cells. The chromomembrins represent a class of water insoluble membrane associated proteins. The medulla also contains high concentrations of neuron specific enolase, the most acidic isoenzyme of the glycolytic enzyme, enolase (protein 14-3-2) (Schmechel et al.).

Synthesis and Inactivation of Catecholamines

Following active transport into cells, tyrosine undergoes a series of transformations to DOPA (dihydroxyphenylalanine), dopamine, norepinephrine, and epinephrine (fig. 31). The formation of epinephrine is almost entirely restricted to chromaffin cells within or just adjacent to the adrenal glands. A number of studies have indicated that the location of the adrenal medullary chromaffin cells within the cortex is associated with ability of the cells to form epinephrine. Animals with anatomically separate cortical tissues have low levels of medullary epinephrine, and exogenously administered steroids have been shown to have an enhancing effect on epinephrine

synthesis. Wurtman and Axelrod have shown that the enzyme phenylethanolamine-methyltransferase is inducible by glucocorticoids. The methylation system required for epinephrine formation appears to be lacking in fetal tissues. After birth, the proportion of epinephrine rises gradually and attains normal levels by two to three years of age.

The catecholamine molecule is inactivated by two major pathways (fig. 31). Meta-O-methylation is catalyzed by catechol-O-methyl transferase, which is present in highest concentrations in liver and kidney. Monoamine oxidase, which is widely distributed in a variety of tissues is responsible for oxidative deamination. Catecholamines and their metabolites may be excreted free in the form of glucuronide or sulfate conjugates. The normal urinary levels of catecholamines and their metabolites are summarized in Table 2. In the plasma, total catecholamines measure less than 1 μg/1. Upper limits of normal plasma norepinephrine and epinephrine are 0.2 $\pm$ 0.08 and 0.05 $\pm$ 0.03 μg/1, respectively. The plasma and urinary levels of free catecholamines and their metabolites may be markedly increased by a variety of drugs, dietary modifications, and emotional and physical stresses. Although catecholamines traditionally have been regarded as the only hormonal products of the adrenal medulla, recent studies have indicated that normal medullary cells have the capacity to synthesize a variety of regulatory peptide products. These include calcitonin, vasoactive intestinal peptide, somatostatin, substance P and leu- and met-enkephalin (DeLellis et al.; Kaplan et al.; Linnoila et al.; Lundberg et al.). The physiologic significance of these products within the medulla, however, remains unknown.

SYNTHESIS and METABOLISM of CATECHOLAMINES

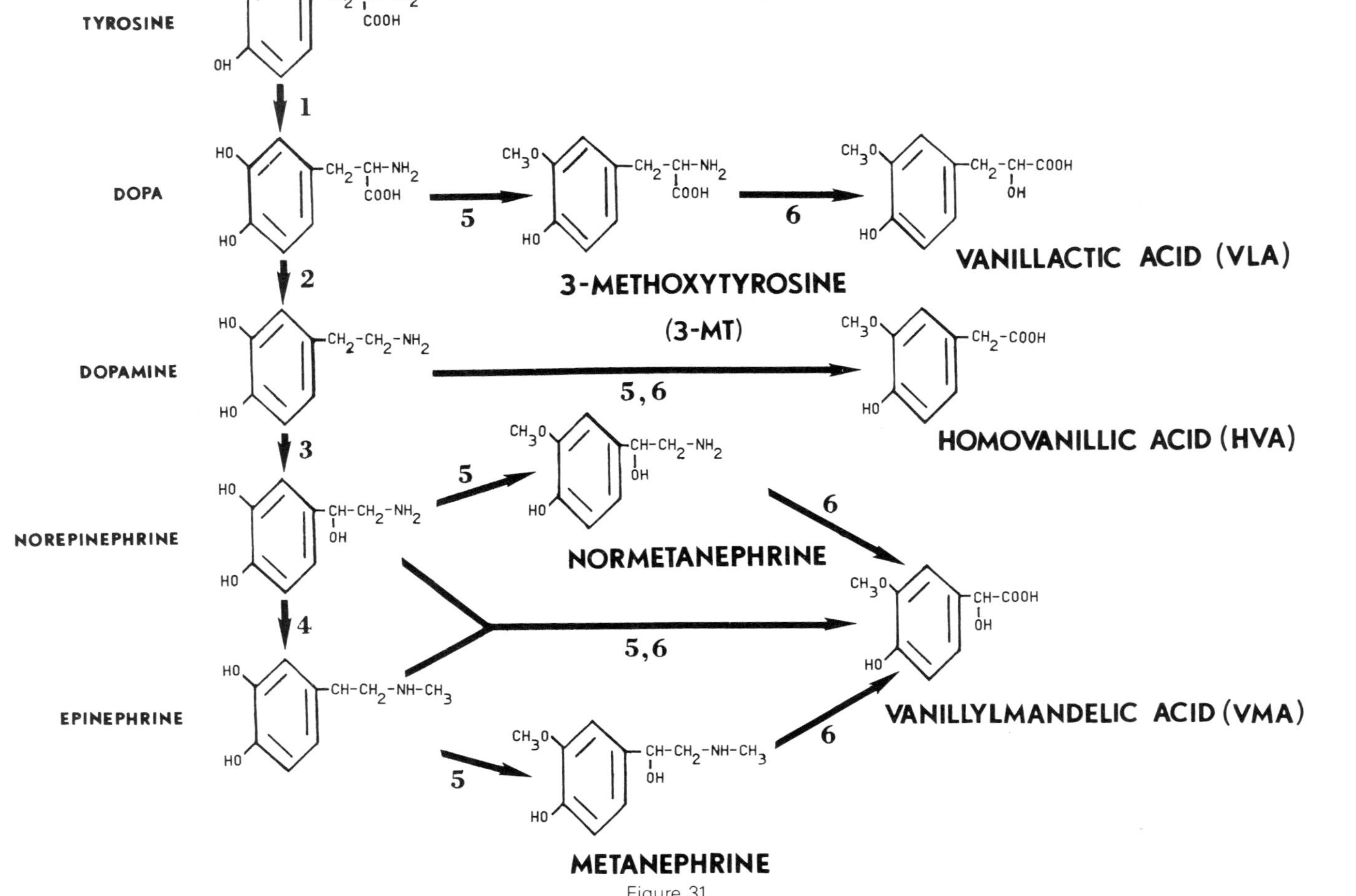

Figure 31
BIOCHEMISTRY

The synthesis and metabolism of catecholamines is summarized in this chart. The various enzymes involved in the synthesis and metabolism of the catecholamines are indicated by the number 1 through 6, as follows: (1) tyrosine hydroxylase; (2) DOPA decarboxylase; (3) dopamine-beta hydroxylase; (4) phenylethanolamine N-methyl transferase; (5) catechol-o-methyl-transferase; (6) monoamine oxidase and aldehyde dehydrogenase.

Table 2
URINARY CATECHOLAMINES AND METABOLITES

	Upper limit of normal (mg/24 hrs.)	Range (μg/mg of creatinine)
Catecholamines		
Epinephrine	0.02	
Norepinephrine	0.08	
	0.10 (total)	
Dopamine	0.20	0.08 to 0.23
Metanephrines		
Metanephrine	0.4	
Normetanephrine	0.9	
	1.3 (total)	0.001 to 2.2
Vanillylmandelic acid (VMA)	6.5	0.2 to 3.5
Homovanillic acid (HVA)	8.0	0.2 to 3.5

References

DeLellis, R. A., Tischler, A. S., Lee, A. K., Blount, M., and Wolfe, H. J. Leu-enkephalin-like immunoreactivity in proliferative lesions of the human adrenal medulla and extra-adrenal paraganglia. Am. J. Surg. Pathol. 7:29-37, 1983.

Hinson, J. P., Vinson, G. P., Whitehouse, B.J., and Price, G. Control of zona glomerulosa function in the isolated perfused rat adrenal gland in situ. J. Endocrinol. 104:387-395, 1985.

Kaplan, E. L., Arnaud, C. D., Hill, B. J., and Peskin, G. W. Adrenal medullary calcitonin-like factor: A key to multiple endocrine neoplasia, type 2? Surgery 68:146-149, 1970.

Kirshner, N. Biosynthesis of the Catecholamines, pp. 341-355. In: Handbook of Physiology. Endocrinology, Section 7, Vol 6. Greep, R. O. and Astwood, E. B. (Eds.). Washington: American Physiological Society, 1975.

Liddle, G. W. The Adrenal Cortex, pp. 233-283. In: Textbook of Endocrinology. Williams, R. H. (Ed.). Philadelphia: W. B. Saunders Company, 1974.

Linnoila, R. I., Diaugustine, R. P., Hervonen, A., and Miller, R. J. Distribution of (met[5])- and (leu[5])-enkephalin-, vasoactive intestinal polypeptide- and substance P-like immunoreactivities in human adrenal glands. Neuroscience 5:2247-2259, 1980.

Lloyd, R. V. and Wilson, B. S. Specific endocrine tissue marker defined by a monoclonal antibody. Science 222:628-630, 1983.

Lundberg, J. M., Hamberger, B., Schultzberg, M., et al. Enkephalin- and somatostatin-like immunoreactivities in human adrenal medulla and pheochromocytoma. Proc. Natl. Acad. Sci. USA 76:4079-4083, 1979.

Manger, W. M. and Gifford, R. W., Jr. Pheochromocytoma. New York: Springer-Verlag, 1977.

Martin, J. B., Reichlin, S., and Brown, G. M. Regulation of ACTH Secretion and its Disorders, pp. 179-200. In: Clinical Neuroendocrinology. Philadelphia: F. A. Davis Co., 1977.

Mazzocchi, G., Meneghelli, V., and Nussdorfer, G. G. Effects of angiotensin II on the zona glomerulosa of sodium-loaded dexamethasone treated rats administered or not with maintenance doses of ACTH: stereology and plasma hormone concentrations. Acta Endocrinol. 102:129-135, 1983.

Melby, J. C. Diagnosis and Treatment of Hyperaldosteronism and Hypoaldosteronism, pp. 1225-1234. In: Endocrinology, Vol. 2. DeGroot, L. J. et al. (Eds.). New York: Grune and Stratton, 1979.

Nussdorfer, G. G. Cytophysiology of the adrenal zona glomerulosa. Int. Rev. Cytol. 64:307-369, 1980.

Schmechel, D., Marangos, P. J., and Brightman, M. Neurone-specific enolase is a molecular marker for peripheral and central neuroendocrine cells. Nature 276:834-836, 1978.

Temple, T. E. and Liddle, G. W. Inhibitors of adrenal steroid biosynthesis. Ann. Rev. Pharmacol. 10:199-218, 1970.

Tischler, A. S., DeLellis, R. A., Biales, B., Nunnemacher, G., Carabba, V., and Wolfe, H. J. Nerve growth factor-induced neurite outgrowth from normal human chromaffin cells. Lab. Invest. 43:399-409, 1980.

Wurtman, R. J. and Axelrod, J. Control of enzymatic synthesis of adrenaline in the adrenal medullary adrenal cortical steroids. J. Biol. Chem. 241:2301-2305, 1966.

LOCALIZATION OF ADRENAL DISEASE

PLAIN FILM RADIOGRAPHY

Anteroposterior projection of the abdomen may reveal adrenal masses larger than 3 cm. Calcification of an adrenal mass when it is smaller than 3 cm may enable visualization, and this also may suggest a specific diagnosis, as 25 percent of adrenal carcinomas, 50 percent of neuroblastomas, and 5 percent of pheochromocytomas have patchy calcification which is virtually never seen in adenomas (Sutton; McAlister and Koehler). As detection with this technic depends on large size, the characteristically small lesions of primary aldosteronism will remain undetected. Adrenal cysts may occasionally be seen on the plain films and have a characteristic ringlike "egg shell" calcification in about 15 percent of cases (Palubinskas et al.). Pheochromocytoma may show a similar ringlike calcification (Neilson and Smith). Thus, only the characteristically bulky lesions of carcinoma and neuroblastoma can regularly be seen on plain film of the abdomen.

INTRAVENOUS UROGRAPHY AND NEPHROTOMOGRAPHY

These technics have an advantage over plain film radiography because the adrenals, along with the kidney, become more radiopaque following the injection of the contrast material. Nephrotomography is also important in excluding overlying soft tissue shadows which can simulate or hide adrenal masses on the plain films (Hartman et al). The intravenous urogram also allows the ureters and bladder to be visualized.

When the regional lymph nodes contain metastatic lesions, one or both ureters may be displaced. As with plain film radiography, the size of the lesions remains the critical factor in diagnosis. Tumors 2 to 5 cm in diameter or larger can be seen by these technics, while smaller adrenal lesions usually will not be identified. Cystic or poorly vascularized lesions may appear as relative radiolucencies during contrast nephrotomography. Mainly, diagnostic usefulness of the urogram depends on displacement of the kidney, renal pelvis, ureters, or bladder.

RETROPERITONEAL PNEUMOGRAPHY

Retroperitoneal pneumography is a technic little used at the present time. Gas is introduced into the retroperitoneal space, enabling the adrenals to be seen on plain radiographs if the gas dissected around the adrenals and kidneys. McLachlan and Beales reviewed 56 patients with this technic; 35 percent were false positive diagnoses. Thus, inconsistency in the ability of the gas to dissect about the gland makes determination of normal size and outline of the adrenal gland by this technic difficult. In general, adrenal masses must be almost 3 cm in diameter before they can be seen clearly by this technic. Other radiographic technics, such as venography and computerized axial tomography scanning, have virtually supplanted retroperitoneal pneumography in the preoperative localization of adrenal tumors.

ARTERIOGRAPHY

Arterial injection of contrast material is useful in the diagnosis of large lesions of the adrenal and the definition of blood supply to lesions already localized. The vascularity of neuroblastomas, pheochromocytomas, and adrenal carcinomas is such that lesions are usually seen with ease (Siekavizza et al.), and tortuous, irregular vessels with shunting to veins are characteristic of carcinoma. Small adenomas and nodules are often missed by arteriography. The reason for this inadequacy of arteriography in defining small lesions is probably related to the complexity of arterial supply to the adrenal.

VENOGRAPHY AND VENOUS SAMPLING

The presence of a single, relatively constant adrenal vein on each side makes this technic of visualization by venous injection more reliable for small lesions than arteriography. The retrograde injection of contrast material into the major adrenal vein may demonstrate mass lesions as small as 1 cm or less, primarily by showing a rounded deformity of adjacent veins "draped" over the surface of the mass. Positive evidence of the presence of a normal adrenal may also be obtained by this technic (fig. 32). Venacavography may visualize extension of adrenal carcinoma into the vena cava (Martorana et al.).

The selective sampling of the adrenal venous effluent is a highly sensitive and specific technic in the diagnosis of many functioning adrenal conditions. The venous samples may be analyzed for steroid hormones or catecholamines, usually to provide evidence for the location of a suspected tumor. This technic is particularly valuable in patients with pheochromocytoma and hyperaldosteronism, where the tumors may be small. The combined analysis of cortisol aids in determining the specificity of the sample as regards defining the sample as coming from the adrenal (Weinberger et al.).

ULTRASONOGRAPHY

Ultrasound evaluation of the adrenal glands is a sensitive modality for the detection of adrenal masses when performed using newer gray-scale ultrasound technics (Ferrucci). The advantages of this technic are that no ionizing radiation is used and the method is easily tailor-made to the individual patient's body characteristics. A careful systematic evaluation of the anatomy by a well trained individual is required to avoid incomplete or erroneous image formation. Given the proper environment, an overall accuracy of 90-95 percent can be attained. Adrenal masses smaller than 2.0, as found commonly in hyperaldosteronism, have not been detected with any degree of certainty, and extremely large tumors (10 cm or greater) so distort the anatomy that misinterpretation of the image can easily occur (Yeh et al.; Sample). Cystic versus solid tissue characterization can be easily performed, thereby refining the differential diagnosis in many cases.

COMPUTED TOMOGRAPHY

Computed tomography is a very sensitive means for studying mass lesions of the adrenal glands because of (1) the sensitivity of the method to changes in different tissue x-ray absorption properties and (2) the cross-sectional display of body anatomy.

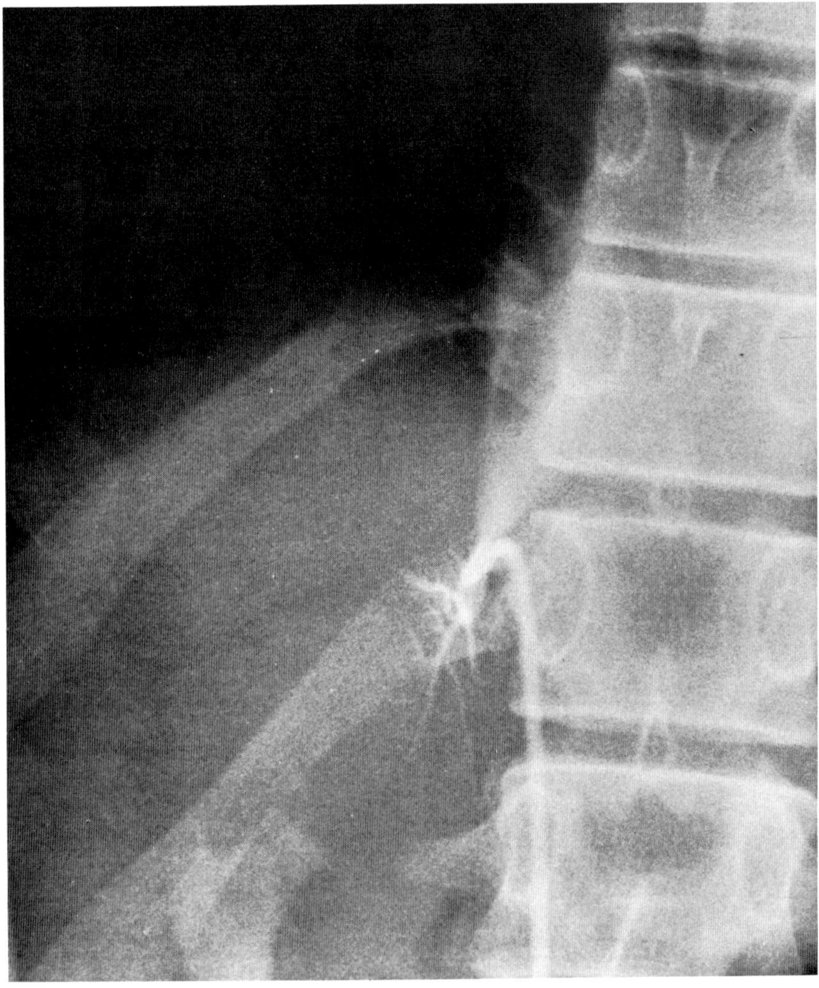

Figure 32
NORMAL ADRENAL
Retrograde injection of contrast material fills the major branches of the right adrenal vein in this venogram. A regular branching pattern is present without rounded contours produced by tumors. (Courtesy of Dr. A.J. Gerlock, Nashville, TN.)

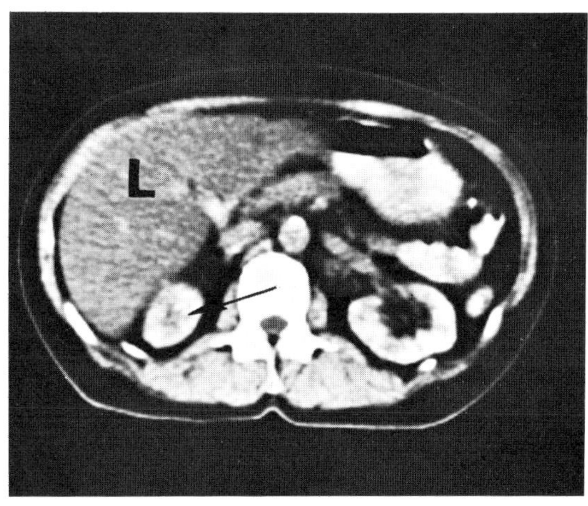

Figure 33
CORTICAL ADENOMA
Computed tomographic image demonstrates a rounded and enlarged right adrenal (arrow) between vertebral column in low central portion of picture and liver (L) at upper left of picture. The adenoma measured 5.5 cm in diameter at operation. (Courtesy of Dr. C. Coulam, Nashville, TN.)

Tumors 1.5-2 cm in diameter and larger are generally easily discerned, because the masses tend to completely replace the normal CT adrenal anatomy and lie as discreet masses in their characteristic position superior and anteromedial to the superior poles of both kidneys (fig. 33). The evaluation of small adrenal tumors or bilateral hyperplastic changes requires that the glands be surrounded by at least 3-5 mm of adipose tissue so the gland contours can be easily discerned. Normal adrenal glands can have overall diameters of 1 cm before they may be considered enlarged (Montagne et al.). Furthermore, since each gland images as a "comma shaped," "inverted V or Y," or "arrowhead" structure, with the thickness of each limb measuring up to 3-5 mm (El-Sherief and Hemmingsson), detection of subtle alterations in the gland configuration is required to identify the small adenomas. Depending upon the inherent spatial resolution of the CT scanner employed (i.e., 1.0 to 1.5 mm or less full-width-half-maximum point source response); the scanner's speed (i.e., five seconds or less); the ability of patients to cooperate by uniform breath holding episodes during the scanning period (i.e., to reposition their diaphragms and therefore adrenal gland positions to nearly the same spatial location); and the use of multiple, thin cross-sectional slice widths (i.e., 5 mm slice widths made every 5 mm through the glands) should allow for detection of 1 cm diameter nodules 50 percent of the time and 2-3 cm diameter masses 85-90 percent of the time (Karstaedt et al.). Central tumor necrosis may also be detected by computed tomography (Dunnick et al.).

NUCLEAR MEDICINE

The uptake of a radioactive tracer of a compound normally concentrated or metabolized by the adrenal gland forms the basis of adrenal scintigraphy. [131]I-19-Iodo-cholesterol is the compound most widely used currently (Seabold et al., 1976), while a newer agent [131]I-6β-Iodomethyl-19-nor-cholesterol (NP-59) has shown greater adrenal uptake and less in vivo deiodination (Sarkar et al.; Miles, et al.; Ryo et al.). Since the adrenal gland will normally concentrate the tracer material to some extent, adenoma formation is expected to show unilaterally increased uptake relative to the contralateral gland (Schteingart et al.). Using this increased activity as a criterion, adenomas 2-3 cm in diameter have been detected (Conn et al.). Quantitative evaluation of uptake by this agent may differentiate between various lesions producing Cushing's syndrome (Gross et al.) Following dexamethasone suppression in patients with Cushing's syndrome, adenomas continue to concentrate the tracer material while the hypoplastic glands cease their metabolic ability, thereby allowing for differentiation. Adenomas 1-2 cm in diameter have been detected following glandular suppression (Seabold et al, 1976). Adrenal gland scintigraphy may detect any type of functioning adenoma and has also demonstrated nodular adrenals (Rizza et al). Accuracy rates for detection and lateralization range from 100 percent (4) to 75 percent (1). Metastases of adrenal carcinoma have also been visualized with scintigraphy (Seabold et al., 1977).

NEEDLE ASPIRATION BIOPSY

The usefulness of diagnostic cytology with material obtained by aspiration has been more widely accepted in recent years. As with other body sites (particularly the thyroid), many diagnoses may be rendered with a high degree of accuracy (Nosher et al.), while other cases will produce indefinite evidence in borderline lesions. Definite diagnosis of adrenal carcinoma with this technic has been reported recently (Levin) and we have confirmed a metastatic seminoma.

MAGNETIC RESONANCE IMAGING

Nuclear magnetic resonance is currently (1984) being evaluated as a diagnostic technic (Moon et al.). Images of the adrenals obtained by this technic will have to be compared to the clarity of those found with computed tomography.

References

Conn, J. W., Morita, R., Cohen, E. L., Beierwaltes, W. H., McDonald, W. J., and Herwig, K. R. Primary aldosteronism. Arch. Int. Med. 129:417-425, 1972.

Dunnick, N. R., Heaston, D., Halvorsen, R., Moore, A. V., and Korobkin, M. CT appearance of adrenal cortical carcinoma. J. Comput. Assist. Tomogr. 6:978-982, 1982.

El-Sherief, M. A. and Hemmingsson, A. Computed tomography of the normal adrenal gland. Acta Radiol. 23:433-442, 1982.

Ferrucci, J. T., Jr. Body ultrasonography. N. Engl. J. Med. 300:590-602, 1979.

Gross, M. D., Valk, T. W., Freitas, J. E., Swanson, D. P., Schteingart, D. E., and Beierwaltes, W. H. The relationship of adrenal iodomethylnorcholesterol uptake to indices of adrenal cortical function in Cushing's Syndrome. J. Clin. Endocrinol. Metab. 52:1062-1066, 1981.

Hartman, G. W., Witten, D. M., and Weeks, R. E. The role of nephrotomography in diagnosis of adrenal tumors. Radiology 86:1030-1034, 1966.

Karstaedt, N., Sagel, S. S., Stanley, R. J., Melson, G.L., and Levitt, R. G. Computer tomography of the adrenal gland. Radiology 129:723-730, 1978.

Kehlet, H., Blichert-Toft, M., Hancke, S. et al. Comparative study of ultrasound, ^{131}I-19-iodocholesterol scintigraphy, and aortography in localising adrenal lesions. Br. Med. J. 2:665-667, 1976.

Levin, N. P. Fine needle aspiration and histology of adrenal cortical carcinoma. Acta Cytol. 25:421-424, 1981.

Martorana, G., Giberti, C., Pescatore, D., and Giuliani, L. Preoperative evaluation of adrenal cortical carcinoma extending into the inferior vena cava. J. Urol. 128:792-793, 1982.

McAlister, W. H. and Koehler, P. R. Diseases of the adrenal. Radiol. Clin. North Am. 5:205-220, 1967.

McLachlan, M. S. F. and Beales, J. S. M. Retroperitoneal pneumography in the investigation of adrenal disease. Clin. Radiol. 22:188-197, 1971.

Miles, J. M., Wahner, H. W., Carpenter, P. C., Salassa, R.M., and Northcutt, R. C. Adrenal scintiscanning with NP-59, a new radioiodinated cholesterol agent. Mayo Clin. Proc. 54:321-327, 1979.

Montagne, J., Kressel, H. Y., Korobkin, M., and Moss, A. A. Computed tomography of the normal adrenal glands. Am. J. Roentgenol. 130:963-966, 1978.

Moon, K. L., Jr., Hricak, H., Crooks, L. E., Gooding, C. A., Moss, A. A., Engelstad, B. L., and Kaufman, L. Nuclear magnetic resonance imaging of the adrenal gland: A preliminary report. Radiology 147:155-160, 1983.

Neilson, J. and Smith, S. M. Egg shell calcification in phaeochromocytoma. J. R. Coll. Surg. Edinb. 18:183-187, 1973.

Nosher, J. L., Amorosa, J. K., Seiman, S., and Plafker, J. Fine needle aspiration of the kidney and adrenal gland. J. Urol. 128:895-899, 1982.

Palubinskas, A. J., Christensen, W. R., Harrison, J. H., and Sosman, M. C. Calcified adrenal cysts. Am. J. Roentgenol. 82:853-861, 1959.

Rizza, R. A., Wahner, H. W., Spelsberg, T. C., Northcutt, R. C., and Moses, H. L. Visualization of nonfunctioning adrenal adenomas with iodocholesterol: Possible relationship to subcellular distribution of tracer. J. Nucl. Med. 19:458-463, 1978.

Ryo, U. Y., Johnston, A. S., Kim, I., and Pinsky, S. M. Adrenal scanning and uptake with ^{131}I-6B-Iodomethyl-Nor-Cholesterol. Radiology 128:157-161, 1978.

Sample, W. F. Adrenal ultrasonography. Radiology 127:461-466, 1978.

Sarkar, S. D., Beierwaltes, W. H., Ice, R. D. et al. A new and superior adrenal scanning agent, NP-59. J. Nucl. Med. 16:1038-1042, 1975.

Schteingart, D. E., Seabold, J. E., Gross, M. D., and Swanson, D. P. Iodocholesterol adrenal tissue uptake and imaging in adrenal neoplasms. J. Clin. Endocrinol. Metab. 52:1156-1161, 1981.

Seabold, J. E., Cohen, E. L., Beierwaltes, W. H. et al. Adrenal imaging with ^{131}I-19-Iodocholesterol in the diagnostic evaluation of patients with aldosteronism. J. Clin. Endocrinol. Metab. 42(1):41-51, 1976.

———, Haynie, T. P., DeAsis, D. N. et al. Detection of metastatic adrenal carcinoma using ^{131}I-6-B-Iodomethyl-19-Norcholesterol total body scans. J. Clin. Endocrinol. Metab. 45:788-797, 1977.

Siekavizza, J. L., Bernardino, M. E., and Samaan, N. A. Suprarenal mass and its differential diagnosis. Urology 18:625-632, 1981.

Sutton, D. The radiological diagnosis of adrenal tumours. Br. J. Radiol. 48:237-258, 1975.

Weinberger, M. H., Grim, C. E., Hollifield, J. W. et al. Primary aldosteronism. Ann. Intern. Med. 90:386-395, 1979.

Yeh, H. C., Mitty, H. A., Rose, J., Wolf, B. S., and Gabrilove, J. L. Ultrasonography of adrenal masses: Usual features. Radiology 127:467-474, 1978.

ENDOCRINOLOGIC ASPECTS OF ADRENOCORTICAL DISEASE

HYPERCORTISOLISM

SYNONYMS AND RELATED TERMS: Cushing's syndrome.

Definition and Endocrinologic Features

Cushing's syndrome is the result of excess glucocorticoids. Patients with endogenous or spontaneous Cushing's syndrome are characterized by adrenal hyperproduction of the principal human glucocorticoid, cortisol. There are several distinct types, including those due to pituitary overproduction of ACTH (with consequent adrenal hyperplasia), ectopic ACTH production, and autonomous adrenal production of cortisol by neoplasms of adrenal cortex. The syndrome is also commonly caused by exogenous glucocorticoid or ACTH administration and is characterized clinically by some combination of the following signs and symptoms: truncal obesity; hypertension; weakness and easy fatigability; amenorrhea; hirsutism; purple abdominal striae; edema; glucosuria; and osteoporosis (Nelson). Diagnosis of Cushing's syndrome is established by the demonstration of increased cortisol production in the absence of stress (Liddle, 1972). This may be accomplished in several ways (Table 3) and will depend upon local laboratory capabilities and preferences. Documentation of elevated glucocorticoid excretion by measurement of 17-OH corticosteroids in urine or elevated plasma cortisol are used most often. In the latter instance particularly, knowledge of the usual diurnal variation in cortisol production is imperative. In the morning, normal cortisol values may be in the same range as in Cushing's syndrome, but during the evening, normal individuals experience a fall in plasma cortisol, while those with Cushing's syndrome maintain values in the same high range observed earlier in the day. Disturbance of the normal homeostatic feedback control between pituitary ACTH release and adrenal cortisol release is definitively shown by the failure of dexamethasone in low dosage to suppress endogenous cortisol release, usually measured as urinary 17-hydroxycorticosteroids. Dexamethasone is a powerful synthetic glucocorticoid, extremely effective in reducing ACTH release when given in such low quantities that it does not interfere with chemical measurements of cortisol, its precursors or metabolites.

Further clinical tests often are able to define the underlying cause of excess adrenocortical hyperactivity. Basically, these tests rest on demonstrating the autonomy of steroid release at the adrenal level, as opposed to dependence of steroid release upon ACTH from the pituitary. The most helpful test is the response to dexamethasone, using a daily dose of 8 mg ("high dose"); pituitary dependent Cushing's syndrome (Cushing's disease) will regularly demonstrate suppression of cortisol release at this level. In contradistinction, tumors that release ACTH ectopically almost never demonstrate suppression in response to dexamethasone (Liddle et al). Adrenal tumors that secrete cortisol autonomously are never reproducibly suppressible with dexamethasone. Carcinoma is strongly suggested by elevation of both 17-OH corticosteroids and 17-ketosteroids. Carcinoma is most often associated with an elevated excretion of metabolites in the intermediary pathway of steroid synthesis, suggesting inefficient conversion of intermediates to cortisol. In hyperplasia and adenoma, metabolites of cortisol itself account for most of the released steroids as ordinarily measured. Adenomas may respond to exogenous ACTH with increased corticoid secretion, but carcinomas do not (Bertagna and Orth).

Metyrapone is a compound blocking 11β-hydroxylation, the last step in the formation of cortisol from its precursors. In the normal condition, this blocking of cortisol production will greatly increase ACTH production, stimulating cortisol precursor production consisting primarily of 11-deoxycortisol (fig. 29), the tetrahydro metabolite of which is measurable as a 17-hydroxycorticoid in the urine (West and Meikle). Unlike cortisol, 11-deoxycortisol lacks the capacity to block the secretion of ACTH by the pituitary. Normal or hyperactive responses to this test are usually seen in adrenal hyperplasia. Autonomous hyperproduction of glucocorticoids in adrenal tumors is usually not affected (Liddle, 1972).

Various radiologic, ultrasonographic, and venous sampling technics are often critical in establishing the site of excess corticoid production. Even intraoperatively at the time of removal of an apparent unilaterally enlarged adrenal, the presence of inactive or atrophic adrenal cortex adjacent to an adenoma should be documented, so that one is confident that one of the unusual cases of multinodular hyperplasia is not present.

Incidence. The great majority of cases of endogenous hypercortisolism are caused by pituitary ACTH overproduction, comprising up to 80 percent of cases of Cushing's syndrome (Cushing's disease or pituitary-based hypercortisolism). Up to 10 percent of these cases may present nodular adrenals associated with hyperplasia of the internodular cortical elements. Individual adrenal weight in this situation may rarely reach 50 g (see section on Hyperplasia). A small number of these greatly enlarged, hyperplastic, nodular glands differ from other cases of pituitary-dependent Cushing's disease by being resistant to acute dexamethasone suppression, thus mimicking autonomous adrenal function demonstrated by neoplasms.

Only about 4 percent of cases of Cushing's syndrome are caused by primary adrenal carcinoma and another 5 to 10 percent by a primary adrenal adenoma (Gold; Orth and Liddle). Ten to 15 percent of patients with endogenous hypercortisolism have production of ACTH by nonpituitary tumors (ectopic ACTH production), most often a small cell carcinoma of the lung.

A unique and rare type of endogenous hypercortisolism is associated with multiple small, usually pigmented nodules in adrenals which are of approximately normal weight. The condition is regularly bilateral and, because of the absence of adrenal enlargement, has been given almost as many diagnostic terms as there are case reports. The many nodules mimic adenoma with an intervening cortex which is inactive or atrophic. This differs greatly from the multinodular hyperplasia mentioned above, in which internodular adrenal tissue is both hypertrophic and hyperplastic. This rare and poorly understood subtype of Cushing's syndrome is associated with low ACTH levels, negative response to metyrapone, and resistance to dexamethasone suppression. Although ACTH levels have

Table 3

DIFFERENTIAL DIAGNOSIS

	NORMAL	ADRENAL NEOPLASM
Adrenal appearance[1]		
Usual weight of single adrenal	4-5 g	Greater than 20 g
Plasma cortisol	Normal daily rhythm	High — no rhythm
Plasma ACTH	Normal	Low
Glucocorticoid response to ACTH	3-5-fold rise	Usually none
Response to metyrapone[2]	2-4-fold rise	Usually none
Response to dexamethasone[3]	Fall with low dose	No fall
Plasma ACTH after adrenalectomy with normal cortisol replacement	Normal	Low
Response to pituitary ablation	—	None

[1] Presented in the same relative scale except for adrenal neoplasm and multinodular hyperplasia, where much larger sizes are usually attained. Shaded areas are active compact cells, diffusely increased in hyperplasia. Rounded mass lesions are nodules or neoplasms, actively releasing cortisol in these conditions.

[2] Metyrapone inhibits the formation of cortisol by blocking the preceding enzymatic step of 11β-hydroxylation. The rise in steroid precursors of cortisol consequent to ACTH release elevation caused by decreased plasma cortisol concentrations is measured as serum 11-deoxycortisol or its primary metabolite tetrahydro-11-deoxycortisol is measured as excretion of larger quantities in the urine as 17-hydroxycorticosteroids (Porter-Silber chromogens) or as 17-ketogenic steroids (17-KGS).

PITUITARY-BASED HYPERPLASIA[4]	ECTOPIC ACTH SYNDROME	MULTINODULAR ADRENAL HYPERPLASIA	MICROADENOMATOUS ADRENAL
6-12 g	12-20 g	30-50 g	Normal
High — no rhythm	High — no rhythm	High — no rhythm	High — no rhythm
High	High	Variable	Very low or undetectable
Rise	Usually none	Variable, often some rise	No response
Rise	Usually none	Often a rise	None
Partial fall (fall with high dose)	No fall	Usually no response	None
High	High	Variable, often high	Unknown
Remission	None	Some remissions	No remissions

[3]Dexamethasone is highly effective in producing the same negative feedback effect upon the pituitary normally accomplished by cortisol. Lowered production of glucocorticoids if ACTH production falls and the adrenal responds by lowering glucocorticoid production is measured either by plasma cortisol, urinary 17-OHCS, or 17-KGS.

[4]May be an occasional nodule present of the type seen in the multinodular adrenal with no hormonal abnormality.

been demonstrated to rise following bilateral adrenalectomy, one case demonstrated no response to pituitary ablation (see microadenomatous adrenal), thus proving autonomy of adrenal cortisol overproduction at least at the time the diagnosis was established. This anatomic and endocrinologic mimicry of adenoma has led us to suggest the terms "adenoma-like" or "microadenomatous adrenal" for this condition.

HYPERALDOSTERONISM

SYNONYMS AND RELATED TERMS: Primary aldosteronism; hyperaldosteronism with low plasma renin.

Definition and Incidence. Hyperaldosteronism defines a condition of elevated aldosterone production which results in hypertension, potassium depletion, and suppression of plasma renin activity.

Primary aldosteronism is conceptually analogous to hypercortisolism produced by adrenal cortical neoplasms in that aldosterone is inappropriately released independent of the renin-angiotensin system. Most patients with primary aldosteronism have unilateral cortical adenoma (Conn's syndrome) associated with hypertension, marked suppression of renin activity, and excessive aldosterone production. Many of the remainder have bilateral disease with a diffusely prominent zona glomerulosa.

Because as many as one-quarter of the population with hypertension may have suppressed or low renin levels, additional studies demonstrating inappropriate aldosterone production are necessary to identify a small percentage of this population (as many as 1 percent of hypertensives) with primary aldosteronism. The occurrence of various patterns of anatomic change in primary aldosteronism will depend upon the screening tests that were used to determine patients selected for surgical exploration. Most recent studies have been able to detect smaller adenomas and screen out a larger percentage of patients with bilateral disease. Probably over 80 percent of patients with primary aldosteronism have adenomas, predominantly solitary, with a definite female preponderance (3:1) and an age incidence predominating from 30 to 50 years (Grim et al.). In over 90 percent of patients with hyperaldosteronism associated with adenoma, the anatomy will be clear-cut, with a solitary adenoma present. Most of the remainder, however, will have multiple adenomas, usually only two, on one side only, leaving room for debate whether they are true adenomas or nodules (see section on Adenomas). Aldosterone secreting adenomas in ectopic locations have not been reported. Patients with bilateral adrenal disease tend to be older and the sex ratio approaches unity. Carcinoma of the adrenal associated with hyperaldosteronism is rare, with less than 20 cases reliably documented. Also, in many of these cases the likely possibility that other steroids such as 18-OH corticosterone or DOC might be responsible was not ruled out. Some carcinomas associated with clinical signs and symptoms of Conn's syndrome may well be producing mineralocorticoid hormones other than aldosterone (Melby), a finding appropriate to the greatly altered function associated with malignant adrenocortical tumors.

An important, although rare, cause of primary aldosteronism is familial and is relieved by dexamethasone. Surgical extirpation of a slightly enlarged adrenal (7 g) with several 1-4 mm nodules of clear cells in the fasciculate zone did not relieve the hypertensive state (Sutherland et al.; New and Peterson).

Clinical Diagnosis. Disease in this condition is recognized by weakness, which may accompany the lowered serum potassium level. Some patients will have asymptomatic hypertension. As in the case of hypercortisolism, the first diagnostic step is to detect the presence of primary aldosteronism and then proceed to a definition of adrenal status and localization of the lesion(s). Hyperaldosteronism occurring in a setting of bilateral adrenal hyperplasia does not often respond to surgical extirpative treatment (Melby). Therefore, the preoperative differentiation of the diffuse and hyperplastic disease from the unilateral form of the the disease seen with adenoma formation is of great importance.

Diagnostic technics in primary aldosteronism are still being developed. The recent availability of radioimmunoassay technics for measuring plasma renin activity and plasma aldosterone, as well as refinement of tests evaluating manipulation of the renin-angiotensin-aldosterone feedback system have enhanced the precision of diagnosis (Weinberger et al.). It must be noted that prior antihypertensive therapy may alter the expected finding of low renin levels. Hypokalemia is a highly suggestive finding in a hypertensive patient, as is elevated aldosterone secretion rate, but neither finding is specific for this syndrome. The finding of serum potassium levels less than 4.0 milliequivalents per liter is a sensitive screening test (Bravo et al.). Intravenous infusion of saline normally suppresses plasma aldosterone levels; if this maneuver does not suppress plasma aldosterone levels into the normal range, the

diagnosis of primary aldosteronism is almost assured. Similarly, the inability to stimulate plasma renin activity by measures which will deplete effective blood volume (upright posture, sodium restriction, or diuretic administration) is quite specific for this syndrome. Some indication of adrenal status may be predicted from these studies, particularly the tendency for patients with anomalous fall of aldosterone level with upright posture to have unilateral adenomas, but more specific localizing procedures are necessary.

No single localizing technic is infallible, because the adenomas associated with this condition are small, rarely over 3 cm in diameter and often less than 1 cm. The sensitivity of arteriography is such that it is almost useless in finding the smaller lesions, and isotopic technics with labelled cholesterol will detect only the larger lesions. Adrenal venography is the most sensitive imaging technic (Javadpour et al.), but cannot identify mass lesions less than 1 cm in diameter (Yune et al.). Computerized axial tomography has a similar sensitivity (Ganguly et al.). It must be noted also that detection of lesions less than 1 cm in diameter may not be more precise at time of surgical exploration unless the lesion is at the periphery of the adrenal, and their final detection may await slicing of the gland in the surgical pathology laboratory. The most reliable method of preoperative assessment of unilateral disease is sampling of the blood from the adrenal veins for aldosterone and comparing the two sides. Aldosterone production by one adrenal seven times greater than the other will regularly predict that surgical removal of the adrenal with elevated production will ameliorate the clinical state (Weinberger et al.).

VIRILIZATION

The appearance of adult masculine characteristics in prepubertal males or females of any age constitutes the syndrome of virilization. Virilization is regularly associated with the common types of congenital adrenal hyperplasia. Adrenal neoplasms producing androgens or androgen precursors may also produce virilization. These may present at any period of life. However, there are almost no reported cases occurring immediately after birth, which is of help in differentiating neoplasms from congenital adrenal hyperplasia (Migeon). In childhood, some of these neoplasms producing virilization may follow a benign clinical course. In adults, however, the majority of these neoplasms are malignant. Total 17-ketosteroid excretion is elevated in most of the neoplasms producing this syndrome. Some cases, however, produce primarily testosterone, which is often not associated with elevation of 17-ketosteroid excretion. Virilizing adrenal neoplasms show no suppression of plasma androgens or urinary 17-ketosteroids during dexamethasone suppression.

FEMINIZATION

Although rarely described in adult males, feminization of adrenal origin is almost always due to a malignant adrenal neoplasm (Harrison et al.). This syndrome is recognized clinically by the presence of gynecomastia, testicular atrophy, feminizing hair changes, and loss of libido. Feminization due to an adrenal lesion in children is more likely to be caused by a benign adrenal neoplasm (Leditschke and Arden; Stewart et al.). Lesions elsewhere than in the adrenal, particularly the ovary in the female, may produce feminization. When caused by an adrenal neoplasm, feminization is usually associated with increased 17-ketosteroid excretion, with greatly elevated levels most likely to be seen with carcinoma (Wolf et al.). Elevation of urinary estrogen excretion should be considered mandatory diagnostic evidence for the syndrome (Gabrilove et al.; Greenwood).

MIXED ENDOCRINE SYNDROMES

Any of the above described syndromes occurring in combination is termed a mixed syndrome. In general, the appearance of a mixed syndrome is associated with a malignant adrenal neoplasm. Elevated excretion of sex hormones and their precursors may accompany hypercortisolism occurring in settings other than malignant tumor, but clinical signs of virilization or feminization occurring with Cushing's syndrome are regularly an indication of adrenal carcinoma.

A startling demonstration of the instability of function in adrenal carcinoma is demonstrated in the case report of a young girl presenting with hypercortisolism and virilization. Her clinical features changed to feminization during the course of her disease (Halmi and Lascari).

References

Bertagna, C. and Orth, D. N. Clinical and laboratory findings and results of therapy in 58 patients with adrenocortical tumors admitted to a single medical center (1951 to 1978). Am. J. Med. 71:855-875, 1981.

Bravo, E. L., Tarazi, R. C., Dustan, H. P., Fouad, F. M., Textor, S. C., Gifford, R. W., and Vidt, D. G. The changing clinical spectrum of primary aldosteronism. Am. J. Med. 74:641-651, 1983.

Gabrilove, J. L., Sharma, D. C., Wotiz, H. H., and Dorfman, R. I. Feminizing adrenocortical tumors in the male. Medicine 44:37-79, 1965.

Ganguly, A., Pratt, J. H., Yune, H. Y., Grim, C. E., and Weinberger, M. H. Detection of adrenal tumors by computerized tomographic scan in endocrine hypertension. Arch. Int. Med. 139:589-590, 1979.

Gold, E. M. The Cushing syndromes: Changing views of diagnosis and treatment. Ann. Int. Med. 90:829-844, 1979.

Greenwood, R. H. Selective feminization due to an adrenal carcinoma. Proc. R. Soc. Med. 67:671-672, 1974.

Grim, C. E., Weinberger, M. H., Higgins, J. T., and Kramer, N. J. Diagnosis of secondary forms of hypertension. J.A.M.A. 237:1331-1335, 1977.

Halmi, K. A. and Lascari, A. D. Conversion of virilization to feminization in a young girl with adrenal cortical carcinoma. Cancer 27:931-935, 1971.

Harrison, J. H., Mahoney, E. M., and Bennett, A. H. Tumors of the adrenal cortex. Cancer 32:1227-1235, 1973.

Javadpour, N., Woltering, E. A., and Brennan, M. F. Adrenal neoplasms. Curr. Probl. Surg. 17:3-52, 1980.

Leditschke, J. F. and Arden, F. Feminizing adrenal adenoma in a five year old boy. Aust. Paediatr. J. 10:217-221, 1974.

Liddle, G. W. The Adrenal Cortex, pp. 233-283. In: Textbook of Endocrinology. Williams, R. H. (Ed.). Philadelphia: W. B. Saunders Company, 1974.

————. Pathogenesis of glucocorticoid disorders. Am. J. Med. 53:638-648, 1972.

————, Nicholson, W. E., Island, D. P., Orth, D. N., Abe, K., and Lowder, S. C. Clinical and laboratory studies of ectopic humoral syndromes. Recent Prog. Horm. Res. 25:283-305, 1969.

Melby, J. D. Diagnosis and Treatment of Hyperaldosteronism and Hypoaldosteronism, pp. 1225-1234. In: Endocrinology, Vol. 2. DeGroot, L. J. et al. (Eds.). New York: Grune and Stratton, 1979.

Migeon, C. J. Diagnosis and Treatment of Adrenogenital Disorders, pp. 1203-1224. In: Endocrinology, Vol. 2. DeGroot, L. J. et al. (Eds.). New York: Grune and Stratton, 1979.

Nelson, D. H. Cushing's Syndrome, pp. 1179-1191. In: Endocrinology, Vol. 2. DeGroot, L. J. et al. (Eds.). New York: Grune and Stratton, 1979.

New, M. I. and Peterson, R. E. A new form of congenital adrenal hyperplasia. J. Clin. Endocrinol. Metab. 27:300-305, 1967.

Orth, D. N. and Liddle, G. W. Results of treatment in 108 patients with Cushing's syndrome. N. Engl. J. Med. 285:243-247, 1971.

Stewart, D. R., Morris Jones, P. H., and Jolleys, A. Carcinoma of the adrenal gland in children. J. Pediatr. Surg. 9:59-67, 1974.

Sutherland, D. J. A., Ruse, J. L., and Laidlaw, J. C. Hypertension, increased aldosterone secretion and low plasma renin activity relieved by dexamethasone. Can. Med. Assoc. J. 95:1109-1119, 1966.

Weinberger, M. H., Grim, C. E., Hollifield, J. W. et al. Primary aldosteronism. Ann. Intern. Med. 90:386-395, 1979.

West, C. D. and Meikle, A. W. Laboratory Tests for the Diagnosis of Cushing's Syndrome and Adrenal Insufficiency and Factors Affecting those Tests, pp. 1157-1177. In: Endocrinology, Vol. 2. DeGroot, L. J. et al. (Eds.). New York: Grune and Stratton, 1979.

Wolf, E. T., Mills, L. C., Newton, B. L. et al. Adrenocortical carcinoma causing feminization in an adult male: hormonal consideration and results of heterotransplantation of the tumor in guinea pigs. J. Clin. Endocrinol. 18:310-317, 1958.

Yune, H. Y., Klatte, E. C., Grim, C. E. et al. Radiology in primary hyperaldosteronism. Am. J Roentgenol. 127:761-767, 1976.

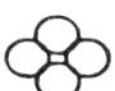

ADRENAL CORTICAL TUMORS AND TUMOR-LIKE CONDITIONS

HYPERPLASIA

The term **hyperplasia** is defined as an increased number of cells in an organ. It is a change usually associated with increased function or compensatory change. We reserve the term hyperplasia, as it relates to the adrenal, for clinicopathologic situations in which increased functional status is present and there is anatomic evidence of generalized increase in cortical cells. A large group of patients with enlarged and nodular adrenal glands lack convincing clinical, biochemical, or anatomic evidence for hypersteroidism. The pathogenetically and functionally noncommittal descriptive term **nodule** is used for these focal increases in adrenal cortical cell numbers where altered functional status is unproved. Diagnostic terms applied to these irregularly enlarged nodular adrenal glands are analogous to those in other glands of the endocrine system, particularly the thyroid, where the use of the terms **nodular** or **multinodular thyroid** are well accepted. It is regrettable that there is no term analogous to **goiter** referrable to the adrenal — the term is noncommittal, denoting only enlargement of the thyroid.

CONGENITAL ADRENAL HYPERPLASIA

Definition. The various forms of congenital adrenal hyperplasia (CAH) are the result of dyshormonogenesis — congenital errors in the biosynthesis of cortisol, androgens, and/or aldosterone consequent to the absence or reduced effectiveness of various enzymatic steps in the sequence of steroid synthesis (Table 4; fig. 29). Common to all is the reduced production of cortisol with compensatory hypersecretion of ACTH, in an attempt to maintain cortisol synthesis in the face of the deficiency (Migeon, 1972, 1979; New and Levine). Virilization, in both males and females, is common to most of these diseases due to the overproduction of cortisol precursors with androgenic activity.

By far the most common of the various types of congenital adrenal hyperplasia results from the impairment of 21-hydroxylation which, when severe, involves life threatening mineralocorticoid deficiency as well. The salt-losing form is much less common than the simple virilizing form. The defect in 21-hydroxylation activity, when complete, prohibits the formation of desoxycorticosterone and aldosterone (fig. 29). The less severe form (termed simple virilizing CAH) involves salt loss only during times of stress, due to partial absence of 21-hydroxylation activity. This simple or virilizing type of CAH is an allelic form of 21-hydroxylase deficiency, as is an even milder or "attenuated" form (Migeon et al.). There is evidence that 21-hydroxylation is present in the glomerular zone in milder forms, accounting for production of mineralocorticoids (Biglieri et al.). The clinical features of the rare forms of this disease are shown in Table 4.

Combined 21- and 11β-hydroxylase deficiency may be seen in familial congenital adrenal hyperplasia (Hurwitz et al.).

Gross. In the severe syndrome, most commonly seen at autopsy, there is a highly characteristic cerebriform appearance of

Table 4

CONGENITAL ADRENAL HYPERPLASIA

Enzyme Defect	Relative Frequency	Clinical Features
21-Hydroxylase	95%	
Mild (compensated)		Virilism
Severe		Virilism and salt losing
11β-Hydroxylase	5%	Virilism and hypertension
17-Hydroxylase	Rare	Immature female phenotype and hypertension
3β Ol-Dehydrogenase	Rare	Sexual ambiguity and salt losing
20-22 Desmolase	Rare	Complete adrenal insufficiency

the adrenal, which is diffusely brown (fig. 34). The very rare enzyme deficiency of 20-22 desmolase (responsible for producing pregnenolone from cholesterol) produces adrenocortical incompetence and is seen with a specific gross appearance (Sandison) of a greatly enlarged, coarsely nodular adrenal with yellow areas due to extensive storage of cholesterol (congenital lipoid adrenal hyperplasia).

As most of the more common types of these diseases are now identified and treated with success, the glands are not usually available for examination. The appearance of the treated glands is not known, but may resemble glands in patients treated with full replacement doses of cortisol.

Histologic Appearance. Histologically, most of the cases are associated with extensive infolding of the cortex producing a cerebriform appearance, with a predominence of compact cells extending throughout the cortical thickness (fig. 35). This appearance is, in reality, an ACTH effect. A few lipid-rich cells may separate these cells from glomerulosa cells or the capsule. Adrenal changes in the salt-losing

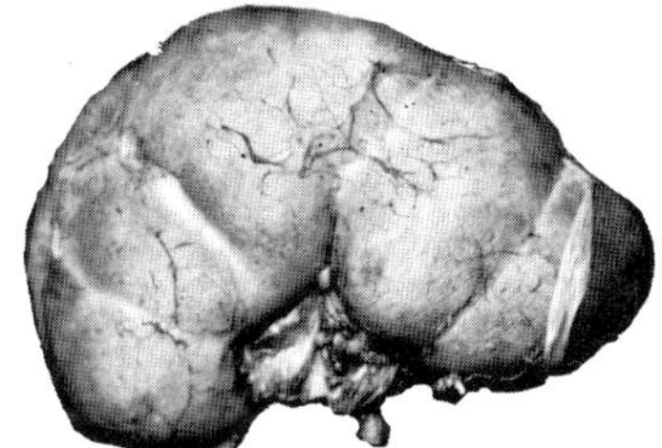

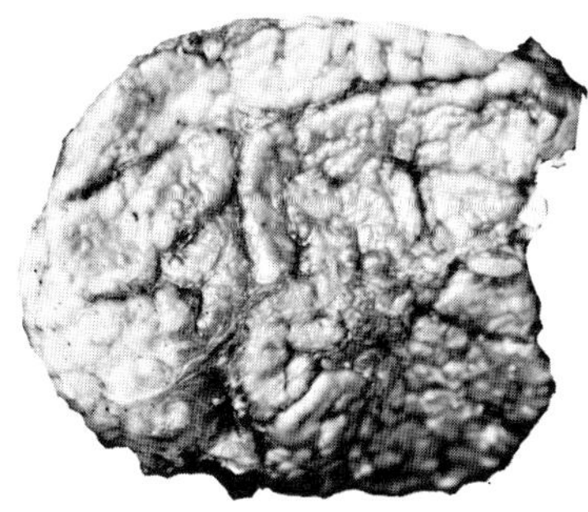

Figure 34
(Figures 34 and 35 from same patient)
CONGENITAL ADRENAL HYPERPLASIA
Gross photograph of kidney and adrenal from a patient with congenital adrenal hyperplasia who died at the age of 6 weeks. Combined adrenal weight was 22 g. 17-ketosteroid urinary excretion in 24 hours was increased to greater than 10 times normal. This is probably an example of severe 21-hydroxylase defect. Actual size. (Courtesy of the Department of Pathology, University of Leeds, Leeds, England.)

syndromes (due to specific defect in aldosterone production from corticosterone) have not been well described (Hamilton). Histology of glands in patients treated with corticoid replacement is also unknown. Changes of myelolipoma may be seen in the adrenals (Boudreaux et al.) in these states, as well as in other syndromes with ACTH excess (Bennett et al.).

Natural History and Therapy. Most cases of congenital adrenal hyperplasia are detected at birth or soon thereafter, some presenting with virilism and others with salt-losing syndrome and/or virilization. When the enzyme defect is mild, some do not present until puberty. Treatment consists in replacing cortisol so that ACTH release is returned to physiologic levels (Brook et al.; Ross et al.).

Testicular enlargement with prominence of interstitial cells indistinguishable from adrenal cells is well described in adults with the 21-hydroxylase defect (Fore et al.; Kirkland et al.; Newell et al.). This condition is dependent upon elevated levels of ACTH and may be relieved by increasing steroid replacement doses.

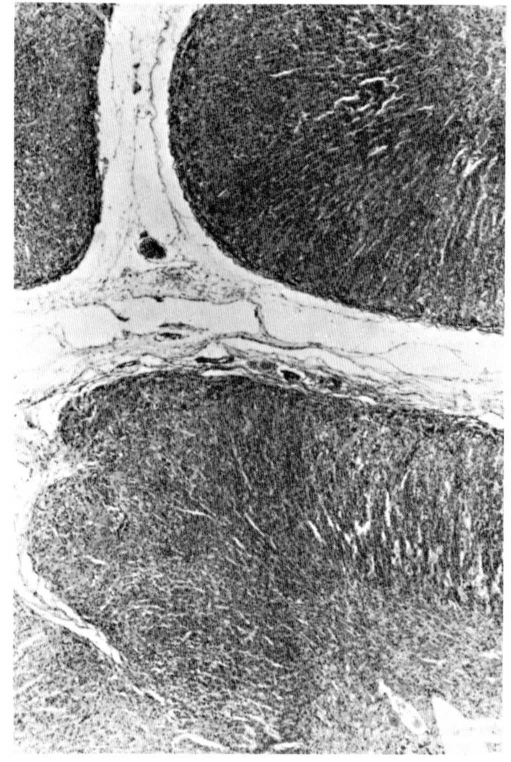

Figure 35
CONGENITAL ADRENAL HYPERPLASIA
Convoluted cortex made up of compact cells from the same patient with congenital hyperplasia shown in figure 34. X10.

SIMPLE DIFFUSE HYPERPLASIA WITH PITUITARY-BASED HYPERCORTISOLISM
(Cushing's Disease)

Definition and Incidence. Diffuse and symmetrical enlargement of the adrenals with hypercortisolism due to pituitary overproduction of ACTH is the most common cause of spontaneous (endogenous) hypercortisolism, accounting for almost 80 percent of clinical diagnoses. Most cases present in the third and fourth decades, with a female predominence of 3 to 1. Children with this condition are usually above the age of 10, and in childhood the sex ratio is about equal. Pituitary adenomas in this condition are much more common than previously realized (Tyrrell et al.) and are now thought to be directly responsible for most cases of Cushing's disease (Fitzgerald et al.; Orth).

Gross. Adrenal enlargement is not impressive, with most cases having approached a doubling of normal size (fig. 36). Weights, then, are usually between 6 and 8 g for each adrenal. Occasionally they approach 12 g for each adrenal and here the adrenals

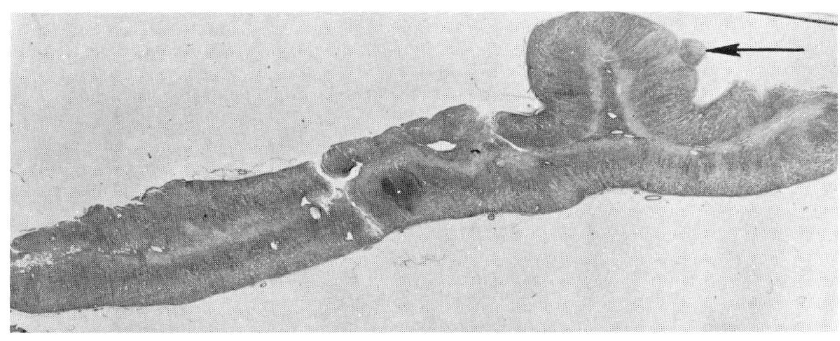

Figure 36
SIMPLE DIFFUSE HYPERPLASIA
This adrenal is from a patient with pituitary based hypercortisolism (Cushing's disease). The diffusely broadened cortex is evident on each side of the gland. A cortical extrusion (arrow) is seen at the upper right of the rounded protuberant area. X3.

regularly demonstrate some degree of nodularity.

Close examination of the cut surface reveals a prominent brown inner cortical layer, with an outer yellow layer of approximately equal thickness. Small nodules, if present, are irregularly distributed and are yellow or yellow with interspersed brown regions, and the term nodular hyperplasia has been used (Neville and Symington, 1972), particularly when nodules of 2.5 cm in diameter are present (Symington, 1982). Smals and associates have shown that nodules of 0.5 to 5.3 cm in size are more commonly found in older patients with longer duration of disease than in others with Cushing's disease. More minute microscopic nodules also are not uncommon. These nodules may present above the capsular surface, are 1-3 mm in diameter, and probably represent hyperplastic extracapsular nodules or extrusions of hyperplastic adrenal cells through the cortex.

Microscopic. A widened inner zone of compact zona reticularis cells (Cohen et al.) is usually sharply demarcated from an outer

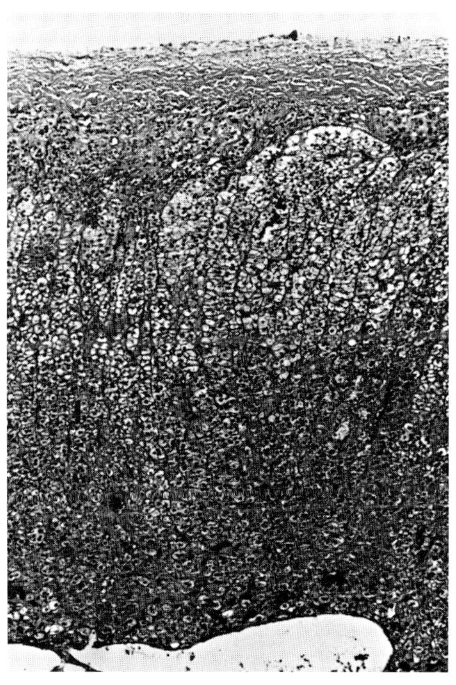

Figure 37
SIMPLE DIFFUSE HYPERPLASIA,
MILD
Full thickness of the cortex is seen from capsule above to central vein below, in a patient with Cushing's disease. Compact cells make up more than 50 percent of the thickness of the cortex, despite the fact that the cortex is not greatly broadened. In a surgical specimen, as in this case, even these mild changes, in the presence of positive biochemical finding (Table 3), are confirmatory evidence for pituitary based hypercortisolism. X75.

zone of clear cells (fig. 37). The occasional nodules or nodular arrangements (Neville and Symington, 1972) are often made up of clear cells which may have interspersed collections of compact cells (figs. 38, 39). The broadening of the compact cell containing zona reticularis is a particularly important confirmatory histologic finding in cases falling within the normal weight range (Cohen et al.).

Diagnosis of this condition at time of autopsy without premortem hormonal studies is difficult. Prolonged illness regularly produces similar adrenal alterations.

Ultrastructural studies are few, but have tended to confirm changes similar to those seen in experimental animals treated with excess amounts of ACTH (Neville and Mackay). Decrease in lipid globule size,

increase in prominence of smooth endoplasmic reticulum, and mitochondrial alterations are present (Reidbord and Fisher). These studies must be carefully structured and interpreted with regard to control of area sampled and understanding of pharmacologic manipulation which may have preceded surgery.

Treatment and Natural History. The ideal treatment goal is to eliminate hypercortisolism and restore the function of the pituitary-adrenal axis. Partial removal of the pituitary, ideally removing cells releasing supraphysiologic amounts of ACTH as well as pituitary irradiation may accomplish this task (Burke et al.). Bilateral adrenalectomy with corticoid replacement is also often used (Scott et al.; Prinz et al.) and is, of course, the source of most adrenals de-

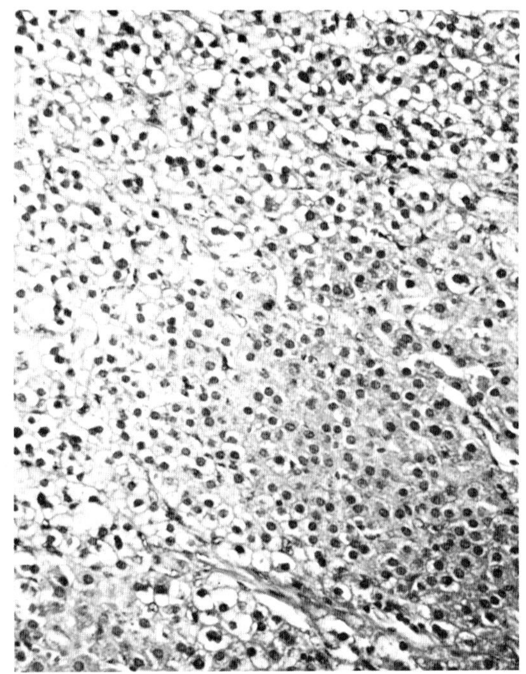

Figure 38
SIMPLE DIFFUSE HYPERPLASIA
A suggestion of nodularity is given by this intermixing of compact, clear, and intermediate cell types in this adrenal removed at bilateral adrenalectomy as definitive treatment for Cushing's disease. X190.

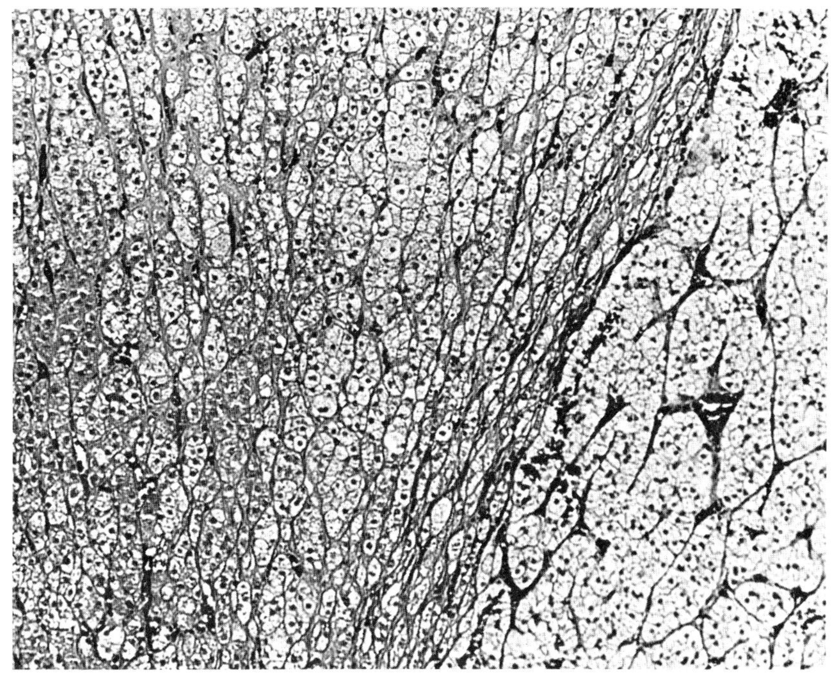

Figure 39
NODULES IN HYPERPLASIA WITH HYPERCORTISOLISM
A nodule of clear cells is seen at right in an adrenal from a 34 year old woman with pituitary dependent hypercortisolism cured by total adrenalectomy after failure of pituitary irradiation. Only three or four nodules were apparent in adrenals, weighing 9 g each, otherwise characteristic of Cushing's disease. X100.

scribed anatomically in this section. Pharmacologic treatment with cortisol blocking agents and cytolytic agents has also been employed (Luton et al.).

The evolution of disease production in this entity varies widely from case to case, with some evolving in a period of months and others over years (Plotz et al.; Smals et al.).

SIMPLE DIFFUSE HYPERPLASIA WITH ECTOPIC ACTH EXCESS
(Ectopic ACTH Syndrome)

Definition. Diffuse and symmetrical adrenal enlargement due to ACTH production from a tumor other than in the pituitary.

Gross. The appearance of the adrenal glands in this condition is quite characteristic, with symmetric enlargement and a diffusely widened cortex, greater than that seen in any other condition. The glands usually weigh at least 12 g each and may rarely reach over 30 g. There is a regularly thickened cortex, usually of at least 4 mm thickness, appearing brown throughout (pl. III). Thus, the regularity and striking degree of cortical expansion constitute the characteristic features of the hyperplastic adrenal in this condition (Singer et al.; Mason et al.).

Microscopic. The broadened cortex consists almost exclusively of straight columns of hypertrophied compact cells (figs. 40,

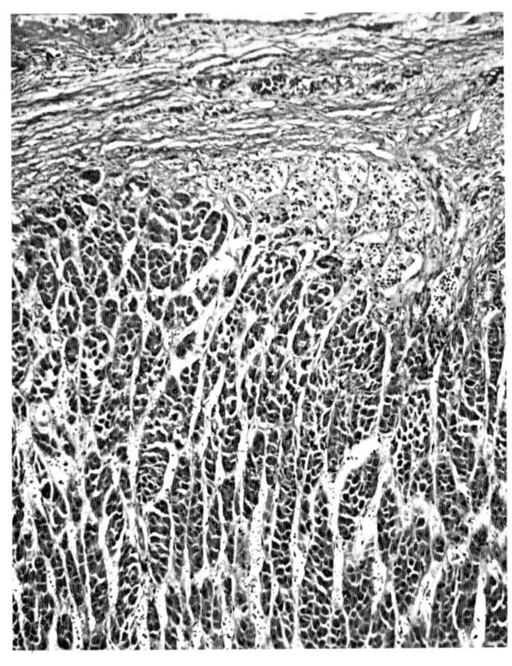

Figure 40
(Figures 40 and 41 from same patient)
HYPERPLASIA FROM
ECTOPIC ACTH PRODUCTION
Hypertrophic compact cells have replaced the entire area of the expanded zona fasciculata due to ACTH production by an oat cell carcinoma of the lung. Centrally, beneath the capsule, a small cluster of glomerulosa cells is evident. The glomerulosa cells have a relatively clear cytoplasm. X160.

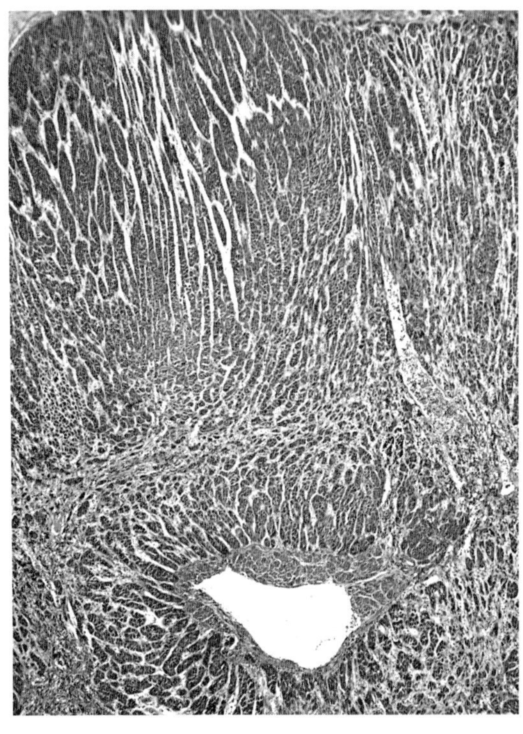

Figure 41
HYPERPLASIA FROM
ECTOPIC ACTH PRODUCTION
All cortical cells have been transformed into enlarged compact cells, including those surrounding the central vein at the lower portion of the picture. X25.

41). Any suggestion of nodule formation is distinctly unusual. Small collections of clear cells may appear at the outer extent of the cortex, but are never prominent, and this is a distinguishing feature from the adrenal in pituitary-dependent Cushing's disease, where clear cells usually constitute at least one-third of the cortical thickness. The zona glomerulosa is normal or difficult to appreciate and metastatic deposits of the ACTH-releasing neoplasm are often seen within the gland (pl. III-B). The adrenal cells adjacent to the metastatic deposits may be greatly enlarged and demonstrate bizarre nuclear patterns (fig. 42). Foci resembling myelolipoma may be seen.

SIMPLE DIFFUSE HYPERPLASIA WITH HYPERALDOSTERONISM

Definition. Hyperplasia with hyperaldosteronism presents anatomic and endocrine features of primary and inappropriate release of excess amounts of aldosterone in which removal of a single adrenal gland will

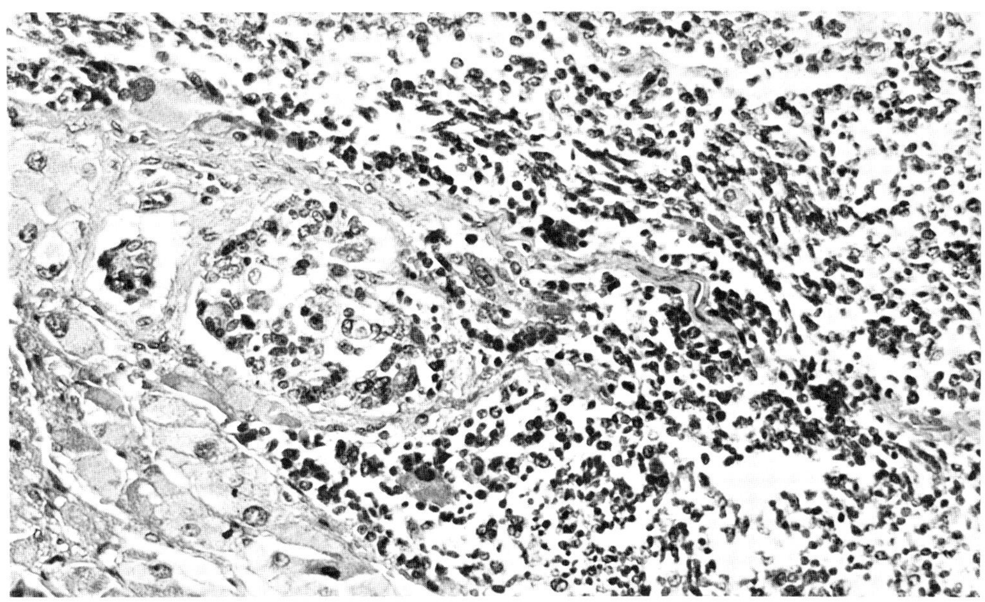

Figure 42
BIZARRE CORTICAL CELLS IN ECTOPIC ACTH SYNDROME
Metastatic cells from an oat cell carcinoma of the lung are apparent at the right of this picture, with enlarged
adrenocortical cells to the left. The patient had Cushing's syndrome due to ectopic ACTH production. X250.

not ameliorate the clinical condition and no adenoma is found (Ferris et al.). Adenomas commonly coexist with diffuse hyperplasia of the zona glomerulosa (Neville and Symington, 1966). These patients are similar to those with adenomas alone (see sections on Hyperaldosteronism and Adenomas). The presence of cortical nodules of unknown pathophysiologic significance adds to the difficulty of clinicopathologic correlation (Neville, 1978; Longo et al.).

Gross. Hyperplasia of the zona glomerulosa is rarely grossly apparent. Rare examples may show a slight prominence or folding of the adrenal cortex.

Microscopic. Identification of zona glomerulosa cells in the normal adrenal is often difficult. This is because of their presence in a discontinuous fashion beneath the adrenal capsule and because of the thinness of the cell layer. Hyperplasia of the zona glomerulosa may be diagnosed with confidence when collections of zona glomerulosa-type cells extend in triangular fashion, with the narrow tip toward the central vein (fig. 43). When these hyperplastic collections of cells are prominent, there is increased interstitial fibrous tissue. Spironolactone bodies may be found in the cytoplasm of the zona glomerulosa and, perhaps, adjacent cells of the zona fasciculata (Neville and Mackay) in glands from patients who have been treated with this drug (see Adenoma with Aldosteronism). Diagnosis of zona glomerulosa hyperplasia from histologic evidence alone cannot be accomplished with confidence without the presence of the prominent triangular groupings of zona glomerulosa cells. Even in that situation, an adenoma is frequently present in either adrenal.

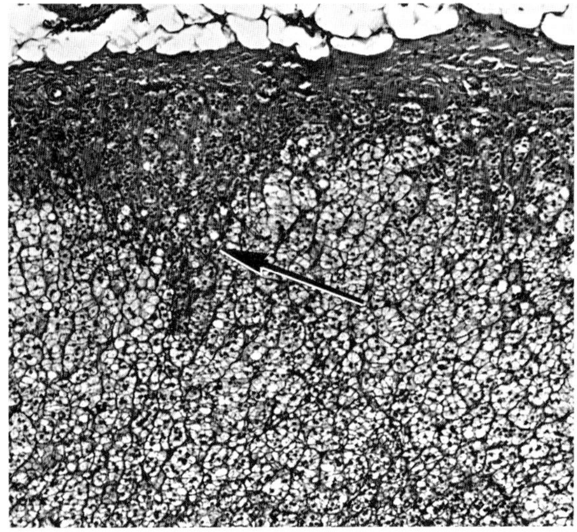

Figure 43
HYPERPLASIA WITH ALDOSTERONISM
Primary hyperplasia of the zona glomerulosa is evidenced by triangular extensions of cells of the zona glomerulosa (arrow) from the capsular region toward central vein just to the left of center. X75.

MULTINODULAR ADRENAL WITH HYPERCORTISOLISM

The few patients who have had bilateral adrenal disease characterized by many nodules and Cushing's syndrome have anatomic features which overlap with adenoma and hyperplasia. As these patients are regularly resistant to dexamethasone suppression, even in high dose, they appear to represent autonomous adrenal hyperfunction, at least by this test. Although there seem to be two types, with a micronodular type (see Microadenomatous Adrenal) more consistently autonomous in its hormonal responses and a macronodular type with greater resemblance to hyperplasia anatomically and functionally, there appear to be some patients falling in an intermediate position between the two types (Bricaire et al.). The common theme in this group of patients, representing either a spectrum of change or two different disease states, is that unilateral adrenalectomy will not effect a cure (Burke).

Although initially confusing, the need or usefulness for these diagnostic categories is due to the fact that there is an occasional case of bilateral disease in which many nodules seem to fill the entire adrenal. The appearance is quite different from that seen in adrenals with nodules in which an intervening cortex is easily identified and may be evaluated. These cases seem to be confined to the functional state of hypercortisolism and are, without exception, bilateral. They are not what was meant, or at least differ substantially from cases described as nodular hyperplasia, by Symington (1982) in which he is referring to cases of pituitary based Cushing's syndrome, where nodules of up to 2.5 cm in diameter are found in the adrenal. The remainder of the cortex, in cases described as nodular hyperplasia by Symington, have the appearance found in diffuse hyperplasia. Neville and O'Hare (1982) agree with Symington's approach and group together cases of Cushing's disease with nodules, marked multinodular hyperplasia, and the micronodular variety. Cases referred to by us as multinodular hyperplasia are very large and have so many nodules that the definition of an intervening cortex is difficult. When defined in this way, such cases are rare, comprising less than 5 percent, and probably less than 2 percent, of Cushing's syndrome. The possibility of misinterpretation of these cases as neoplasms warrants their consideration as a separate diagnostic category because of their unique anatomic presentation, as well as the fact that their functional status often mimics that of neoplasms as well (Table 4). We accept the fact that a precise diagnostic division of simple hyperplasia with nodules from multinodular disease is not possible. However, we suggest that the term multinodular hyperplasia be reserved for cases in which the cortex between nodules is difficult to identify because of the many nodules. The micronodular "hyperplastic" disease is probably a separate disease entity.

Multinodular Hyperplasia with Hypercortisolism
(Pseudoadenomatous Hyperplasia)

Definition. Irregularly distributed nodules producing gross enlargement of the adrenal are present throughout each gland, with identification of intervening cortex difficult because of the complexity and large numbers of nodules. These patients are regularly resistant to dexamethasone suppression, but usually respond to administered ACTH as well as metyrapone. The condition is appropriately termed **hyperplasia,** as the cortex within and between the nodules is histologically active and hyperplastic.

Gross. Prominent nodules ranging in size from a few mm to about 3 cm in diameter seem to make up the entire gland, producing adrenals of 30-50 g in weight each, but reported to reach 100 g (Hidai et al.; figs. 44, 45). The nodules have mixed yellow and brown areas. The many nodules are more discrete when evaluated in three dimensions than those seen at autopsy in a nodular adrenal with hypercortisolism (fig. 46).

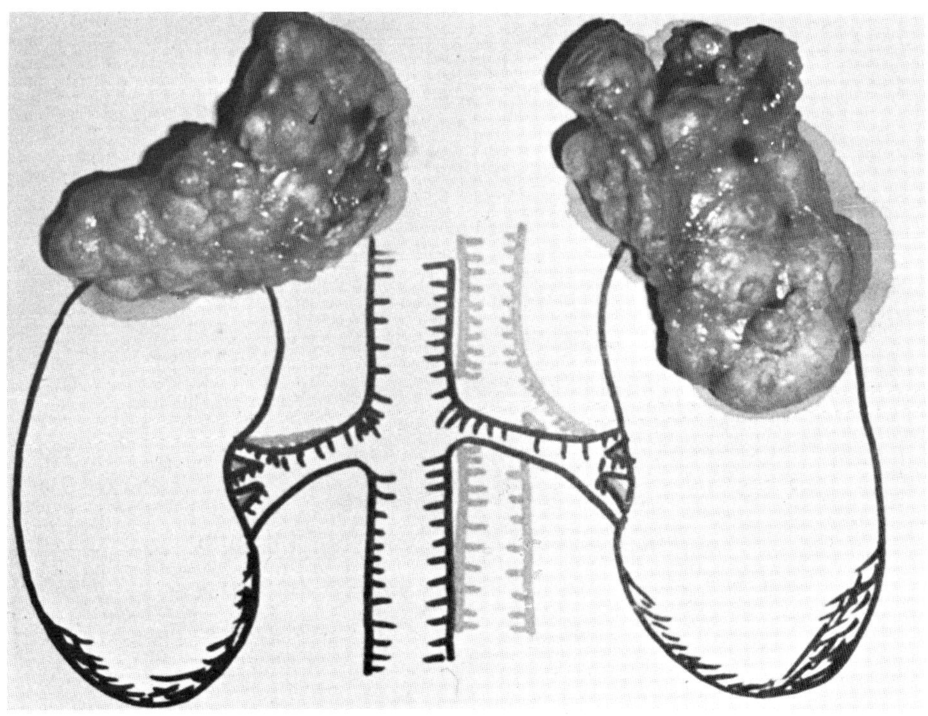

Figure 44
(Figures 44 and 45 from same patient)
MULTINODULAR HYPERPLASIA WITH HYPERCORTISOLISM
Combined weight was 161 g. Bilateral adrenalectomy cured a Cushing's syndrome of two years' duration. One-half actual size. (From Hidai, H., Fujii, H., Otsuka, K., Abe, K., and Shimizu, N. Cushing's syndrome due to huge adrenocortical multinodular hyperplasia. Endocrinol. Japn. 22:555-560, 1975.)

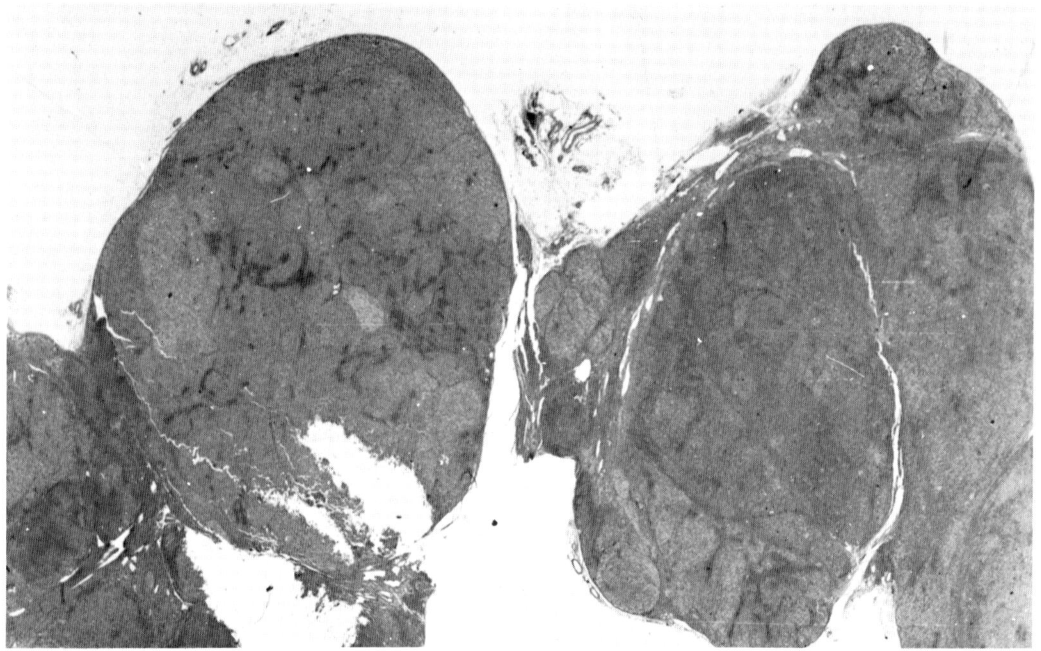

Figure 45
MULTINODULAR HYPERPLASIA WITH HYPERCORTISOLISM
Cross section of adrenals for case illustrated in figure 44. Entire adrenal is transformed into nodules,
which were brown and yellow grossly. X10.

Microscopic. The various nodules are alternating collections of compact and clear cells, with some appearing intermediate between these two cytoplasmic characteristics (figs. 47–49). The defining anatomic feature of this condition is the irregularly hyperplastic intervening cortex which presents elongated cords of compact cells between small nodules that appear histologically similar to the many cells in the larger nodules (fig. 50). Occasional collections of cells have deeply eosinophilic and broadened granular cytoplasm, as well as enlarged and somewhat bizarre nuclei (fig. 51). These bizarre cells may occur between or within nodules. Some nodules may be composed primarily of clear cells (fig. 52), but extensive sampling of these glands will reveal the characteristic mixture of clear, compact, and intermediate cells (fig. 53) through much of the greatly enlarged glands. In contrast, cases of simple hyperplasia (Cushing's disease) with several defined nodules will demonstrate regular, clear cells in the nodules (fig. 39).

Natural History and Incidence. This condition is distinctly unusual, with only seven cases reviewed by Burke (1978). Although the pathogenesis of this condition is unknown, it is certainly more closely related to pituitary dependent hyperplasia than to adrenal neoplasm. ACTH levels tend to be high in reported cases (Choi et al.), with the patient of Burke and Beardwell demonstrating remission following

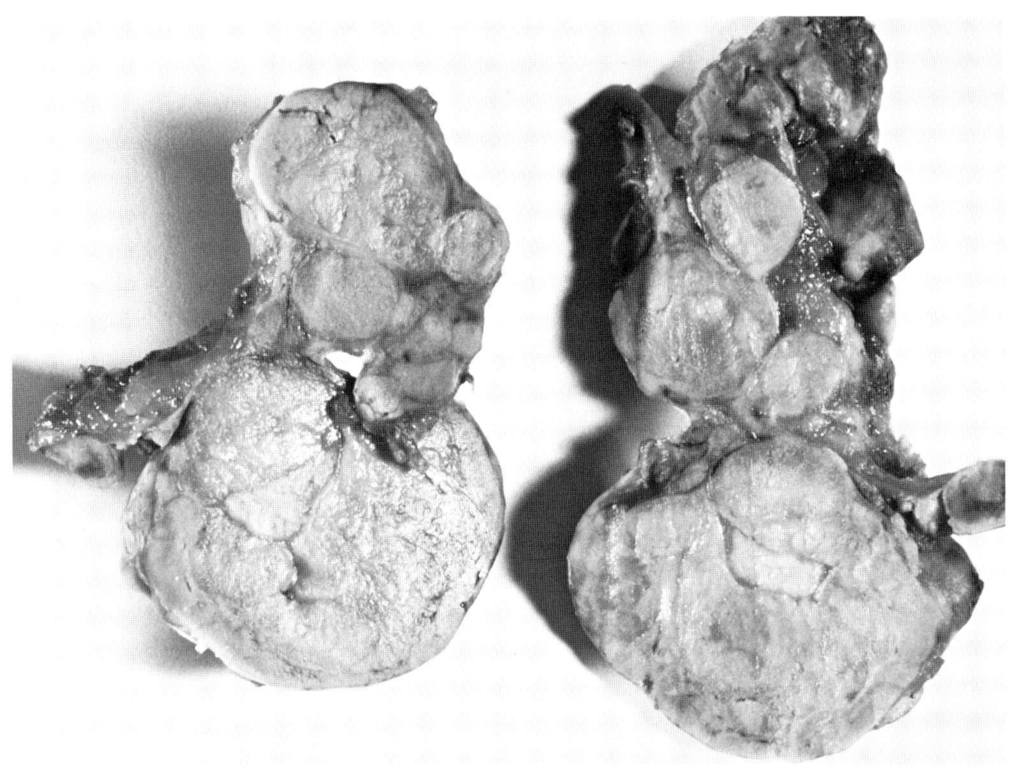

Figure 46
(Figures 46, 47, and 51 from same patient)
MULTINODULAR HYPERPLASIA WITH HYPERCORTISOLISM
Cross section of adrenal from a 44 year old woman who had Cushing's syndrome and multinodular hyperplasia. Bilateral adrenalectomy was required to effect a cure. (Courtesy of Department of Pathology, University of Leeds, Leeds, England.)

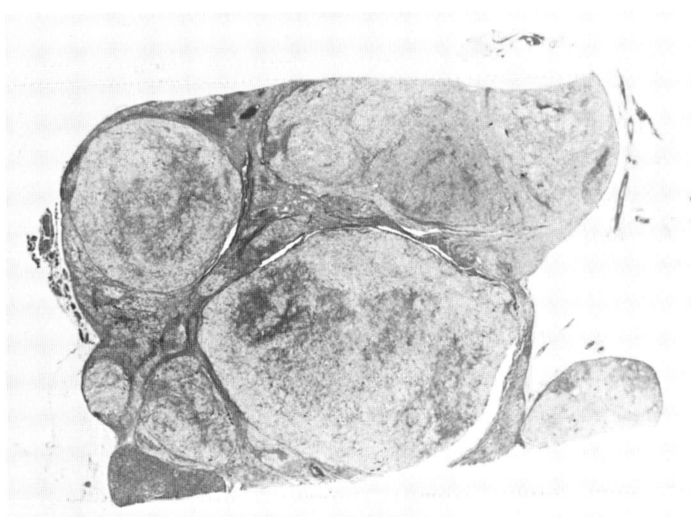

Figure 47
MULTINODULAR HYPERPLASIA
WITH
HYPERCORTISOLISM
Note apparent encapsulation of the nodules. Internodular cells are also hypertrophic. X3.

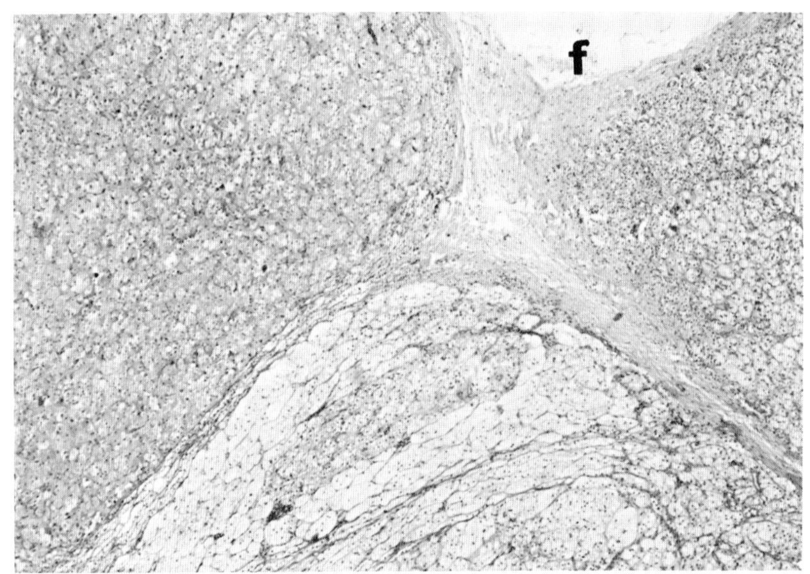

Figure 48
MULTINODULAR HYPERPLASIA WITH HYPERCORTISOLISM
Bilateral adrenalectomy was required to effect cure of Cushing's syndrome. Note deformed capsular region under fat (f), at top of the picture. X15. (Courtesy of Department of Pathology, Radcliffe Infirmary, Oxford, England.)

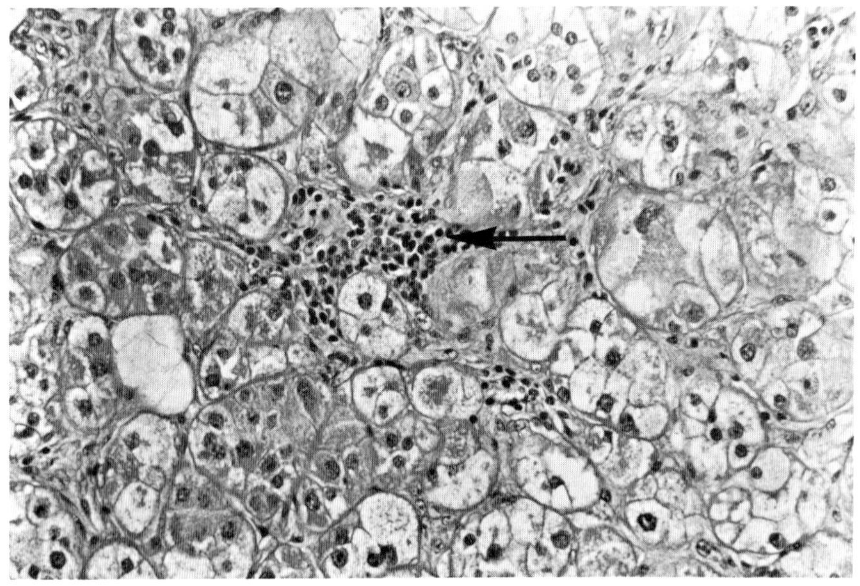

Figure 49
(Figures 49 and 50 from same patient)
MULTINODULAR HYPERPLASIA WITH HYPERCORTISOLISM
Large, irregular cells with mixed clear and granular eosinophilic cytoplasm are seen in a case of multinodular hyperplasia and hypercortisolism. Bilaterally enlarged adrenals were revealed preoperatively and removed simultaneously. Note collection of lymphocytes (arrow) centrally. X180. (Courtesy of Dr. A. Graber and Dr. L. Graham, Jr., Nashville, TN.)

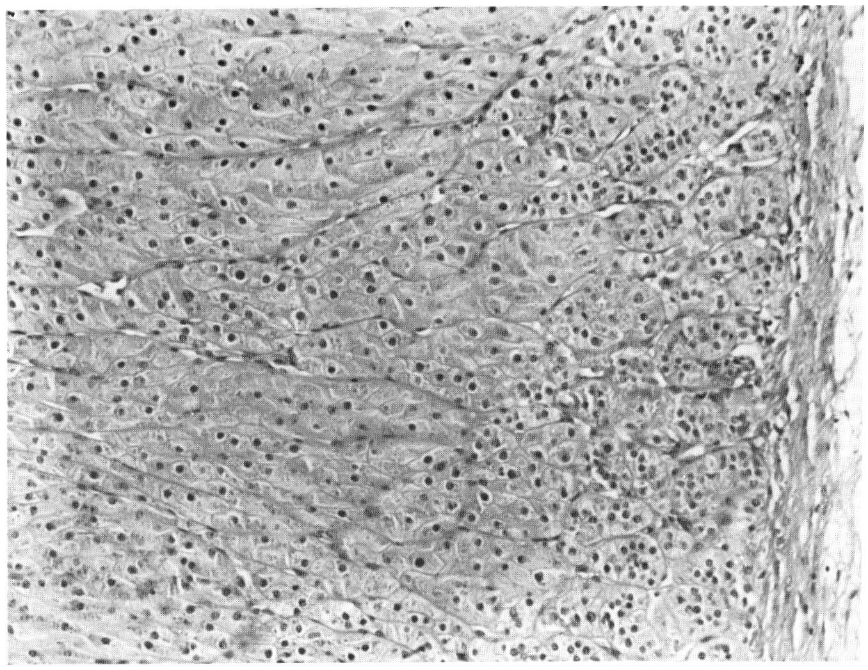

Figure 50
MULTINODULAR HYPERPLASIA WITH HYPERCORTISOLISM
Subcortical and internodular region demonstrates enlarged hyperfunctioning cells. Note the large granular cells arranged perpendicular to the capsular surface. This resembles the zona fasciculata cells of ectopic ACTH syndrome, with complete alteration of adrenal cortex to large granular cells. X60. (Courtesy of Dr. A. Graber and Dr. L. Graham, Jr., Nashville, TN.)

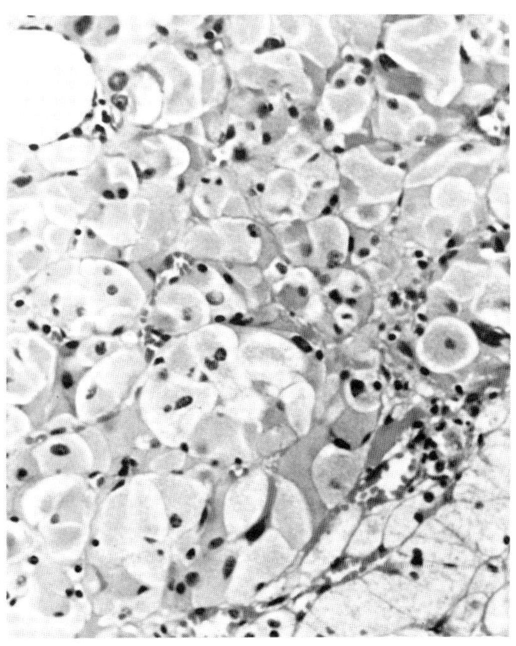

Figure 51
MULTINODULAR HYPERPLASIA
WITH HYPERCORTISOLISM
Extreme irregularity of cellular appearance is seen in multinodular adrenal hyperplasia. X140.

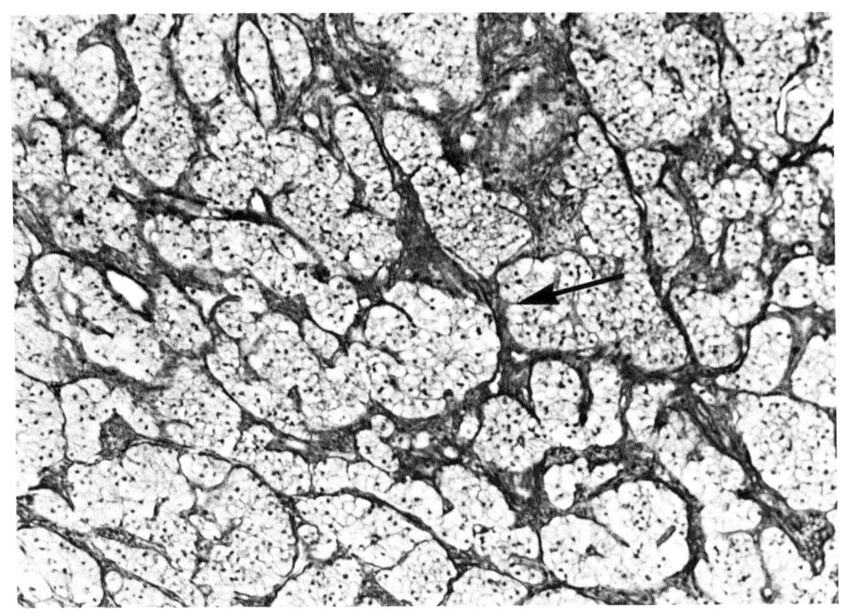

Figure 52
(Figures 52 and 53 from same patient)
MULTINODULAR HYPERPLASIA WITH HYPERCORTISOLISM
This area within a nodule is from a patient with multinodular hyperplasia with total adrenal weight of 137 g. Cortisol secretion was not affected by high dose dexamethasone or metyrapone. ACTH administration did increase 17-hydroxysteroid secretion. Many nodules, such as this one, had primarily clear cells with some faint cytoplasmic eosinophilia and increased collagen (arrow) between rounded cellular masses. X100.

pituitary ablation. These cases also tend to respond to metyrapone and ACTH administration with an increase in production of cortisol or its precursors. Most of the reported cases have been in adults, although the case of Mosier and associates may represent such a case in a child.

Microadenomatous Adrenal with Hypercortisolism

SYNONYMS AND RELATED TERMS: Nodular dysplasia; micronodular adrenal disease; polymicroadenomatosis; micronodular cortical adenomatosis.

Definition. Adrenals of near normal weight with many almost evenly dispersed small nodules associated with hypercortisolism, combined with small and inactive appearing internodular cells, define this condition. The patients have hypercortisolism without response to any hormonal manipulative tests and have low plasma ACTH levels (Burke), endocrinologically characteristic of adrenal neoplasm. These cases have been recognized by various terms attempting to denote these unusual features. Although no classification system yet proposed adequately explains these peculiar cases, we prefer a term relating the small size of the gland and mimicry of adenoma. "Micronodular cortical adenomatosis" is also a useful term (Williams et al.). Shenoy and associates have proposed "bilateral primary pigmented nodular adrenocortical disease."

Gross. The adrenals are usually within normal weight range or slightly greater, with many nodules of 1-5 mm diameter throughout each gland. The nodules are

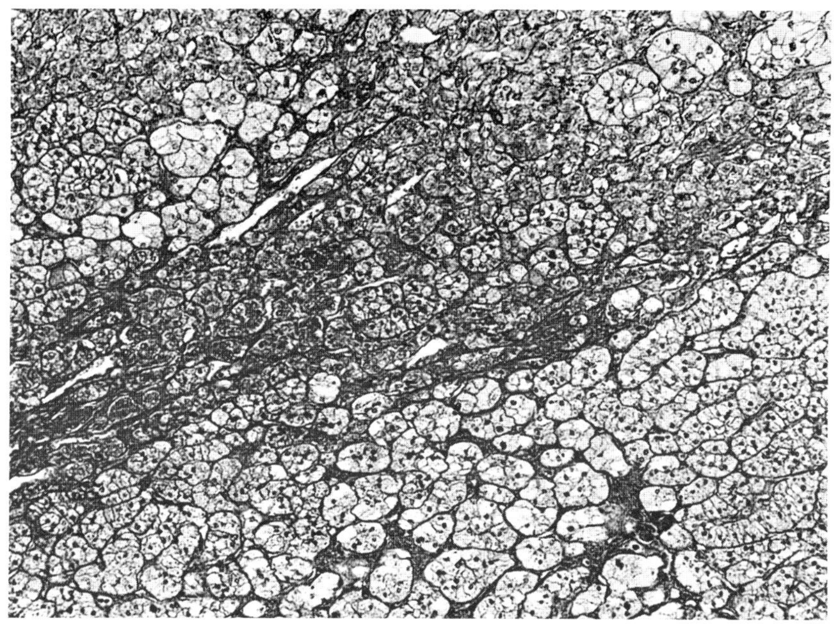

Figure 53
MULTINODULAR HYPERPLASIA WITH HYPERCORTISOLISM
Internodular cortex is demonstrated from same patient as figure 52. Note intermixture of
compact cells and enlarged cells which have almost clear cytoplasm. The groups of clear
cells to either side of the more compact cells could be interpreted as poorly demarcated
nodules. X100.

usually brown or black (pl. III-A), and are more likely to have this pigmented appearance and to be larger in older patients (McArthur et al.).

Microscopic. The nodules are made up of large cells with eosinophilic cytoplasm containing brown pigment which is probably similar to that seen in "black adenomas" (q.v.). The nuclei are also frequently enlarged and present some variation in size and shape. Electron microscopic studies in one case (Hasleton et al.) demonstrated predominating fasciculate features. The adjacent nonnodular cortex is composed of small regular cells with clear cytoplasm (fig. 54) — the type of cells seen in an inactive or atrophic adrenal.

Incidence and Natural History. This is a rare condition occurring primarily in chil-

dren, including infants (McArthur et al.) and young adults, with less than 20 reported cases. Clinical features are similar to Cushing's disease, except that osteopenia may be more prominent (Ruder et al.).

ACTH is low or undetectable at time of diagnosis (DeGennes et al.), indicating autonomous adrenal hyperfunction, and did not rise above normal levels, in one patient, seven months after bilateral adrenalectomy (Meador et al.). Dexamethasone is not able to suppress the hypercortisolism, even in high doses, and there is no response to metyrapone administration.

Recent reports document the familial occurrence of this rare condition (Arce et al.; Schweizer-Cagianut et al., 1980, 1982). This is strong evidence for considering this disease a distinct entity, accepting the fact that pathogenesis is unknown.

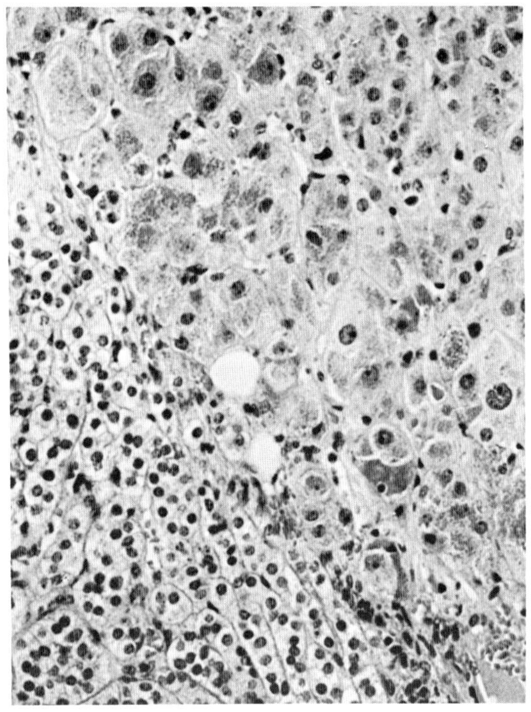

Figure 54
MICROADENOMATOUS ADRENAL
WITH HYPERCORTISOLISM
Enlarged cells with pigmented granules are in a nodule at upper right. Small inactive cells with clear cytoplasm comprise the internodular cellular population and are seen at lower left. X180.

Treatment. Because of the autonomy of cortisol release and bilateral abnormality, bilateral adrenalectomy has been the treatment chosen in most cases. o,p'-DDD may be effective.

RELATIONSHIP OF HYPERPLASIA TO NEOPLASIA

There is little evidence that adrenal hyperplasia of any type other than the congenital varieties progresses to the development of true neoplasia. Because individual nodules may mimic adenomas, evidence for neoplastic development in the setting of hyperplasia must be more than histologic. Thus, despite the encapsulation that may occur around nodular collections of cells in the adrenal gland (Cohen), they cannot be interpreted as neoplasms without the demonstration of functional autonomy or metastasis.

Despite the evident rarity, there are reported cases of neoplasms developing in adrenals of patients with congenital adrenal hyperplasia. The case reported by Hamwi and associates probably represents the development of a locally infiltrating adrenal carcinoma, weighing 228 g, in the setting of untreated congenital adrenal hyperplasia (21-hydroxylase deficiency). Bauman and Bauman present a case of virilizing adrenocortical carcinoma in an 11 year old girl with treated salt-losing congenital hyperplasia. An adenoma is reported to have developed in an adrenal of a 60 year old woman with untreated mild 21-hydroxylase deficiency, but the evidence is not completely convincing (VanSeters et al.). The case of a unique patient reported by Anderson and associates is best explained as adrenal cortical carcinoma developing in the setting of hyperplasia with Cushing's disease. A basophilic adenoma of the pituitary was demonstrated with radiographic findings consistent with its presence for at least seven years. Virilization developed rapidly in this patient and was relieved by removal of a 450 g unilateral adrenal carcinoma. At autopsy three months later, there were metastases, although death was caused by a myocardial infarction. Removal of the carcinoma had ameliorated the virilization, but other hormonal findings were consistent with continuing pituitary based hypercortisolism. Other cases, such as that of Dluhy and associates, are as easily explained by the assumption that there was a slowly evolving carcinoma, rather than the assumption that the tumor arose in the background of hyperplasia.

THE MULTINODULAR ADRENAL
(Nodular Adrenal, Nodular Hyperplasia)

"Nodules . . . represent one of the principal remaining enigmas of adrenocortical pathology" (Neville and O'Hare, 1979).

Definition and Natural History. Rounded masses of adrenocortical cells stand out as individual clusters distinct from surrounding tissue (Cohen). The term "nodular adrenal" probably describes this change equally well (Neville, 1978), but the term "multinodular" accepts the fact that the nodules are rarely, if ever, solitary. A solitary nodule cannot be distinguished from an adenoma anatomically without evaluation of the surrounding adrenal, although nodules tend to be made up of clear cells with no variation from one cell to another (Neville and O'Hare, 1982). The smallest nodules are barely perceptible and, as they are of unknown clinicopathologic significance, are better left undiagnosed, as is usually the case in milder forms of nodule formation in other endocrine glands.

Neville and O'Hare (1982) emphasize the continuity of simple, diffuse, and nodular hyperplasias, emphasizing the usefulness of the noncommittal term "nodule."

The change described here is the most common type of focal or generalized enlargement of the adrenal recognized by the pathologist, usually at autopsy. The clinical significance of these nodules has recently increased with the wide use of computerized tomography. The incidental nature of these lesions must be understood (Geelhoed and Druy; Copeland). There is an increased incidence of adrenal nodularity with advancing age, unassociated with any evidence of deranged general adrenal function. The number and size of the nodules tend to rise with increasing age, and hypertension and vascular disease are more common in people presenting with this type of adrenal. The change is virtually always bilateral.

These nodules do not seem to be precursors of neoplastic lesions, as the incidence of adrenal neoplasms does not continue to rise with increasing age and their functional significance seems to be a local one, possibly related to relative refractoriness to effects of ACTH when the cells are within the nodule. Disease is not caused by this change, nor is the change an accomplice in production of disease.

Gross. Nodules are rarely larger than 2 or 3 cm in greatest diameter. A disparity in the weights of the glands may be produced by presence of larger nodule(s) on one side or the other. While it is relatively common for only one or two nodules to reach large size, multiplicity of occurrence is the rule. Each nodule, particularly larger ones, may appear sharply demarcated from surrounding structures, but they regularly lack encapsulation, as evidenced by continuity with

PLATE III

A. MICROADENOMATOUS ADRENAL WITH HYPERCORTISOLISM

This adrenal and the contralateral similar gland were removed from a 14 year old girl with no response to hormonal manipulation and low ACTH levels (see, also, figure 54). These cases usually have pigmented nodules. Weight was 4.0 g. X4.5. (Courtesy of Dr. C.K. Meador, Nashville, TN.)

B. HYPERPLASIA WITH ECTOPIC ACTH EXCESS

Cross section of each adrenal at autopsy from a 52 year old woman who had ACTH producing oat cell carcinoma of the lung. Adrenals weighed 28 and 32 g. Note widened, brown cortex and white foci of metastatic oat cell carcinoma. The flecks of yellow in the rounded area at lower left are clear cells histologically, and the area probably represents a nodule almost completely transformed into brown compact cells. X1.25.

C. SIMPLE HYPERPLASIA WITH HYPERCORTISOLISM.

This adrenal demonstrates diffuse adrenocortical hyperplasia with Cushing's disease. The lighter fascicular zone and the darker reticular zone are both increased in thickness. X3.

D. MULTINODULAR ADRENAL WITHOUT KNOWN CLINICAL SIGNIFICANCE

External view of a 17 g multinodular adrenal is shown from an autopsy of a 56 year old woman. Opposite adrenal was similar. X.8. (Courtesy of Dr. A.E. Kalderon, Little Rock, AR.)

E. MULTINODULAR ADRENAL WITHOUT KNOWN CLINICAL SIGNIFICANCE
(Plate III-E and G from same patient)

Section of multinodular adrenal with only slight enlargement of gland is from an autopsy of a 69 year old man with severe atherosclerosis. Light gray medulla is seen at right. Weight, 9 g. X3.5. (Courtesy of Dr. W.A. Gardner, Jr., Nashville, TN.)

F. MULTINODULAR ADRENALS WITHOUT KNOWN CLINICAL SIGNIFICANCE

Note deep brown reticularis and fine nodularity of subcapsular yellow cortex. There is a great increase of yellow cortical cells related to central veins, presenting central to the brown reticular zone. Adrenal weights were 17 and 18 g at autopsy. X.6.

G. MULTINODULAR ADRENALS WITHOUT KNOWN CLINICAL SIGNIFICANCE

Cross section of each adrenal is seen at autopsy in a 69 year old man with a long history of hypertension and severe coronary and aortic atherosclerosis. Note coalescence of nodules with cortex. X1.3.

PLATE III

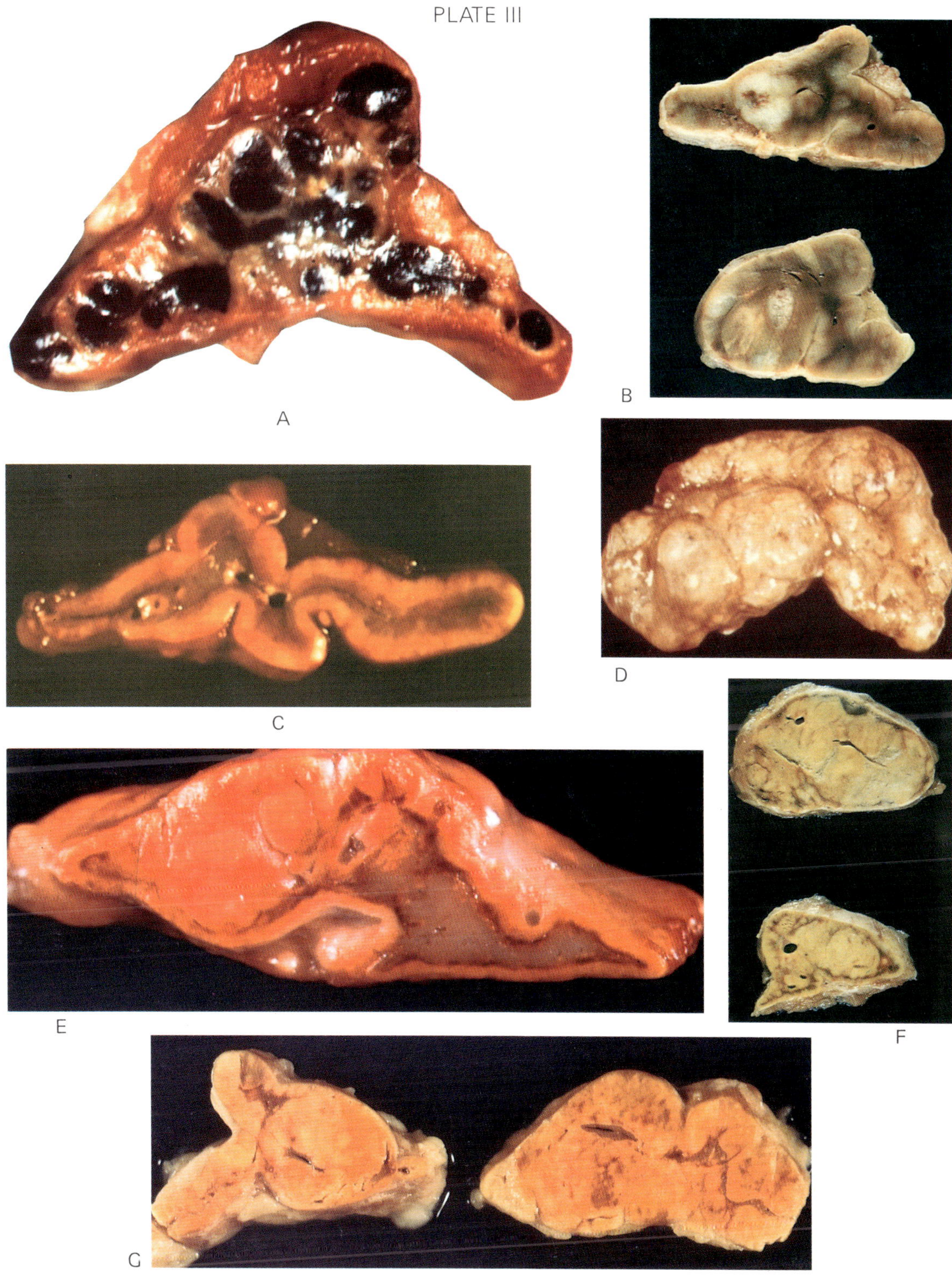

adjacent adrenocortical cells at most edges (pl. III-E—G; fig. 55). A pale yellow color characterizes each nodule, with brown foci present in the clinical setting of prolonged stress preceding death. Most often the cortex adjacent to nodules will appear brown in patients with shorter periods of stress before death, with the nodules retaining their yellow color.

Microscopic. The first noticeable change in the evolution of nodules is an alteration in the radial symmetry of cortical cells, followed by compression of adjacent cells (fig. 56). In the earliest stages, this minimal change is most easily demonstrated with lipid and reticulin stains (Cohen). The former will demonstrate variation in quantity and cytoplasmic pattern of lipid from the surrounding, nonnodular cortex (pl. II); the reticulin stain will show a curvilinear surface about a nodule, with a different pattern of internal reticulin framework from the adjacent cortical cells (fig. 57).

The pale yellow gross appearance correlates microscopically with the regular presence of large, lipid filled cytoplasmic spaces with cells resembling closely those of the unaltered zona fasciculata. The cells are arranged in short cords and rounded masses separated by fibrovascular trabeculae. The change appears to occur in the inner cortex, not involving the glomerulosa. The cortical cells arranged about the central veins are frequently involved in nodular change. The nodules are relatively refractory to the lipid depleting effects of stress, as demonstrated at autopsy when the nodules are commonly rich in lipid and the remaining gland has changed to compact cells. Prolonged stress before death results in conversion of some cells of the nodules into compact, lipid-poor cells. Collagen may be increased between component cell bundles, which tend to be arranged in haphazard, rounded groupings. Larger nodules may seem encapsulated by an encircling collagenous capsule with prominent vessels. Fibrous and myxomatous scars, hemosiderin deposition, myelolipomatous change, and marked cytoplasmic lipofuscin (Feuerstein and Tiamson) may be seen, but all are quite rare.

Pathogenesis. Although the clinical situations in which nodule formation is most likely to occur are well known, the pathogenesis is unclear. The presence of prominent hyaline vessels has led Dobbie to a rationally consistent theory of ischemic atrophy producing compensatory nodular hyperplasia. The origin of some nodules from the cells adjacent to the central vein which presumably have a protected blood supply from the arteriae commitantes is compatible with this theory; but the presence of abnormal vessels in cases without nodules, the presence of abnormal vessels within nodules, and the relative functional inactivity of cells within nodules leaves the theory in doubt. What is clear from the monolayer culture work of O'Hare and associates and Neville is that the cells themselves do not have altered functional capacity (Symington, 1969) and that the position of the cells in nodules vis-a-vis other cells and/or vascular supply may be local determining factors.

Differential Diagnosis. In different forms of hyperplasia, as with adenomas, a careful evaluation of surrounding cortex is essential to accurate diagnosis. Nodules are separated from other conditions because of the absence of histologic signs of inactivity or hyperactivity in the intervening cortex. The coexistence of nodules with hyperfunctioning states (fig. 39) presents problems in diagnosis, and the presence of nodules

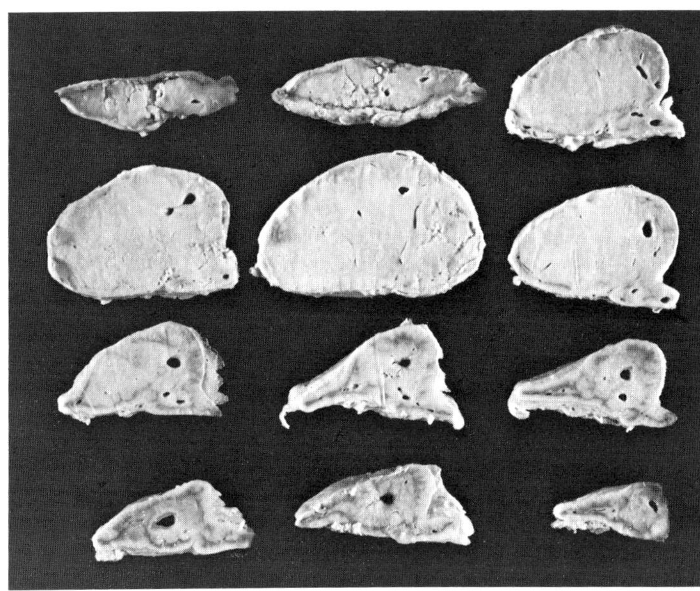

Figure 55
MULTINODULAR ADRENAL
Cross sections of entire nodular adrenal are demonstrated at autopsy. Thin dark line just inside the capsular surface is brown zona reticularis. Note extension of centrally placed cortical tissue throughout length of adrenal, as well as mild nodularity present everywhere and confluence of nodules with remainder of adrenal. Actual size.

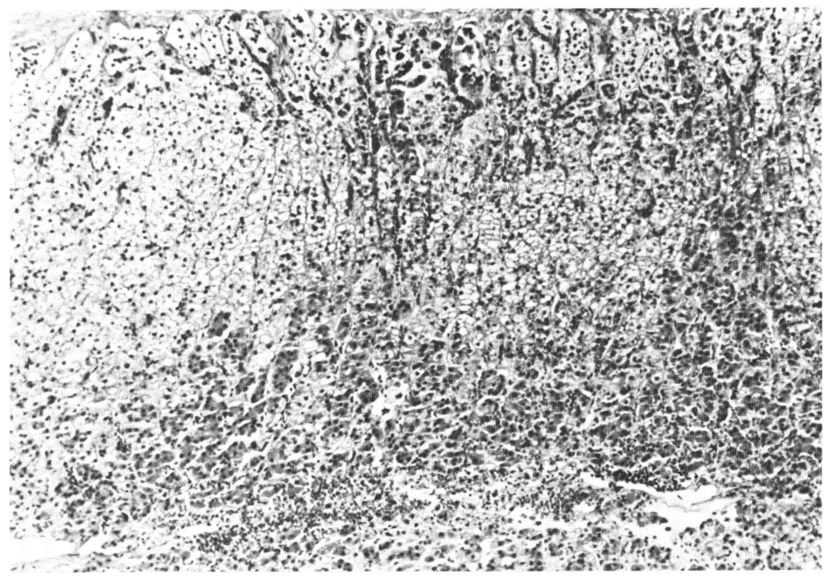

Figure 56
MULTINODULAR ADRENAL
Early nodule formation is seen at autopsy as two rounded collections of clear cells surrounded by compact cells. Entire cortical thickness is shown with capsule above. X100.

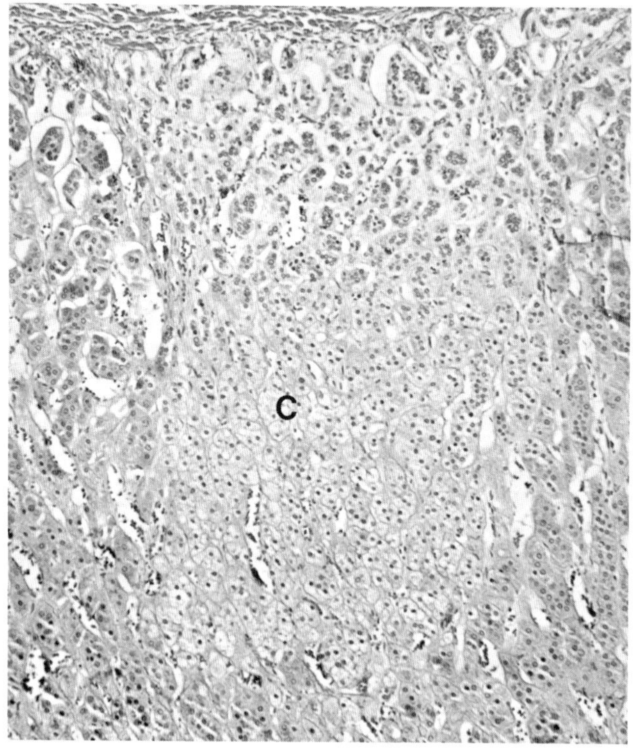

Figure 57
MULTINODULAR ADRENAL
Early nodule formation is demonstrated at autopsy with a light reticulin stain. Clear cells at center (c) represent early nodule formation. Compact cells comprising remainder of the adrenal are "depleted" of lipid, except for clear cells of nodules. X100.

with no pathophysiologic significance is a possibility that must be considered in any hyperfunctioning gland with more than one nodular aggregate of cortical cells.

Nodules are usually made up of a uniform population of large, clear, lipid-rich cells. This is particularly true of the patient who has not experienced prolonged severe illness. The nodules tend to have some continuity with adjacent cortical cells, rather than to be completely encapsulated, and a dominant nodule is often present, extending in continuous fashion through much of the adrenal length (fig. 55).

References

Anderson, D. C., Child, D. F., Sutcliffe, C. H. et al. Cushing's syndrome, nodular adrenal hyperplasia and virilizing carcinoma. Clin. Endocrinol. 9:1-14, 1978.

Arce, B., Licea, M., Hung, S., and Padrón, R. Familial Cushing's Syndrome. Acta Endocrinol. 87:139-147, 1978.

Ashworth, C. T. and Garvey, R. F. The diffuse adrenal lesion in Cushing's disease. Am. J. Pathol. 34:1161-1171, 1958.

Bauman, A. and Bauman, C. G. Virilizing adrenocortical carcinoma. J.A.M.A. 248:3140-3141, 1982.

Bennett, B. D., McKenna, T. J., Hough, A. J., Dean, R., and Page, D. L. Adrenal myelolipoma associated with Cushing's disease. Am. J. Clin. Pathol. 73:443-447, 1980.

Biglieri, E. G., Wajchenberg, B. L., Malerbi, D. A., Okada, H., Leme, C. E., and Kater, C. E. The zonal origins of the mineralocorticoid hormones in the 21-hydroxylation deficiency of congenital adrenal hyperplasia. J. Clin. Endocrinol. Metab. 53:964-969, 1981.

Boudreaux, D., Waisman, J., Skinner, D. G., and Low, R. Giant adrenal myelolipoma and testicular interstitial cell tumor in a man with congenital 21-hydroxylase deficiency. Am. J. Surg. Pathol. 3:109-123, 1979.

Bricaire, H., Luton, J-P., Ghozland, M., and Forest, M. La polymicroadénomatose de la cortico-surrénale dans le syndrome de Cushing. Ann. Med. Interne (Paris) 121:755-777, 1970.

Brook, C. G. D., Zachmann, M., Prader, A., and Mürset, G. Experience with long term therapy in congenital adrenal hyperplasia. J. Pediatr. 85:12-19, 1974.

Burke, C. W. Disorders of cortisol production: diagnostic and therapeutic progress. Recent Adv. Endocr. Metab. 1:61-90, 1978.

_______ and Beardwell, C. G. Cushing's syndrome. Q. J. Med. 42:175-204, 1973.

_______ , Doyle, F. H., Joplin, G. F., Arnot, R. N., Macerlean, D. P., and Fraser, T. R. Cushing's disease. Q. J. Med. 168:693-714, 1973.

Choi, Y., Werk, E. E., Jr., and Sholiton, L. J. Cushing's syndrome with dual pituitary-adrenal control. Arch. Int. Med. 125:1045-1049, 1970.

Cohen, R. B. Observations on cortical nodules in human adrenal glands. Cancer 19:552-556, 1966.

_______ , Chapman, W. B., and Castleman, B. Hyperadrenocorticism (Cushing's disease): a study of surgically resected adrenal glands. Am. J. Pathol. 35:537-561, 1959.

Copeland, P. M. The incidentally discovered adrenal mass. Ann. Surg. 199:116-122, 1984.

DeGennes, J-L., Garnier, H., Calmette Mme., Malinsky, M., and Bertrand, C. Étude clinique, biologique et histologique d'un cas exemplaire de polymicroadénomatose cortico surrénale. Ann. Endocrinol. (Paris) 31:1022-1038, 1970.

Dluhy, R. G., Barlow, J. J., Mahoney, E. M., Shirley, R. L., and Williams, G. H. Profile and possible origin of an adrenocortical carcinoma. J. Clin. Endocrinol. Metab. 33:312-317, 1971.

Dobbie, J. W. Adrenocortical nodular hyperplasia: The ageing adrenal. J. Pathol. 99:1-18, 1969.

Ferris, J. B., Brown, J. J., Fraser, R. et al. Hypertension with aldosterone excess and low plasma-renin: preoperative distinction between patients with and without adrenocortical tumour. Lancet 2:995-1000, 1970.

Feuerstein, I. M. and Tiamson, E. M. Focal cytomegaly of the adult adrenal cortex. Arch. Pathol. Lab. Med. 109:198-200, 1985.

Fitzgerald, P. A., Aron, D. C., Findling, J. W., Brooks, R. M., et al. Cushing's Disease: Transient secondary adrenal insufficiency after selective removal of pituitary microadenomas; evidence for a pituitary origin. J. Clin. Endocrinol. Metab. 54:413-421, 1982.

Fore, W. W., Bledsoe, T., Weber, D. M., and Brooks, R. T. Cortisol production by testicular tumors in adrenogenital syndrome. Arch. Intern. Med. 130:59-63, 1972.

Geelhoed, G. W. and Druy, E. M. Management of the adrenal "incidentaloma." Surgery 92:866-874, 1982.

Hamilton, W. Congenital Adrenal Hyperplasia, pp. 503-547, In: Clinics in Endocrinology and Metabolism, Vol. 1, No. 2. London, Philadelphia, Toronto: W. B. Saunders Co., 1972.

Hamwi, G. J., Serbin, R. A., and Kruger, F. A. Does adrenocortical hyperplasia result in adrenocortical carcinoma? N. Engl. J. Med. 257:1153-1157, 1957.

Hasleton, P. S., Ali, H. H., Anfield, C., Beardwell, C. G., and Shalet, S. Micronodular adrenal disease: a light and electron microscopic study. J. Clin. Pathol. 35:1078-1085, 1982.

Hidai, H., Fujii, H., Otsuka, K., Abe, K., and Shimizu, N. Cushing's syndrome due to huge adrenocortical multinodular hyperplasia. Endocrinol. Japn. 22:555-560, 1975.

Hurwitz, A., Brautbar, C., Milwidsky, A., Vecsei, P., et al. Combined 21- and 11β-hydroxylase deficiency in familial congenital adrenal hyperplasia. J. Clin. Endocrinol. Metab. 60:631-638, 1985.

Jennings, A. S., Liddle, G. W., and Orth, D. N. Results of treating childhood Cushing's disease with pituitary irradiation. N. Engl. J. Med. 297:957-962, 1977.

Kirkland, R. T., Kirkland, J. L., Keenan, B. S. et al. Bilateral testicular tumors in congenital adrenal hyperplasia. J. Clin. Endocrinol. Metab. 44:369-378, 1977.

Longo, D. L., Esterly, J. A., Grim, C. E., and Keitzer, W. F. Pathology of the adrenal gland in refractory low-renin hypertension. Arch. Pathol. Lab. Med. 102:322-327, 1978.

Luton, J. P., Mahoudeau, J. A., Bouchard, P. et al. Treatment of Cushing's disease by o,p'DDD. N. Engl. J. Med. 300:459-464, 1979.

Mason, A. M. S., Ratcliffe, J. G., Buckle, R. M., and Mason, A. S. ACTH secretion by bronchial carcinoid tumours. Clin. Endocrinol. 1:3-25, 1972.

McArthur, R. G., Bahn, R. C., and Hayles, A. B. Primary adrenocortical nodular dysplasia as a cause of Cushing's Syndrome in infants and children. Mayo Clin. Proc. 57:58-63, 1982.

Meador, C. K., Bowdoin, B., Owen, W. C., Jr., and Farmer, T. A., Jr. Primary adrenocortical nodular dysplasia: A rare cause of Cushing's syndrome. J. Clin. Endocrinol. Metab. 27:1255-1263, 1967.

Migeon, C. J. Adrenal androgens in man. Am. J. Med. 53:606-626, 1972.

Migeon, C. J. Diagnosis and Treatment of Adrenogenital Disorders, pp. 1203-1224. In: Endocrinology, Vol. 2. DeGroot, L. J. et al. (Eds.). New York: Grune and Stratton, 1979.

————, Rosenwaks, Z., Lee, P. A., Urban, M. D., and Bias, W. B. The attenuated form of congenital adrenal hyperplasia in an allelic form of 21-hydroxylase deficiency. J. Clin. Endocrinol. Metab. 51:647-649, 1980.

Mosier, H. D., Flynn, P. J., Will, D. W., and Turner, R. D. Cushing's syndrome with multinodular adrenal glands. J. Clin. Endocrinol. Metab. 20:632-640, 1960.

Neville, A. M. The nodular adrenal. Invest. Cell Pathol. 1:99-111, 1978.

————. The Pathology of the Adrenal Gland in Cushing's Syndrome, pp. 12-25. In: Cushing's Syndrome, Diagnosis and Treatment. Binder, C. and Hall, P. (Eds.). London: Heinemann Medical Books, 1972.

———— and Mackay, A. M. The Structure of the Human Adrenal Cortex in Health and Disease, pp. 361-395. In: Clinics in Endocrinology and Metabolism, Vol. 1, No. 2. London, Philadelphia, Toronto: W. B. Saunders Company, 1972.

———— and O'Hare, M. J. Aspects of Structure, Function and Pathology, pp. 1-65. In: The Adrenal Gland. James, V. H. T. (Ed.). New York: Raven Press, 1979.

———— and O'Hare, M. J. The Human Adrenal Cortex. Berlin: Springer-Verlag, 1982.

———— and Symington, T. Bilateral adrenocortical hyperplasia in children with Cushing's syndrome. J. Pathol. 107:95-106, 1972.

———— and Symington, T. Pathology of primary aldosteronism. Cancer 19:1854-1868, 1966.

New, M. I. and Levine, L. S. Congenital adrenal hyperplasia. Adv. Hum. Genet. 4:251-326, 1973.

Newell, M. E., Lippe, B. M., and Erlich, R. M. Testis tumors associated with congenital adrenal hyperplasia: a continuing diagnostic and therapeutic dilemma. J. Urol. 117:256-258, 1977.

O'Hare, M. J., Ellison, M. L., and Neville, A. M. Tissue culture in endocrine research: perspectives, pitfalls, and potentials. Curr. Top. Exp. Endocrinol. 3:1-56, 1978.

Orth, D. N. The old and the new in Cushing's Syndrome. N. Engl. J. Med. 310:649-651, 1984.

Plotz, C. M., Knowlton, A. I., and Ragan, C. The natural history of Cushing's syndrome. Am. J. Med. 13:597-614, 1952.

Prinz, R. A., Brooks, M. H., Lawrence, A. M., and Paloyan, E. The continued importance of adrenalectomy in the treatment of Cushing's disease. Arch. Surg. 114:481-484, 1979.

Reidbord, H. and Fisher, E. R. Electron microscopic study of adrenal cortical hyperplasia in Cushing's syndrome. Arch. Pathol. 86:419-426, 1968.

Ross, G., Jr., Schneider, R. E., Thompson, I. M., Anast, C. S., and Montie, J. E. Our experience with the adrenogenital syndrome. J. Urol. 115:462-464, 1976.

Ruder, H. J., Loriaux, D. L., and Lipsett, M. B. Severe osteopenia in young adults associated with Cushing's syndrome due to micronodular adrenal disease. J. Clin. Endocrinol. Metab. 39:1138-1147, 1974.

Sandison, A. T. A form of lipoidosis of the adrenal cortex in an infant. Arch. Dis. Child. 30:538-541, 1955.

Schweizer-Cagianut, M., Froesch, E. R., and Chr. Hedinger, E. Familial Cushing's syndrome with primary adrenocortical microadenomatosis (primary adrenocortical nodular dysplasia). Acta Endocrinol. 94:529-535, 1980.

————, Salomon, F., and Chr. Hedinger, E. Primary adrenocortical nodular dysplasia with Cushing's syndrome and cardiac myxomas. Virchows Arch. [Pathol. Anat] 397:183-192, 1982.

Scott, H. W., Jr., Liddle, G. W., Mulherin, J. L., et al. Surgical experience with Cushing's disease. Ann. Surg. 185:524-534, 1977.

Shenoy, B. V., Carpenter, P. C., and Carney, J. A. Bilateral primary pigmented nodular adrenocortical disease. Am. J. Surg. Pathol. 8:335-344, 1984.

Singer, W., Kovacs, K., Ryan, N., and Horvath, E. Ectopic ACTH syndrome: clinicopathological correlations. J. Clin. Pathol. 31:591-598, 1978.

Smals, A. G. H., Pieters, G. F. F. M., van Haelst, U. J. G., and Kloppenborg, P. W. C. Macronodular adrenocortical hyperplasia in long-standing Cushing's Disease. J. Clin. Endocrinol. Metab. 58:25-31, 1984.

Symington, T. The Adrenal Cortex, pp. 419-471. In: Endocrine Pathology, 2d. Ed. Bloodworth, J. M. B., Jr. (Ed.). Baltimore: The Williams & Wilkins Company, 1982.

————. Functional Pathology of the Human Adrenal Gland, pp. 150-154. Baltimore: The Williams & Wilkins Company, 1969.

Tyrrell, J. B., Brooks, R. M., Fitzgerald, P. A. et al. Cushing's disease. N. Engl. J. Med. 298:753-758, 1978.

Van Seters, A. P., Van Aalderen, W., Moolenaar, A. J., et al. Adrenocortical tumour in untreated congenital adrenocortical hyperplasia associated with inadequate ACTH suppressibility. Clin. Endocrinol. 14:325-334, 1981.

Williams, E. D., Siebenmann, R. E., and Sobin, L. H. Histological typing of endocrine tumours. International Histological Classification of Tumours, No. 23. Geneva: World Health Organization, 1980.

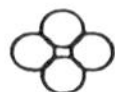

ADRENAL CORTICAL ADENOMA

SYNONYMS AND RELATED TERMS: Adrenal adenoma; adrenocortical adenoma.

Definition. Adrenal cortical adenoma is a benign neoplasm of adrenal cortical cells resembling normal adrenal cells histologically but evidencing physiologic autonomy.

Incidence. When adrenal cortical adenomas are separated (Table 5) from the incidental adrenal cortical nodules frequently seen in autopsies, it becomes apparent that true benign neoplasms of the adrenal cortex are comparatively rare (Neville and O'Hare). Although true nonfunctioning adenomas in the adrenal cortex do occur (Symington), most lesions which can be characterized confidently as adenomas produce a definite clinical syndrome due to overproduction of steroid hormones or precursor substances (Neville and O'Hare). It is difficult to distinguish a nonfunctioning adenoma from the adrenal cortical nodules seen commonly at autopsies in older individuals (see Adrenal Cortical Hyperplasia, the nodular adrenal). In most large series reported (Neville and Mackay; Neville and Symington; Symington), primary hyperaldosteronism is the most common clinical syndrome accompanying adrenal cortical adenomas, followed in decreasing order of frequency by Cushing's syndrome (hypercortisolism), virilism and, very rarely, feminization. In this context, it should be emphasized that bilateral cortical hyperplasia is a far more common finding than adenoma in hypercortisolism (Orth and Liddle), accounting for approximately 80 percent of all cases of this syndrome. The reverse, however, is seen in primary hyperaldosteronism (Conn's syndrome), where adenomas account for the majority of the cases (Neville and O'Hare).

Regardless of the clinical syndrome produced, females outnumber males two to one in series reporting adult patients. However, a more equal sex ratio is seen in children afflicted with adrenal adenoma (Neville and O'Hare). In contrast to adrenal cortical carcinoma, where one of the two periods of peak incidence is in the first decade of life (Hutter and Kayhoe), adrenal adenomas as a whole are less common in children, as compared to adults (Visser; Neville and O'Hare). Exceptions are the benign sex steroid producing tumors, which are more frequent in children than in adults (Symington). The left and right adrenal glands are equally likely to be affected. Familial adrenal cortical tumors are exceedingly rare (Fraumeni and Miller) but have been reported. Bilaterality and ectopic origin have been described, but are also uncommon. Almost all bilateral cases are actually variants of the multinodular adrenal, with or without accompanying hyperplasia. Cases of adrenal adenoma with hypercortisolism may be misinterpreted as unilateral hyperplasia, as in the patient reported by Josse and associates. Evidence of inactivity in the cortex adjacent to the adenoma is manifested in this case by loss of compact cells from all layers, the presence of small clear cells throughout the cortex, and a thickened capsule. These features of atrophy in the cortex surrounding an adenoma define the adenomas as such. (See Multinodular Adrenal and Multinodular Hyperplasia).

Clinical Diagnosis. The clinical diagnosis of adrenal cortical adenomas is accomplished by biochemical and radiologic methods. Since most benign adrenal

Table 5

ADENOMAS OF VARIOUS FUNCTIONAL TYPES COMPARED TO "NODULES"

Clinical Syndrome	Gross Appearance	Microscopic Appearance	Ultramicroscopic Appearance	Remainder of Gland
Hyperaldosteronism	Golden-yellow, usually homogeneous, average 1.5 cm., may not be encapsulated.	Mixtures of clear cells with characteristics of both ZG* and ZF** (hybrid cell). Compact cells may also be present.	Small to intermediate cytoplasmic volume with little SER,*** elongated, tubulo-lamellar mitochondria and few osmiophilic droplets or lysosomes.	Normal or hyperplastic ZG.
Hypercortisolism	Yellow-brown, mottled, usually encapsulated, rarely black, average 4.0 cm.	Mixture of compact and clear cells, myelolipomatous foci common.	Large cytoplasmic volume with tubulo-vesicular mitochondria, variable numbers of lysosomes. Usually many osmiophilic free droplets.	Atrophy of inner zones, especially reticularis, with small, clear cells. Normal ZG.
Virilization	Red-brown encapsulated, average 5 cm. May be as large as 10 cm. without malignant features.	Compact cells arranged in cords or acini.	Intermediate cytoplasmic volume with densely packed SER, few osmiophilic granules and many lysosomes.	Normal
Feminization	Similar to virilization except benignancy rare and average size less.	Similar to virilism.	Similar to virilism.	Similar to virilism.
Nodule	Pale yellow, up to 2 cm., nonencapsulated.	Clear fasciculata type cells, rarely foci of compact reticularis type cells.	Similar to normal ZF.	Normal with fine nodularity.

*ZG: zona glomerulosa
**ZF: zona fasciculata
***SER: smooth endoplasmic reticulum

tumors produce a definite clinical syndrome (Symington; Neville and O'Hare), a constellation of biochemical findings accompanies each type of adenoma. In the case of the most common syndrome, primary hyperaldosteronism, the diagnosis is achieved by demonstrating hypertension with hypokalemia and suppressed plasma renin activity resistant to acute stimulation. Similar biochemical findings may be present in certain rare cases of congenital adrenal hyperplasia (Visser). However, in this latter condition, they are corrected by glucocorticoid administration.

The majority of cases manifesting the syndrome of primary hyperaldosteronism have a unilateral adrenal adenoma (Neville and O'Hare), with or without hyperplasia of the zona glomerulosa of the surrounding gland (figs. 58—60). Not all patients with the syndrome can be so characterized, some having bilateral hyperplasia and, a few, bilateral adenomas (Favre et al.). Due to the small size of these neoplasms (Table 5), preoperative localization may be difficult, conventional radiography and arteriography having little utility. Bilateral adrenal venography (fig. 61) with differential adrenal vein aldosterone:cortisol ratio determinations will usually lateralize the tumor (Lecky et al.). Rarely, the ratios are similar between the tumor and nontumor bearing sides. Venography may also cause intra-adrenal hemorrhage with the formation of misleading pseudotumors (pl. IV). These pseudotumors may lead to erroneous removal of a nontumor-bearing adrenal. Scintillation scans of adrenal uptake of 19-I^{131} cholesterol after dexamethasone suppression of the surrounding adrenal gland have been used to identify aldosterone secreting tumors in the 1 to 2 cm range (Sebold et al). However, results in localization of tumors smaller than 1 cm in diameter have not been as rewarding.

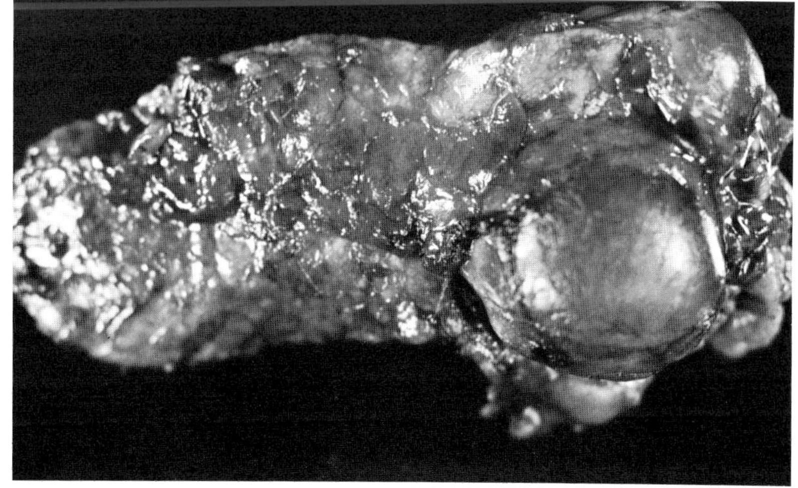

Figure 58
ADRENAL CORTICAL ADENOMA
Surface view of this adrenal gland shows the characteristic localized round swelling of an adrenal cortical adenoma. Atrophy of the attached gland is not present. The patient had primary aldosteronism. X1.5.

PLATE IV
ADRENAL CORTICAL ADENOMA

(Plate IV-A and figures 64, 68, and 79 from same patient)

A. This adrenal gland was removed from a 44 year old woman with Cushing's syndrome. One large red brown adenoma and one smaller nodule are present. The smaller one may represent a second adenoma. The remainder of the gland shows atrophy. X2.

(Plate IV-B, C, and figure 83 from same patient)

B. Atrophy of the cortex is manifested in this case by loss of normal zonation, absence of compact cells of the reticulate zone, and a thick fibrous capsule (c). The patient was a non-Cushingoid woman with elevated plasma cortisol levels failing to show diurnal variation or suppression with dexamethasone. Removal of adenoma restored dexamethasone suppressibility. X12.

C. Typical yellow brown globoid adenoma, shown microscopically in plate IV-B, is seen. The yellow areas represent clear cells, while brown areas are composed primarily of compact cells. Atrophic cortex is reduced to a narrow rim at lower left. X1.5.

D. This bright yellow adenoma, seen in an en face view, measured 1.5 cm in diameter and is typical of those occurring in primary aldosteronism. The patient was an adult male with suppressed plasma renin and hypertension cured by unilateral adrenalectomy. X1.5.

E. This hypertensive patient was thought to have bilateral adrenal adenomas on adrenal venography. The larger apparent mass (above) is a central hemorrhage probably occurring as a complication of preoperative adrenal venography. The actual 0.5 cm adenoma was in the contralateral adrenal (below). The hypertension was abolished by partial adrenalectomy on the side with adenoma. X2.

PLATE IV

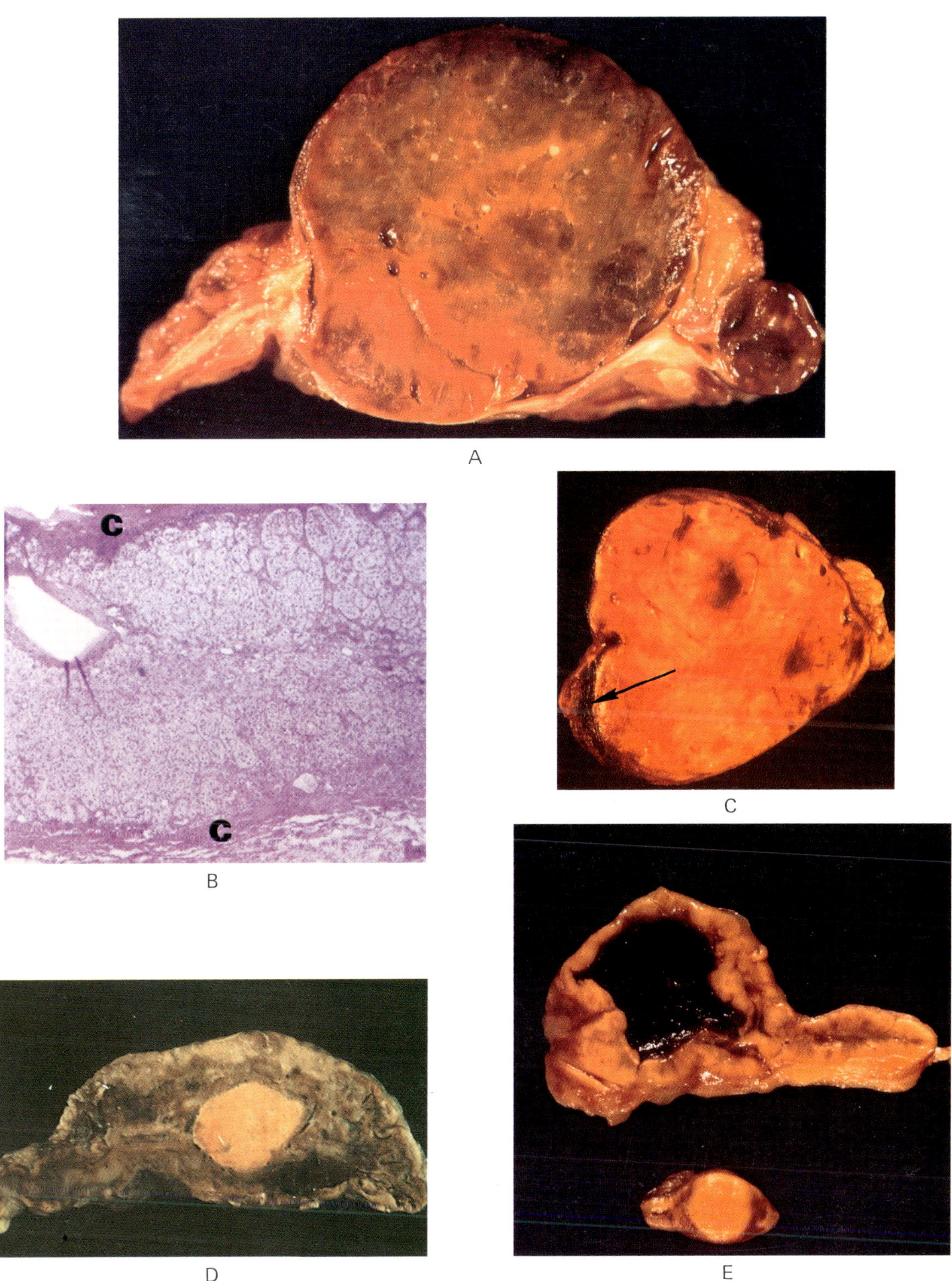

PLATE V
ADRENAL CORTICAL ADENOMA

(Plate V-A and B and figures 62 and 76 from same patient)

A. This adrenal adenoma was removed from a 67 year old woman with mild hypercortisolism. A left adrenal mass was noted on intravenous pyelography and with computerized axial tomography (fig. 62). The tumor, which weighed 130 g, was composed of interspersed yellow and brown areas. Actual size.

B. A macrosection wholemount reveals that the yellow areas are composed of lighter, lipid-containing cells, while the brown areas contain lipid poor cells. The residual cortex (arrow) is compressed and disorganized. X1.6.

C. Multiple sections of single adrenal gland reveal an adenoma which produced aldosterone seen as a 3.0 cm round nodule localized to one end of the gland. Note the prominent zona reticularis (arrow). The patient was cured by adrenalectomy. X.75.

PLATE V

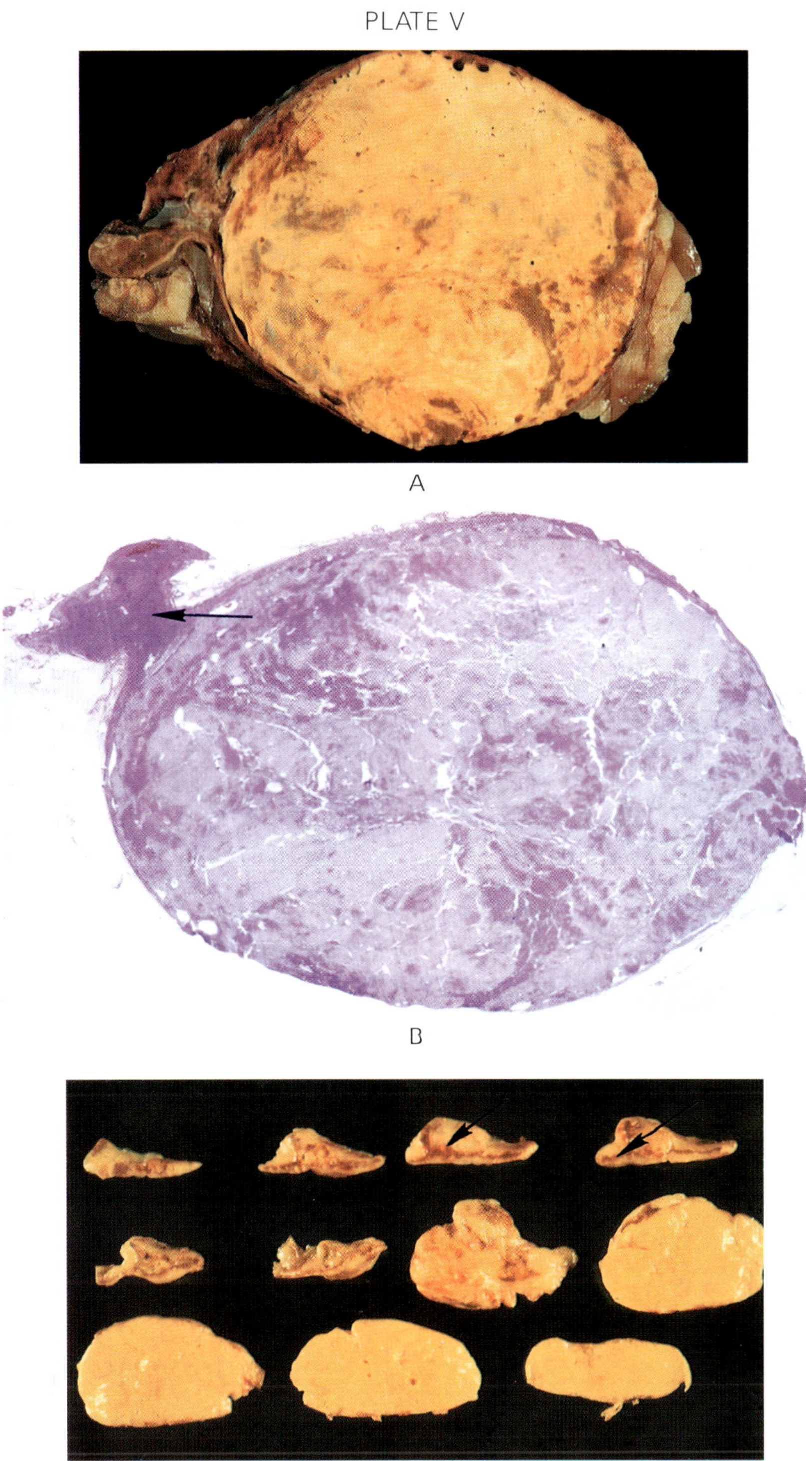

A

B

C

PLATE VI
ADRENAL CORTICAL ADENOMA

(Plate VI-A, B, and figure 84 from same patient)

A. Gross photograph of a typical "black" adenoma of adrenal reveals characteristic pigmentation. Black adenomas may cause any of the common clinical syndromes of adrenal hyperfunction. X2. (Courtesy of Dr. G. Gray, New York, NY.)

B. Histologic appearance demonstrates cells with uniform nuclei and cytoplasm filled with pigment granules. Pigment is much less apparent microscopically than grossly. X400.

C. Laminated cytoplasmic inclusions are seen in this adenoma that produced primary aldosteronism. The patient had been treated with spironolactone prior to operation. X800.

(Plate VI-D, figures 85, and 86 from same patient)

D. An alveolar growth pattern is seen in this ectopic adrenal cortical tumor originating in the pancreas. The patient was a 31 year old man with Cushing's syndrome who was cured by removal of the mass. X160.

PLATE VI

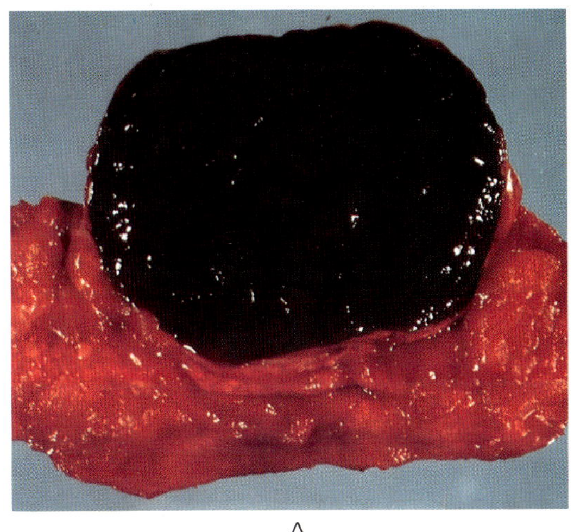

A

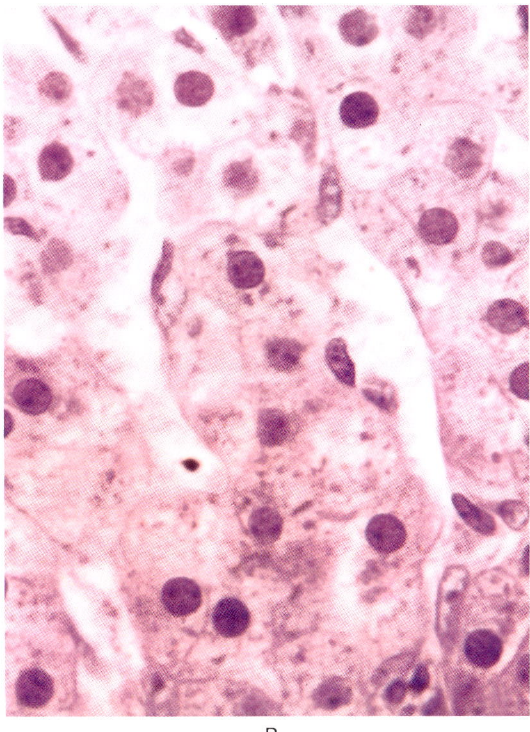

B

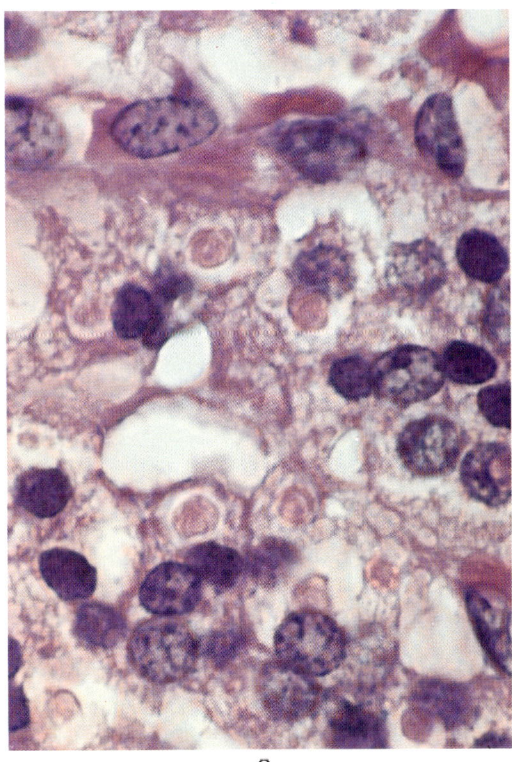

C

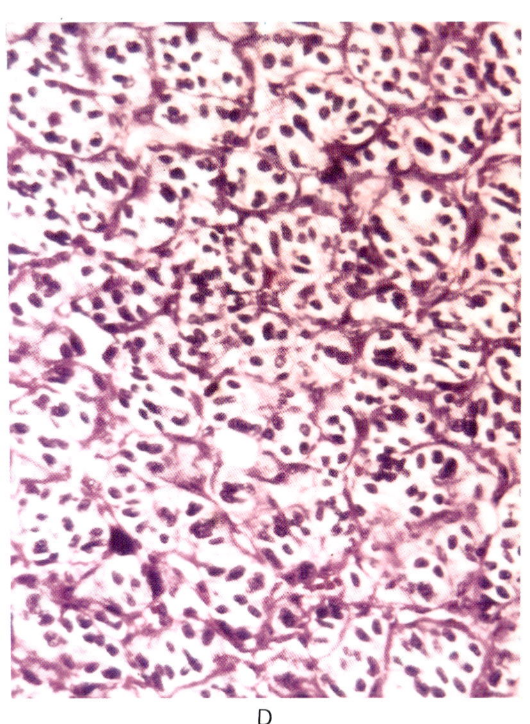

D

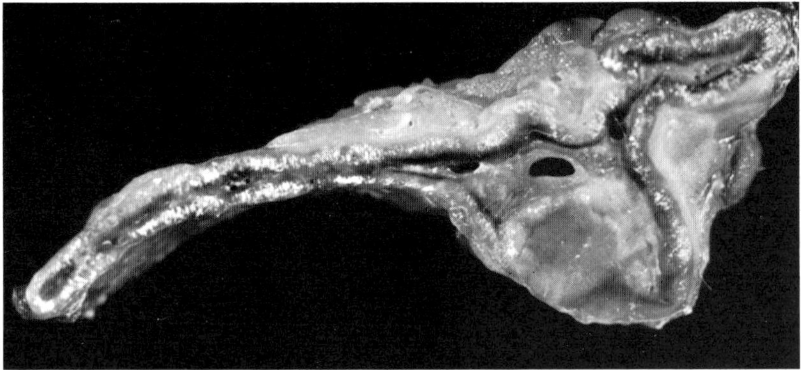

Figure 59
ADRENAL CORTICAL ADENOMA
Adrenal gland of a 48 year old man with primary aldosteronism contains a 6.5 mm
adenoma. The small size is characteristic of these lesions. X2.

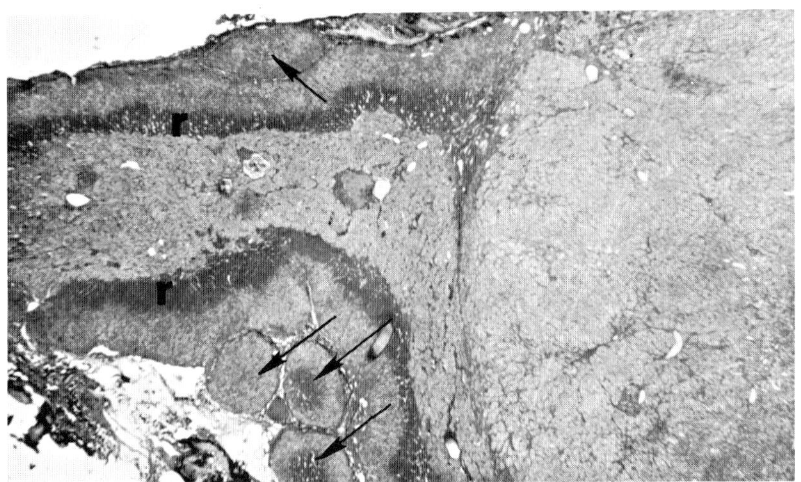

Figure 60
ADRENAL CORTICAL ADENOMA
Adenoma producing primary aldosteronism is demarcated from the surrounding
normal gland. Zona reticularis (r) is well preserved. A rounded configuration is usually
seen. Several capsular extrusions (arrows) are also present. These are incidental findings
without clinical significance. X10.

The clinical picture of hypercortisolism (Cushing's syndrome) may also result from an adrenal adenoma. The differentiation of pituitary from adrenal-based Cushing's syndrome is achieved by biochemical means. Both types of disease produce elevated plasma cortisol and urine 17-hydroxycorticoid values not suppressible by low dose dexamethasone. That due to an adrenal adenoma, however, usually fails to suppress with high dose dexamethasone, while pituitary-based Cushing's syndrome virtually always does (Liddle). Plasma ACTH is usually undetectable in the presence of a cortisol-secreting tumor in contrast to the normal or elevated values associated with pituitary-based Cushing's disease.

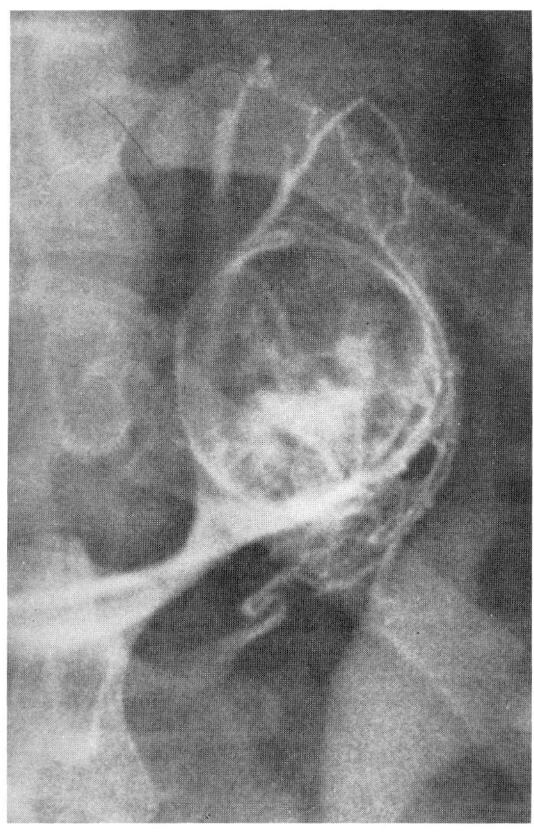

Figure 61
ADRENAL CORTICAL ADENOMA
Venogram of small adrenocortical adenoma associated with primary aldosteronism reveals stretching and displacement of veins about the tumor. Note the round configuration.

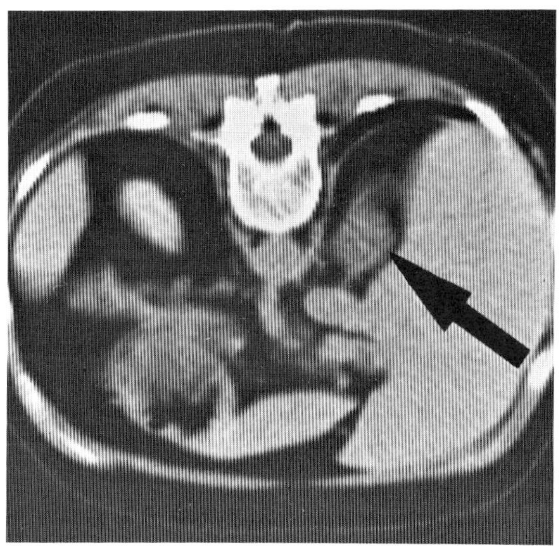

Figure 62
(Figures 62, 76 and plate V-A, B from same patient)
ADRENAL CORTICAL ADENOMA
Computerized axial tomographic (CAT) scan of adenoma seen in plate V-A reveals mass in left adrenal (arrow) with residual adrenal gland spiraling outward in two thin rays.

Localization of an adrenal adenoma in Cushing's syndrome is usually less difficult than in primary hyperaldosteronism due to the larger average size of cortisol-producing adenomas. However, such sensitive means as adrenal venography, computerized axial tomography (fig. 62), and 19-I^{131} cholesterol scans may be required to localize tumors less than 2 cm in diameter. Arteriography and ultrasonography are usually helpful only in lesions over 4 cm in largest dimension.

Adenomas producing the adrenogenital syndrome (virilism or feminization) are rare and often larger than those producing either primary hyperaldosteronism or Cushing's syndrome (Symington). Clinical impressions may be confirmed by plasma and urine steroid determinations. Specific assays are available for androgens such as dehydroepiandrosterone and testosterone, as well as for various estrogens.

Gross. Adrenal adenomas vary remarkably in gross appearance. Although it is difficult to achieve sound generalizations for the entire group of tumors, those applicable to size and color are presented in Table 5. In general, adenomas of primary hyperaldosteronism are bright yellow in color (pl. IV-D, E), often unencapsulated, and small (regularly less than 2.5 cm in diameter and often less than 1 cm). Those producing Cushing's syndrome are usually yellow with brown foci (pl. V) and appear encapsulated, averaging 4 cm in diameter. The relatively uncommon benign tumors producing the adrenogenital syndrome are usually red brown in color, averaging greater than 5 cm in diameter. Although benign tumors as large as 10 cm in diameter associated with the adrenogenital syndrome have been reported (Symington), these are quite rare, and most tumors of this size are malignant. Nodules, common incidental findings at autopsy, are usually pale yellow in color, but may be brown or black (pl. II-C), non-encapsulated, irregular in shape, and usually less than 2 cm in diameter (pl.

III-E — G). Although an encroaching tumor may distort the residual adrenal gland (fig. 63), actual adrenal cortical atrophy accompanies only those adenomas producing glucocorticoids, primarily cortisol (fig. 64). These tumors are almost always associated with some variant of Cushing's syndrome.

Microscopic. Although certain histologic features are associated with each functional type of adrenal cortical adenoma, none is sufficiently pronounced or constant to characterize function from histology alone. A summary of current knowledge is presented in Table 5. Although some

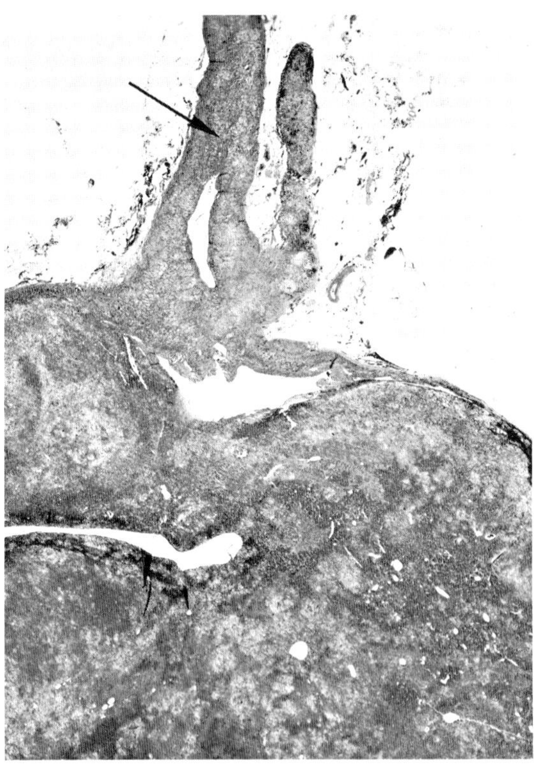

Figure 63
(Figures 63, 67, and 69 from same patient)
ADRENAL CORTICAL ADENOMA
Adrenal cortical adenoma (above) producing primary aldosteronism distorts the surrounding gland, but does not produce atrophy of gland (below). The patient was a 17 year old male who was cured by adrenalectomy. X25.

Figure 64
(Figures 64, 68, 79, and plate IV-A from same patient)
ADRENAL CORTICAL ADENOMA
Adrenal cortical adenoma producing cortisol induces striking atrophy of remainder of gland (arrow) due to suppression of ACTH release. X25.

authors characterize adrenal adenomas by adrenal cell type (Williams et al.), the large number of tumors composed of several varieties of cortical cells and the lack of a clear functional correlation with specific cell types, have prompted our present approach. Paradoxically, and in contrast to the diagnosis of malignancy, the assessment of functional status is best done by careful study of that portion of the adrenal gland uninvolved by the tumor, searching for evidence of hyperplasia or atrophy.

The microscopic pathology of adenomas producing primary hyperaldosteronism is relatively constant. The major portion of these tumors is made up of so-called hybrid cells incorporating characteristics of glomerulosa and fasciculata cells (fig. 65). These cells are clear in appearance but have a slightly larger nucleus than a normal fasciculata cell. Occasionally, small foci of glomerulosa-like cells and compact cells may be present. Nuclear pleomorphism is rare in this group of tumors. The histology of the surrounding gland may be either normal (fig. 66) with clearly defined zonation or demonstrate a hyperplastic glomerulosa (fig. 67). Quantitation of the degree of hyperplasia of the glomerulosa is difficult, however, because it is irregularly distributed in the normal gland.

Adenomas producing Cushing's syndrome (hypercortisolism) are characteristically composed of mixtures of clear (zona fasciculata type) and compact (zona reticularis type) cells (fig. 68). Sasano and associates have reported that clear cell areas were predominant in cortisol-secreting adenomas from patients responding to ACTH stimulation. Some cellular pleomorphism with occasional giant cells may be observed (fig. 69). However, true nuclear pleomorphism is uncommon in these adenomas (see section on Carcinoma).

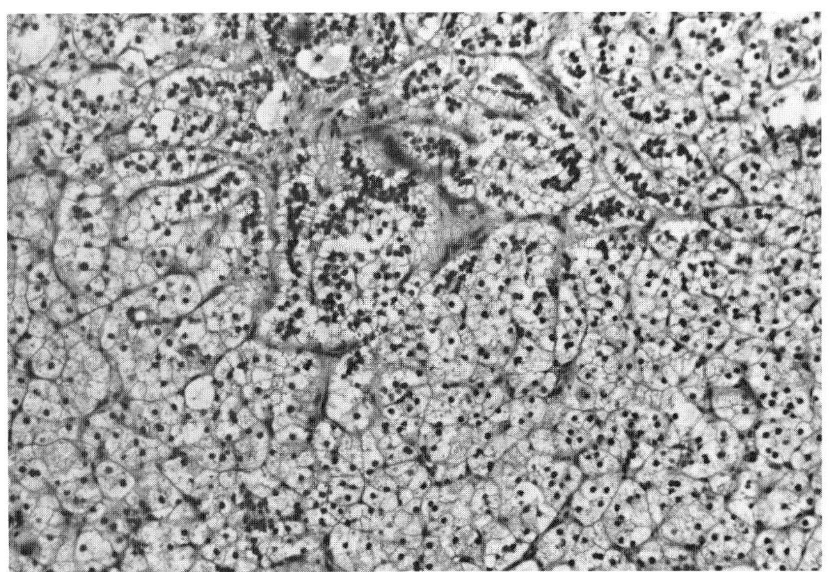

Figure 65
ADRENAL CORTICAL ADENOMA
This adrenal cortical adenoma producing aldosterone is characterized by uniform cells having features of both fasciculata and glomerulosa types. These "hybrid" cells rarely show significant pleomorphism. X100.

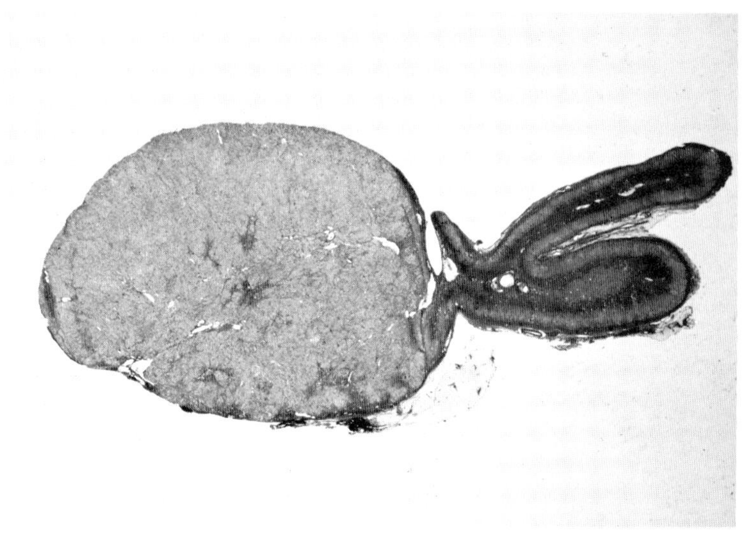

Figure 66
ADRENAL CORTICAL ADENOMA
Low power view of adrenal cortical adenoma producing aldosterone shows clear preservation of normal zonation in the attached adrenal gland. (Compare with figure 64.) X6.

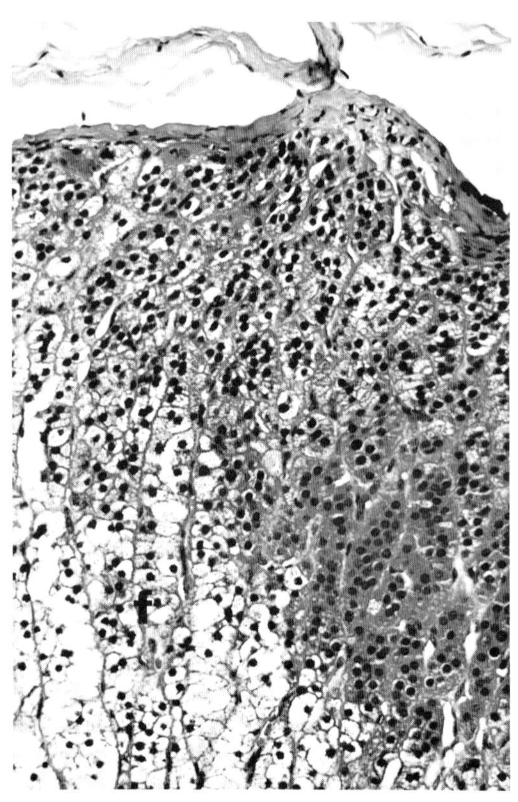

Figure 67
ADRENAL CORTICAL ADENOMA
Wedge of hyperplastic glomerulosa cells (upper right) extends into the fasciculate zone (clearer cells at lower left) in the adrenal gland of a patient with an ipsilateral adenoma producing aldosterone. Hypertension was ameliorated by unilateral adrenalectomy. Hyperplasia of this sort is not uncommon. X160.

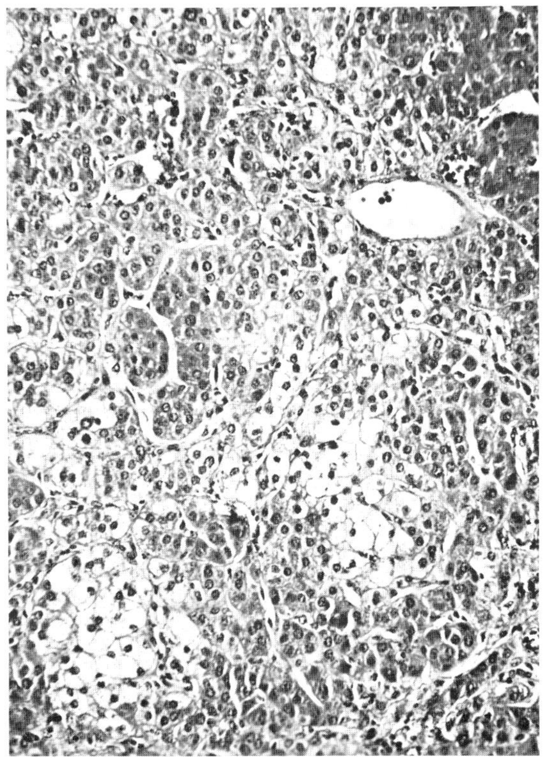

Figure 68
(Figures 64, 68, 79, and plate IV-A from same patient)
ADRENAL CORTICAL ADENOMA
This cortisol secreting adenoma is composed predominantly of compact, lipid poor cells with islands of clear lipid laden cells (center). Such tumors are usually brown. X160.

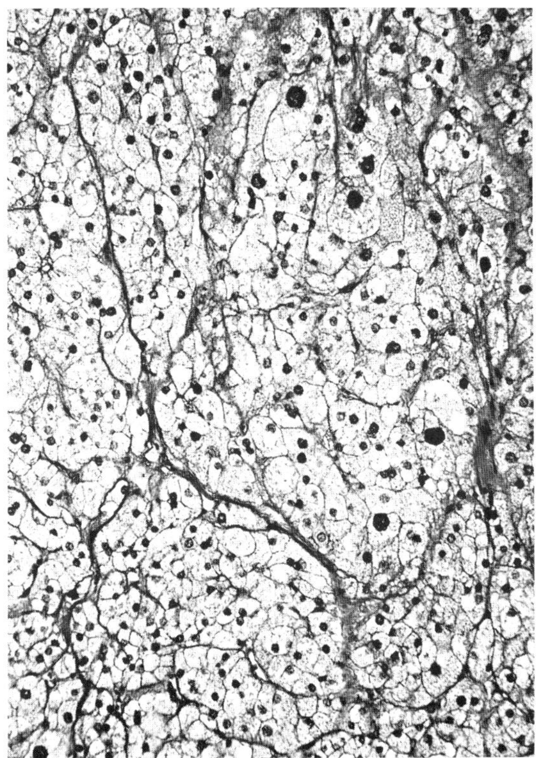

Figure 69
ADRENAL CORTICAL ADENOMA
A mild degree of nuclear enlargement and pleomorphism is seen in this adrenal adenoma producing aldosterone. X160.

Tumor necrosis is rare and is often a complication of thrombosis following adrenal venography (figs. 70, 71). Necrosis should not be regarded as incontrovertible evidence of malignancy and an explanation should be sought in tumors which do not have other characteristics associated with subsequent malignant behavior. Myelolipomatous foci may be seen and have no bearing on prognosis. The adjacent adrenal gland always shows some degree of atrophy in tumors producing Cushing's syndrome. This may take the form of absence or attenuation of compact cells in the zona reticularis, indicating the inactivity resulting

from suppression of ACTH secretion (fig. 72). Alternatively, the atrophy may lead to a rather profound total disorganizaton of the cortex with marked thinning of all layers. Characteristically, the thinned cortex presents a uniform appearance of small cells with clear cytoplasm demonstrating no difference between inner and outer zones (pl. IV-B; fig. 64). The glomerulosa is not affected, and the capsule is thickened.

The adenomas producing the adrenogenital syndrome are perhaps the most difficult to separate reliably from the carcinomas more commonly associated with this condition. This is particularly true for larger

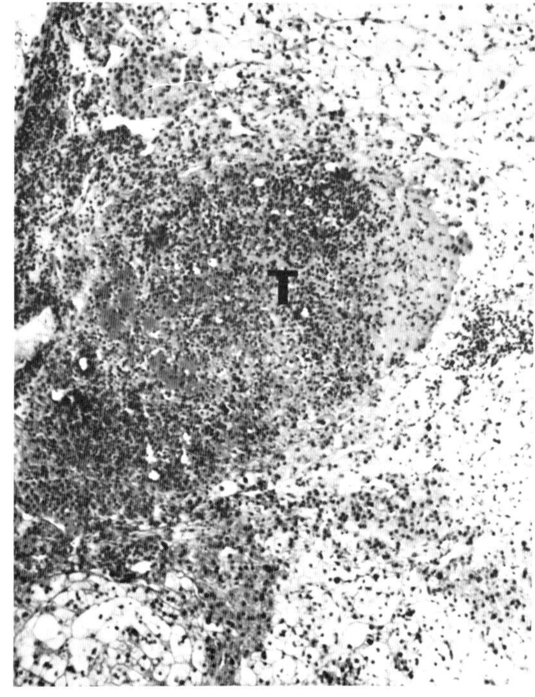

Figure 70
ADRENAL CORTICAL ADENOMA
Thrombosis of adrenal vein following venography is occasionally seen. Acute inflammation and edema are present, surrounding organizing thrombus (lower middle, left). X50.

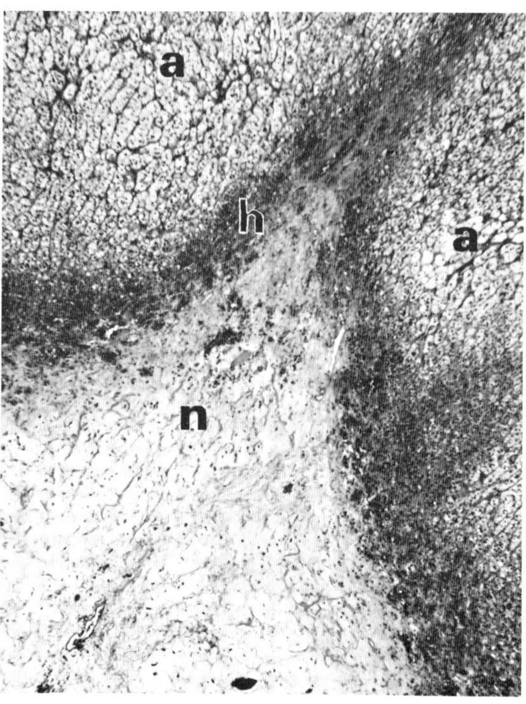

Figure 71
ADRENAL CORTICAL ADENOMA
Late effects of adrenal vein thrombosis are seen in this 104 g adrenal cortical adenoma. Area of organizing necrosis (n) is surrounded by hyperemic zone (h) and adenoma (a). X40.

tumors of 100 g or greater. Half of these adenomas occur before the age of 12, in contrast to benign tumors causing either Cushing's syndrome or primary hyperaldosteronism (Symington), which are relatively rare in childhood. The tumors are commonly composed of compact, reticularis-like cells, although foci of clear (fasciculata-like) cells may be present (fig. 73). However, all adenomas with this appearance are not associated with the adrenogenital syndrome and many will produce instead some variant of Cushing's syndrome. The adrenal cortex adjacent to the adenomas producing the adrenogenital syndrome is not atrophic, nor is the contralateral adrenal gland. Caution must be used in interpreting

any large adrenal tumor producing the adrenogenital syndrome in an adult as benign. Minimal pleomorphism, mitotic activity or tumor necrosis have been associated with subsequent malignant behavior (Symington; Hough et al.; Case Records, Massachusetts General Hospital). Consequently, any degree of true nuclear hyperchromatism and mitotic activity in a large tumor producing the adrenogenital syndrome is strong evidence for aggressive potential (fig. 74).

Benign adrenal cortical tumors producing feminization are extremely rare. Most tumors producing this syndrome in adults are malignant (Case Records, Massachusetts General Hospital; Bhettay and Bonnici)

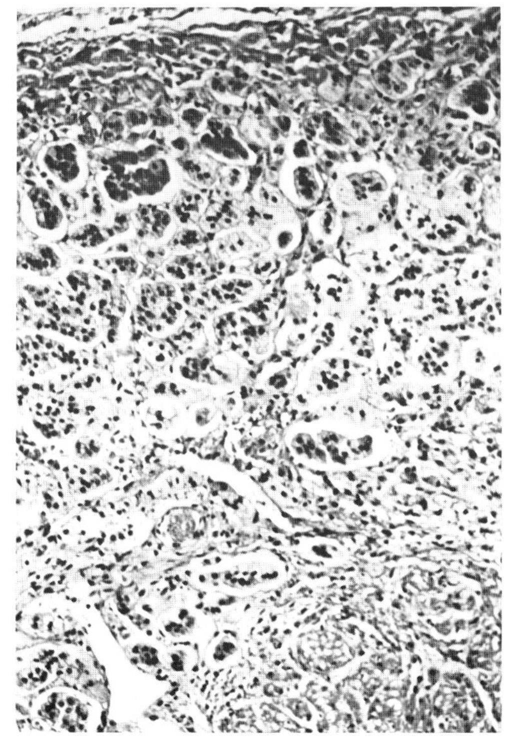

Figure 72
ADRENAL CORTICAL ADENOMA
A severe degree of adrenocortical atrophy is seen accompanying cortisol-secreting adenomas. Here there is disorganization of the cortex, with marked thinning, absence of zonation, and no apparent zona reticularis. Note musculature of adrenal vein at lower right. X100.

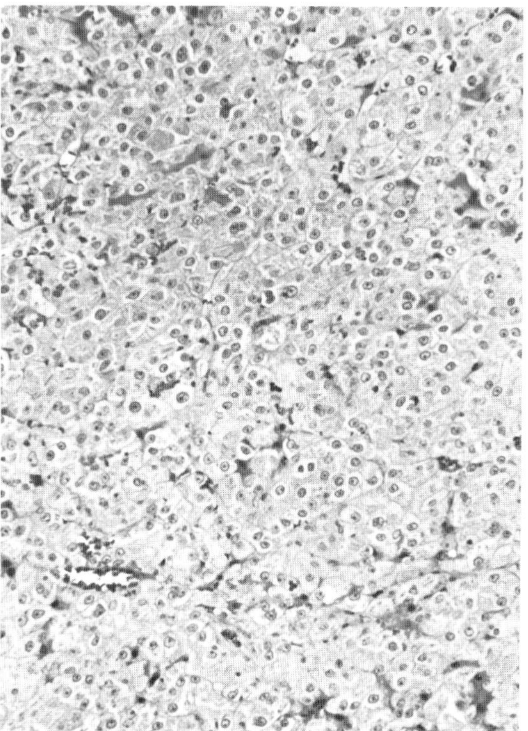

Figure 73
ADRENAL CORTICAL ADENOMA
Adrenal cortical adenomas predominantly producing androgens usually show less pleomorphism than those producing Cushing's syndrome, even when greater than 100 g in weight. This 49 g adenoma produced virilism without Cushing's syndrome in a 27 year old woman. Both plasma testosterone and dehydroepiandrosterone levels were elevated. Note the uniform appearance of the cells, which resemble leuteinized thecal cells. Removal resulted in cessation of symptoms. X100.

with histologic characteristics described in the section on Adrenal Cortical Carcinoma. Small tumors (less than 50 g) producing this syndrome in children have been reported as benign (Howard et al.) and are histologically similar to those causing virilism. However, those feminizing tumors which appear histologically benign are best regarded as malignant in the light of their aggressive natural history. Most cases of benign feminizing tumors reported have been followed for relatively short periods of time.

An unusual variant of the adrenogenital syndrome results not from production of C-19 androgens such as dehydroepiandro-

sterone, but from testosterone itself (Costin et al.; Kable and Yussman). Testosterone, an extremely powerful androgen, may induce a clinical syndrome even when produced in amounts too small to be detected by routine analysis of urinary 17-ketosteroids (Burr et al.; Werk et al.). Although some testosterone-producing tumors have a histologic appearance similar to other virilizing adrenocortical neoplasms, a few have unusual microscopic features best described as plump acidophilic cells resembling ovarian theca-lutein cells (fig. 75).

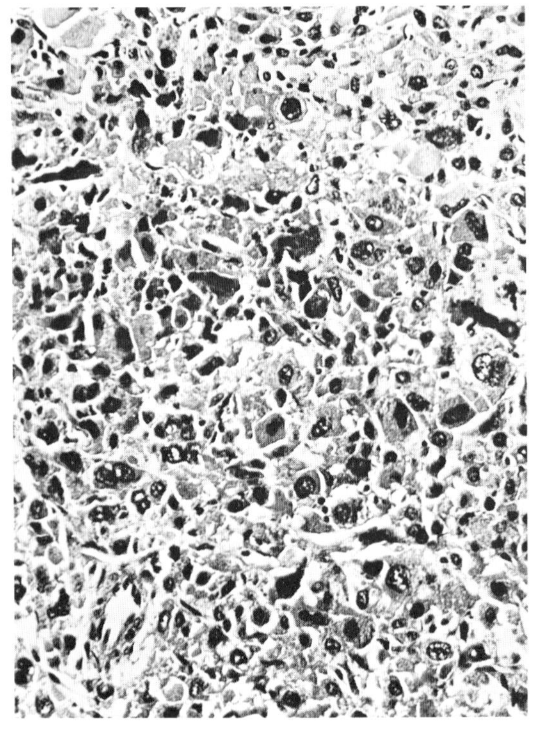

Figure 74
ADRENAL CORTICAL CARCINOMA
Most virilizing adrenal cortical tumors are frankly malignant, with marked degrees of nuclear pleomorphism, as in this patient. (Compare this appearance with figure 73.) X160.

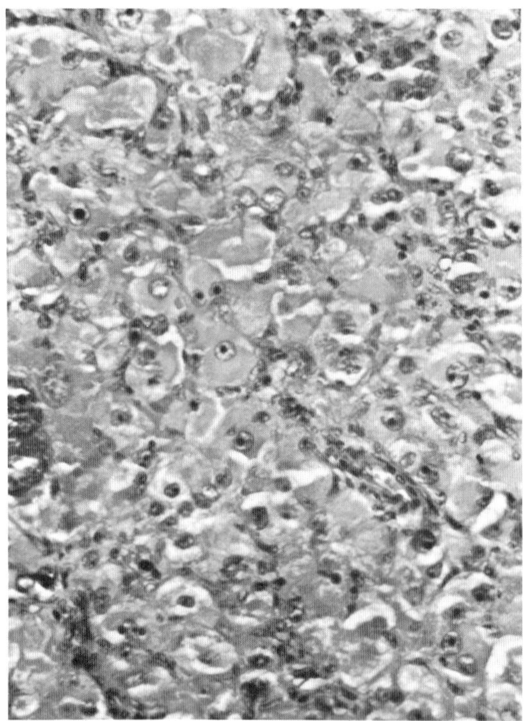

Figure 75
ADRENAL CORTICAL ADENOMA
An unusual variant of virilizing adrenal cortical adenoma is characterized by large and globoid cells with abundant eosinophilic cytoplasm, resembling ovarian theca-lutein cells. Many such cases respond to gonadotrophins. The patient was a 12 year old girl cured by adrenalectomy. X160.

Some of these tumors apparently respond not to ACTH, but to gonadotrophins, although similar responses have been described in tumors resembling zona reticularis-type cells. Any relationship to virilizing tumors of the ovary and testis is unclear, although ovarian thecal metaplasia has been described in adrenal glands of postmenopausal women (Fidler).

Ultrastructure. The electron microscopic appearance of cells comprising adrenal cortical adenomas resembles cells of the normal cortex (fig. 76). Characteristic features of steroid secreting cells are present including tubulovesicular or tubulo-lamellar mitochondria (fig. 77), parallel stacks of rough endoplasmic reticulum (fig. 78), and abundant smooth endoplasmic reticulum (fig. 79). In some cases, intrusions of cytoplasm into the nucleus (nuclear pseudoinclusions) and qualitative and quantitative changes in mitochondria are also present. These mitochondrial changes include increase in number (fig. 80), loss of cristae (fig. 81), and formation of proteinaceous intramitochondrial deposits (fig. 82). Lipid-poor (nonosmiophilic) cells with extremely abundant mitochondria and smooth endoplasmic reticulum are characteristic of androgen producing tumors. However, many tumors composed of osmiophilic cells also produce androgens.

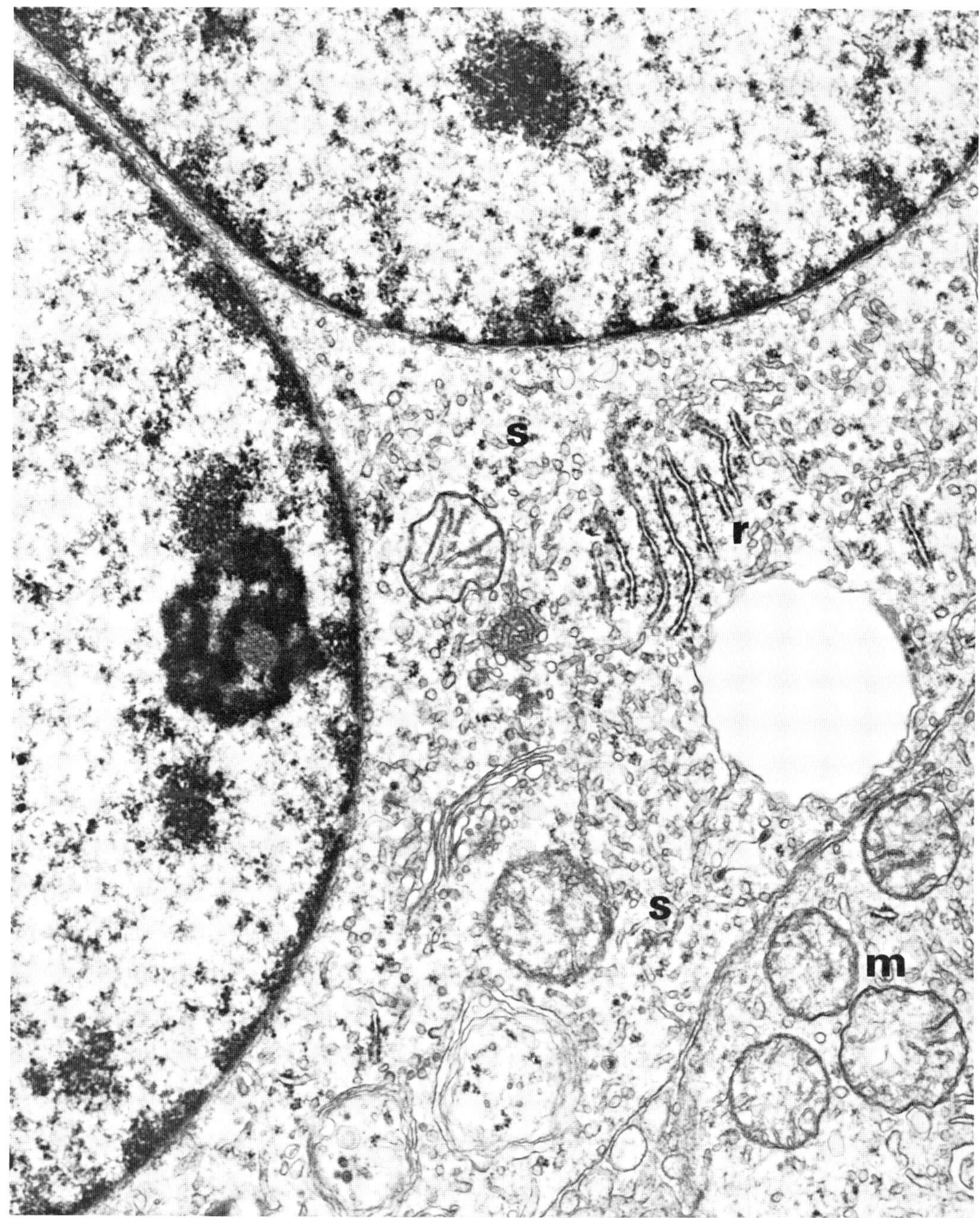

Figure 76
(Figures 62, 76, and plate V from same patient)
ADRENAL CORTICAL ADENOMA
Ultrastructure of typical adrenal cortical adenoma reveals a binucleate cell containing parallel array of rough endoplasmic reticulum (r), spherical vesicular mitochondria (m) in an adjacent cell, and abundant smooth endoplasmic reticulum (s). Material is from the same patient as plate V. Uranyl acetate-lead citrate. X30,000.

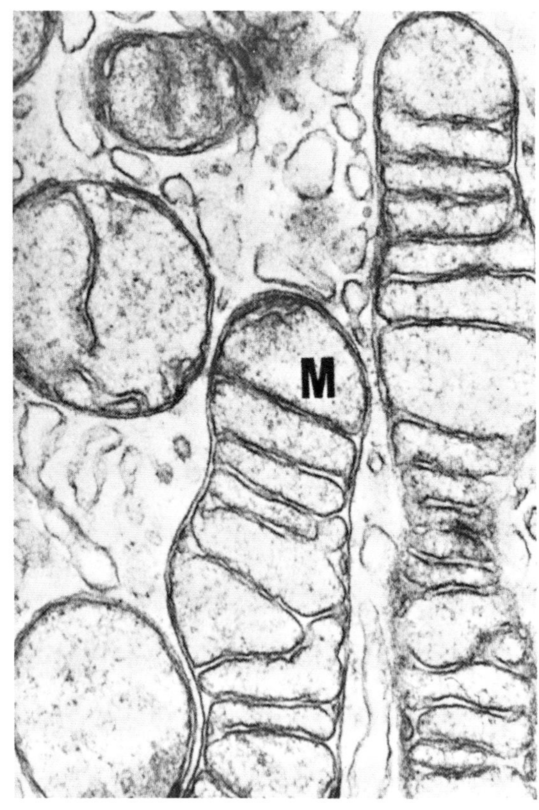

Figure 77
ADRENAL CORTICAL ADENOMA
Electron micrograph is of mitochondria (M) from adenoma
producing Cushing's syndrome. Elongated lamellar cristae
are suggestive of zona glomerulosa. Compare to the mito-
chondria in figure 76. Uranyl acetate-lead citrate. X46,800.
(From Symington, T. In: Functional Pathology of the Human
Adrenal Gland. Edinburgh: Churchill Livingstone, 1969.)

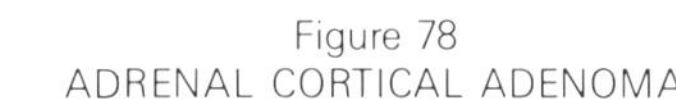

Figure 78
ADRENAL CORTICAL ADENOMA
Ultrastructure of parallel arrays of rough endoplasmic
reticulum reveals continuity with background of smooth
endoplasmic reticulum. Numerous microbodies are present.
The case was of a 6x5x5 cm, virilizing adrenal cortical
adenoma in a two year old boy. X17,000. (Courtesy of Dr.
K. Gorgas, Federal Republic of Germany. Also from Gorgas,
K., Bock, P., and Wuketich, S. Fine structure of a virilizing
adrenocortical adenoma. Beitr. Pathol. 159:371-397, 1976.)

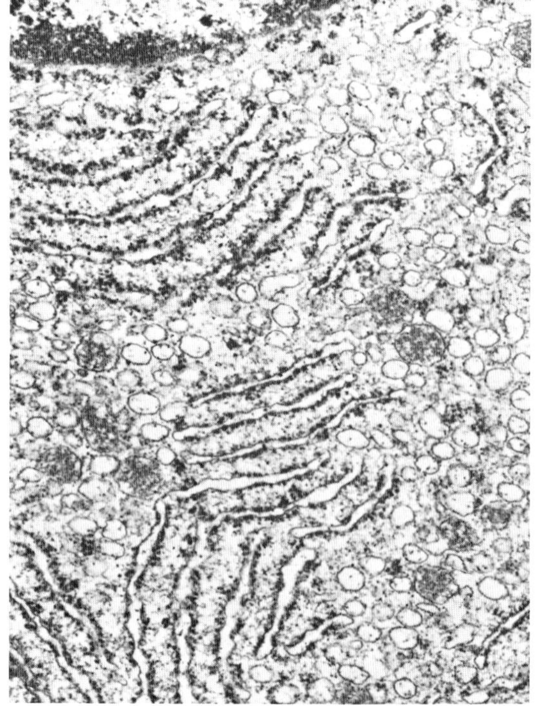

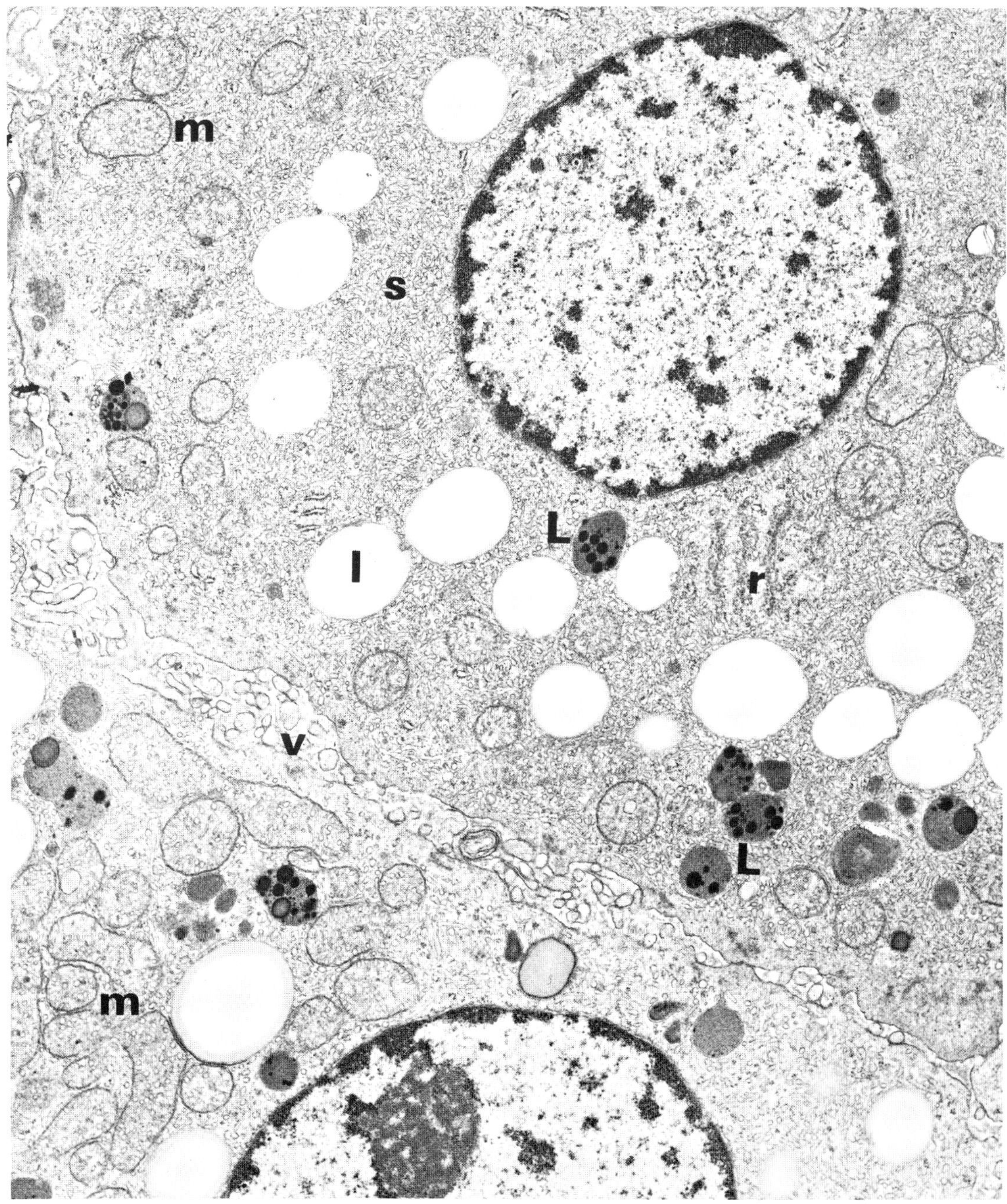

Figure 79
(Figures 64, 68, 79, and plate IV-A from same patient)
ADRENAL CORTICAL ADENOMA
Ultrastructure of a cortisol secreting adenoma shows features typical of cells of inner zona fasciculata. These include abundant smooth endoplasmic reticulum (s), lysozomes with lipofuscin pigment (L), relatively sparse stacks of rough endoplasmic reticulum (r), tubulovesicular mitochondria (m), sparse intracytoplasmic lipid (l), and prominent microvilli (v). Uranyl acetate-lead citrate. X9500.

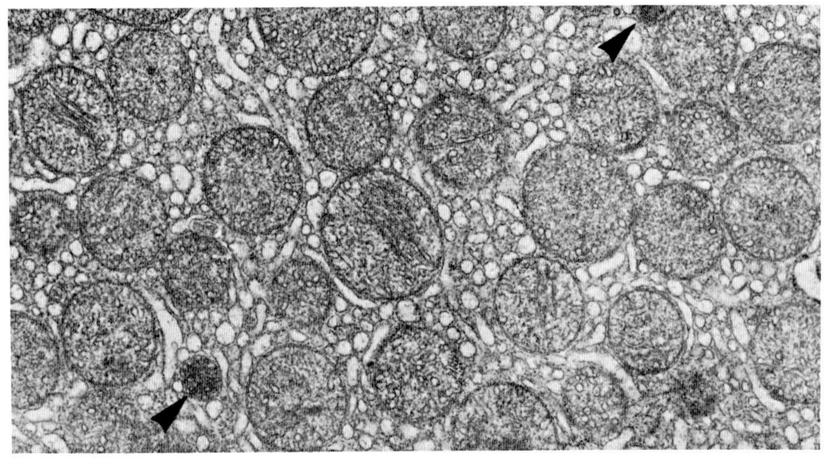

Figure 80
(Figures 80—82 from same patient)
ADRENAL CORTICAL ADENOMA
Mitochondria from adrenal cortical adenomas may show alterations, compared to those seen in normal cells. Several microbodies (arrows) are present in this virilizing tumor; mitochondria are extremely numerous. Diaminobenzidine reaction (DAB) lead nitrate. X17,000. (Courtesy of Dr. K. Gorgas, Federal Republic of Germany. Also from Gorgas, K., Bock, P., and Wuketich, S. Fine structure of a virilizing adrenocortical adenoma. Beitr. Pathol. 159:371-397, 1976.)

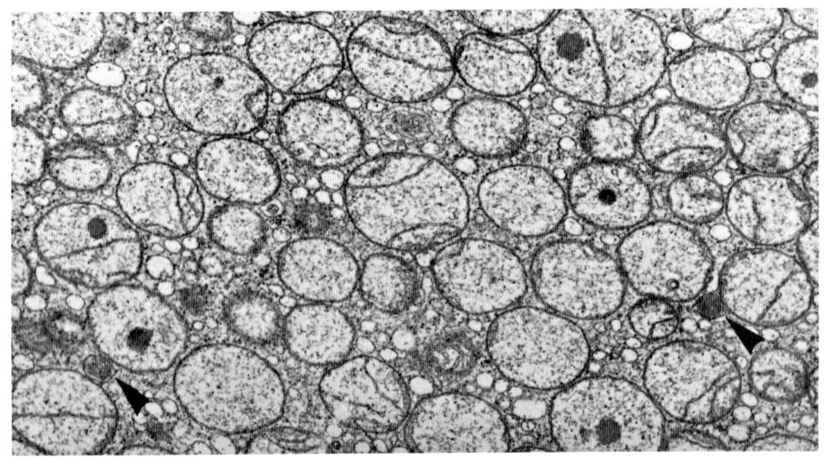

Figure 81
ADRENAL CORTICAL ADENOMA
The internal structure of the mitochondria may become sparse and small, homogenous, intramitochondrial inclusion bodies may develop. DAB-lead citrate. X17,000.

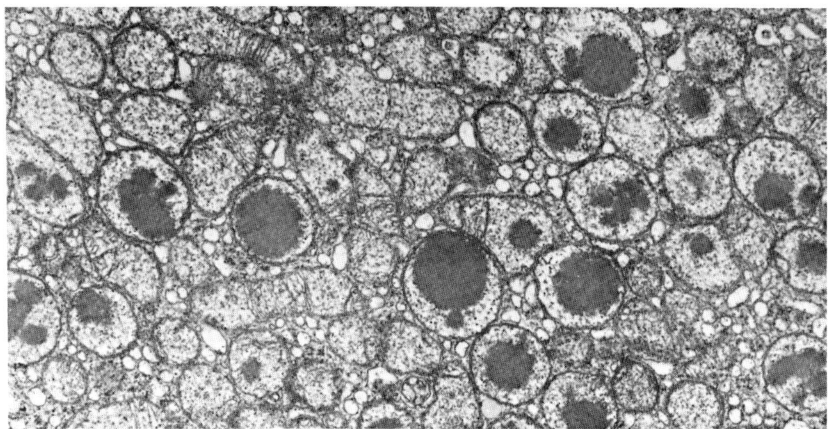

Figure 82
ADRENAL CORTICAL ADENOMA
The extreme loss of internal mitochondrial structure is shown. Many dense inclusions are present. DAB-lead citrate. X17,000.

Cells comprising adrenal cortical adenomas producing Cushing's syndrome show greater ultrastructural deviation from normal than is found in cells from adrenal hyperplasia associated with Cushing's disease (Mackay). These changes include variation in the amount and distribution of various organelles present (Symington; fig. 83) and certain bizarre ultrastructural features such as loss of perivascular and pericellular fibrous connective tissue. Some authors (Tannenbaum) have noted changes in the basement membrane surrounding the neoplastic cells associated with the development of aggressive behavior.

The ultrastructure of tumors producing primary aldosteronism is dominated by the characteristics of the cellular types composing these tumors (Eto et al.). Generally speaking, the cells comprising these aldosterone-producing adenomas contain a more prominent Golgi apparatus than is seen in cells comprising other types of adrenal cortical adenomas. Considerable lipid content is present in vacuoles. The mitochondria are usually elongated, with long tubulovesicular cristae. Less commonly, cells with spherical mitochondria and prominent lipofuscin granulation may also be encountered. Glomerulosa-type cells containing 18-hydroxylase systems are not seen in adrenal nodules (Neville; Reidbord and Fisher).

VARIANTS

Gross and microscopic appearances of adrenal cortical adenomas differ considerably (pl. V). One important variant is the so-called "black adenoma" (Visser et al.; Macadam). These tumors contain abundant lipofuscin pigment (pl. VI) in exaggeration of the phenomenon normally seen in the zona reticularis (fig. 84). These tumors may produce Cushing's syndrome with or without virilism (Kovacs et al.; Zaniewski and Sheeler). Macronodules encountered at autopsy without a clinical syndrome may also be pigmented (pl. II-C) as well as the rare bilateral micronodular adenomatosis seen with variants of Cushing's syndrome (pl. III-A). Rarely, black adenomas have

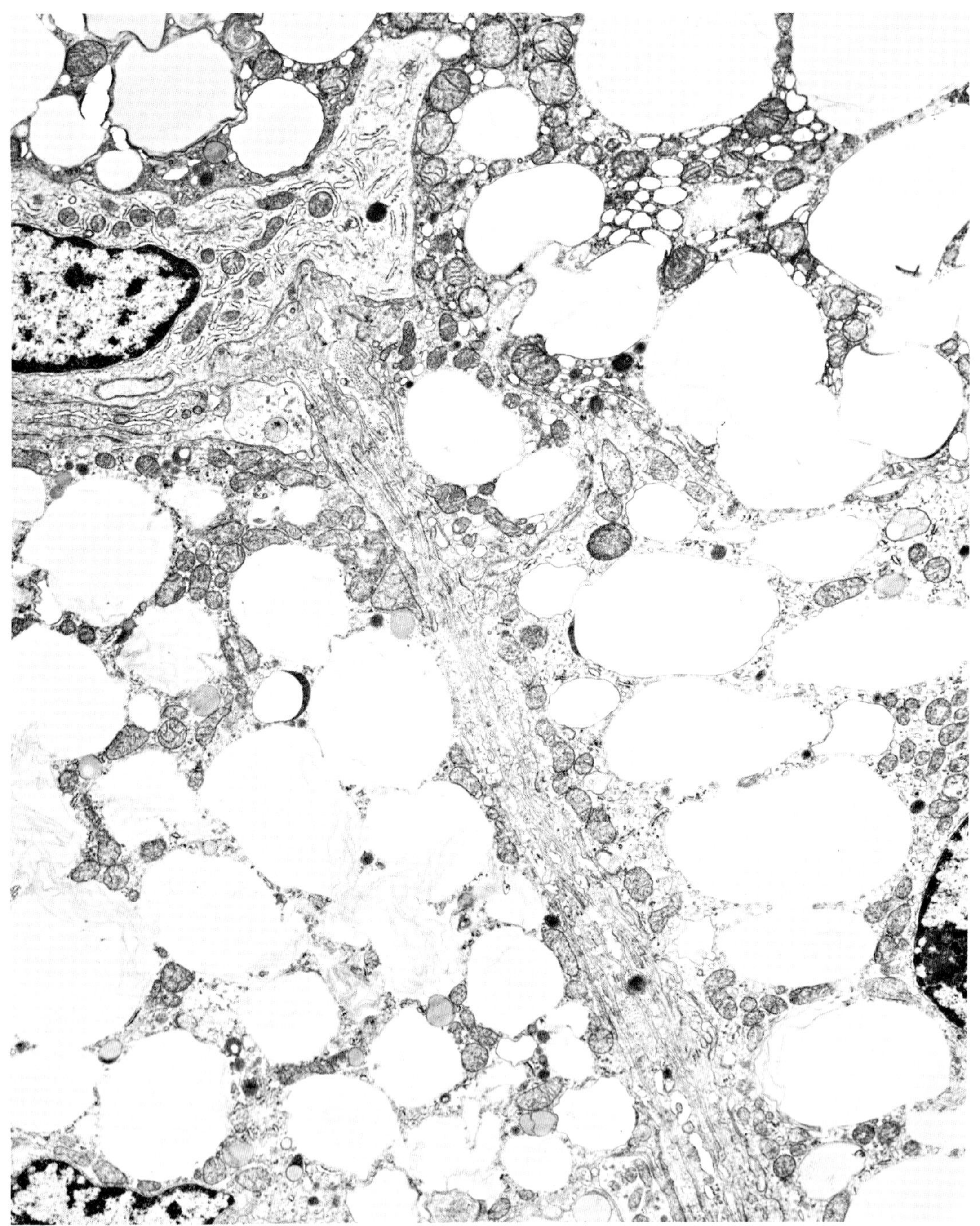

Figure 83
(Figure 83 and plate IV-B, C from same patient)
ADRENAL CORTICAL ADENOMA
Marked variation in organelle content among areas of individual cells and among different cells is characteristic. Lipid filled cells are characteristic of outer zona fasciculata type cells. Uranyl acetate-lead citrate. X10,000.

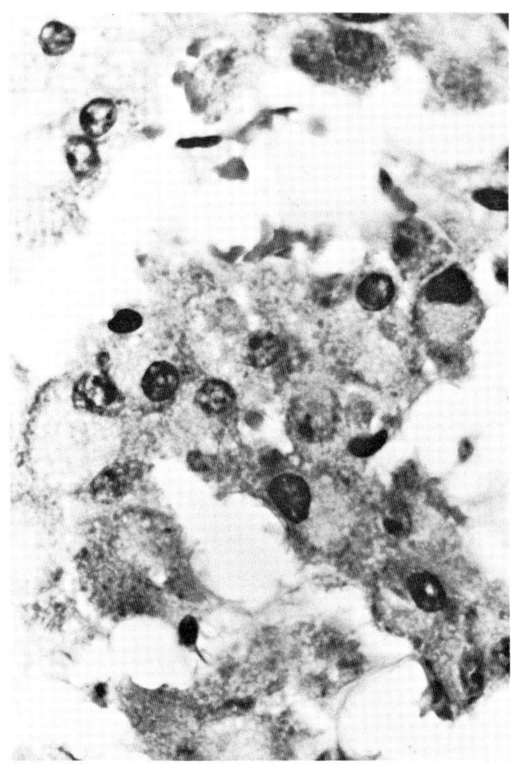

Figure 84
(Figure 84 and plate VI-A, B from same patient)
ADRENAL CORTICAL ADENOMA
Abundant lipofuscin pigment is seen in this "black" adenoma. Pigment tends to be associated with peripheral cytoplasm. This is an exaggeration of the pigment associated with the zona reticularis of the normal adrenal. (Courtesy of Dr. G. Gray, New York, NY.) X400.

been associated with primary hyperaldosteronism (Caplan and Virata; Sienkowsky et al.). Other variants are the previously mentioned virilizing adrenal cortical adenomas resembling ovarian cells, some of which respond to HCG (Werk et al.; fig. 75). Rarely, an adrenal adenoma may occur in an ectopic location (Adashi et al.). This phenomenon is reported most commonly in the liver, the kidney, or gonads, but may occur at any site where ectopic adrenocortical tissue is known to occur (Strauch and Vinnick; Hamwi et al.; Uehling). Rarely, such tumors may occur in the pancreas

causing confusion with islet cell adenoma (figs. 85, 86). Electron microscopy may be necessary for definitive diagnosis in this situation. Equally uncommon is the presentation of a functioning adrenal cortical adenoma in association with an adrenal medullary tumor (Dahms et al.). Although examples of this phenomenon have been reported (Mathison and Waterhouse), most instances are probably cortical hyperplasia with nodules associated with ACTH production due to the adrenal medullary tumor (Spark et al.).

Prognosis and Natural History. The prognosis of an adrenal cortical adenoma in large measure depends upon the type of clinical syndrome produced. Uncomplicated adenomas producing Cushing's syndrome with contralateral adrenal cortical atrophy are characteristically cured by surgical extirpation of the tumor and the involved adrenal gland. Spontaneous remission has been reported (Blau et al.). Care must be taken to avoid contamination of the operative bed with fragments of tumor, since recurrences have been reported with otherwise benign tumors from inadvertent entry into the tumor during removal. Depending upon their severity, the clinical stigmata of Cushing's syndrome disappear relatively rapidly with return to normal body habitus and biochemistry occurring over the course of six months to one year. Of considerably more concern is the relatively common persistence of adrenal insufficiency due to longstanding suppression of the contralateral adrenal gland by the cortisol producing tumor. This state is usually treated by a combination of gluco- and mineralocortocoid replacement and ACTH administration. Relative refractoriness to ACTH is common and recovery periods of one year or greater have been reported.

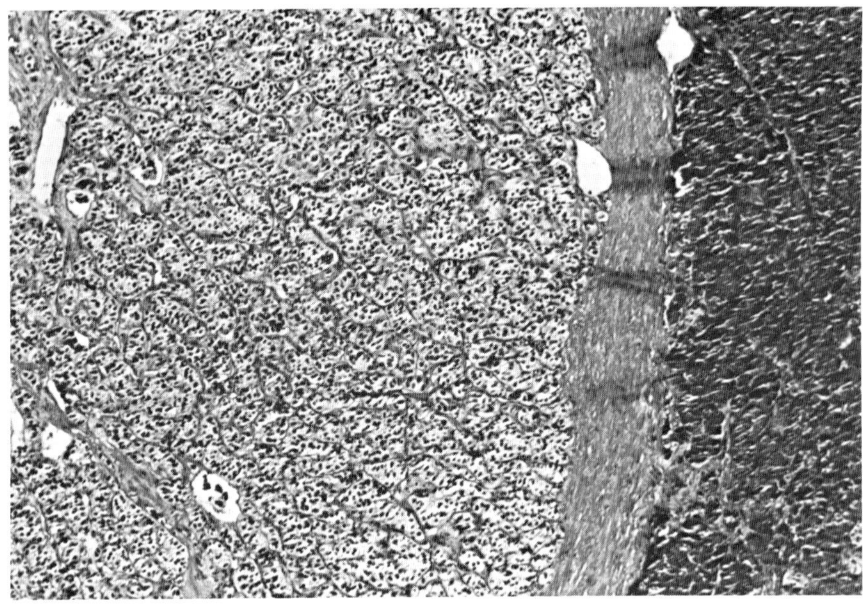

Figure 85
(Figures 85, 86, and plate VI-D from same patient)
ADRENAL CORTICAL ADENOMA
This ectopic adrenal cortical tumor produced Cushing's syndrome. The tumor is entirely
within the pancreas (seen at right) and is composed of alveolar groups of cells. X50.

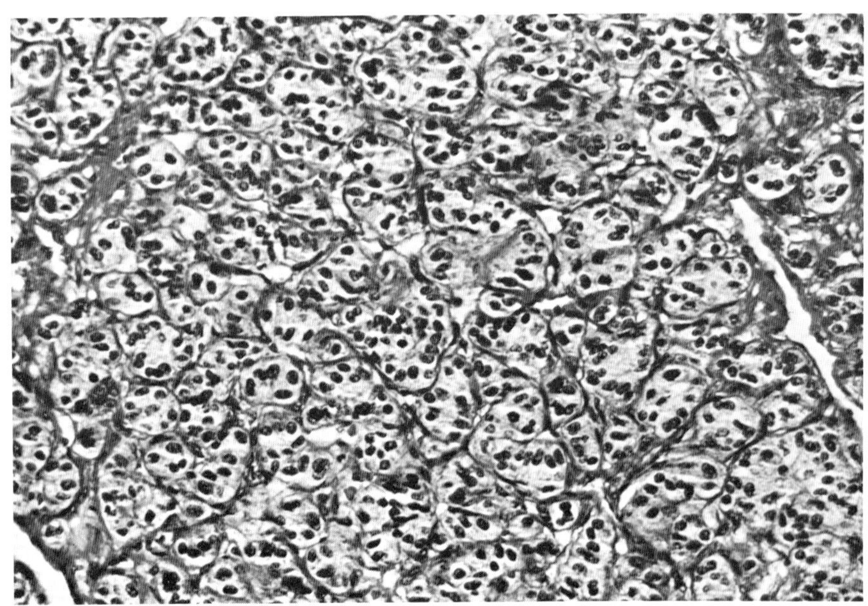

Figure 86
ADRENAL CORTICAL ADENOMA
The tumor cells are uniform, with little evidence of pleomorphism. The patient was alive and
well 12 years later. X300.

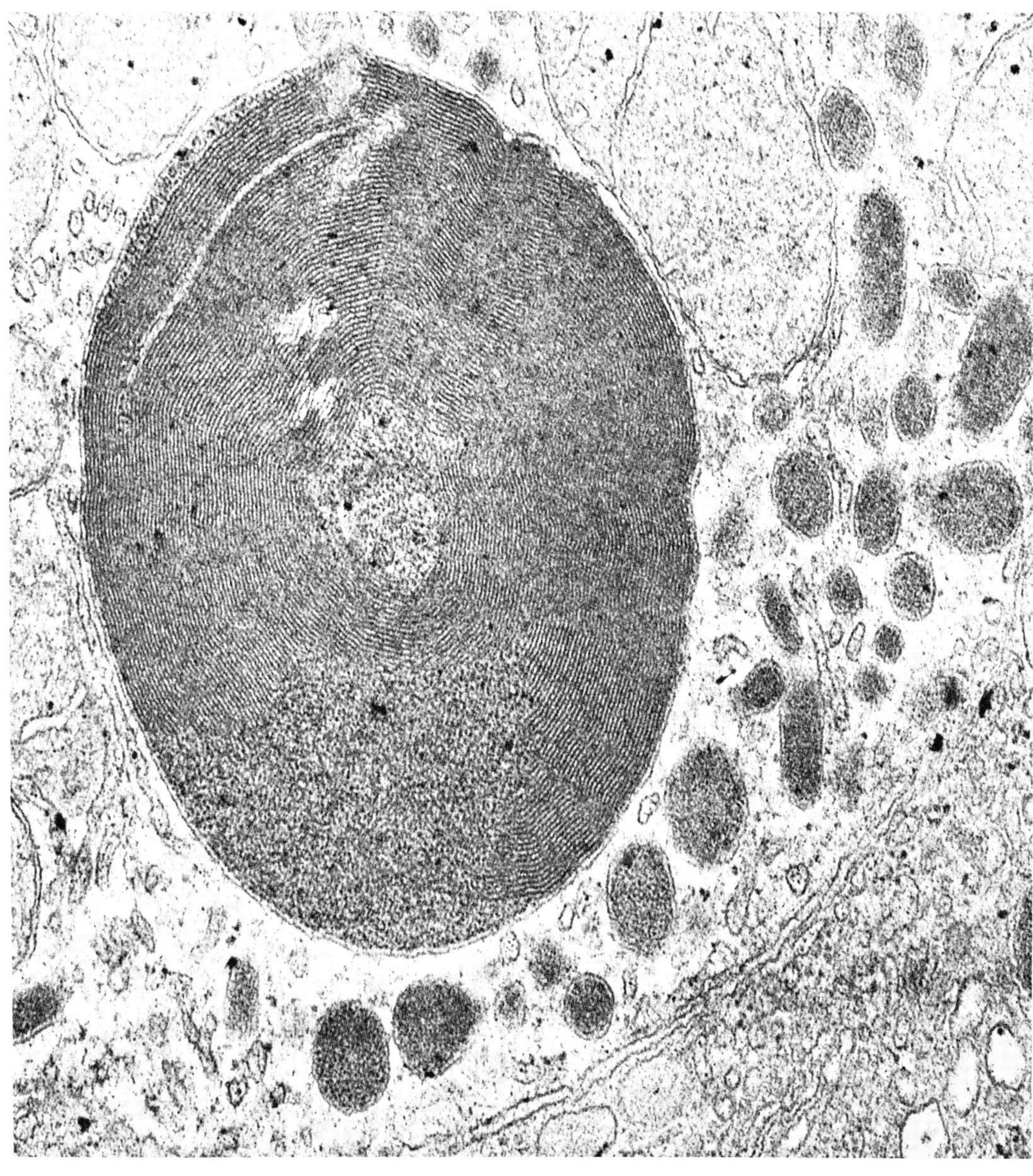

Figure 87
ADRENAL CORTICAL ADENOMA
Typical laminated spironolactone body is seen in adrenal from a 49 year old man with primary aldosteronism. These bodies are usually, but not always, seen after spironolactone therapy. Uranyl acetate-lead citrate. X73,000. (Courtesy of Dr. J. Connolly, Boston, MA.)

Surgical extirpation of a unilateral aldosterone producing tumor and the surrounding adrenal gland is usually followed by a clinical response, characterized by a fall in blood pressure and potassium excretion rate accompanied by the decline in aldosterone secretion. However, patients with bilateral adrenal cortical disease producing aldosteronism, with or without accompanying hyperplasia, are often not cured or substantially improved by surgery, including bilateral adrenalectomy. Consequently, many of these patients are treated medically with antihypertensives and aldosterone antagonists such as spironolactone. In primary aldosteronism, characteristic multilaminated inclusion bodies within the cytoplasm of zona glomerulosa-type cells may be seen in either hyperplastic adrenal cortex (fig. 87)

or within adrenal adenomas (Kovacs et al.; Shrago et al.). There is evidence (Conn et al.) that spironolactone bodies develop only in cells actively synthesizing aldosterone from corticosterone. Thus, finding spironolactone bodies in only one of several nodules supports that one as an autonomously functioning adenoma (Favre et al.). This may be of clinical importance when bilaterally enlarged adrenals are encountered in primary aldosteronism. However, structures resembling spironolactone bodies have been described in other adrenal cortical adenomas (Akhtar et al.) in which the patient had not been treated with spironolactone.

The prognosis and response to therapy of adrenal cortical adenomas producing the adrenogenital syndrome (figs. 88−90) is

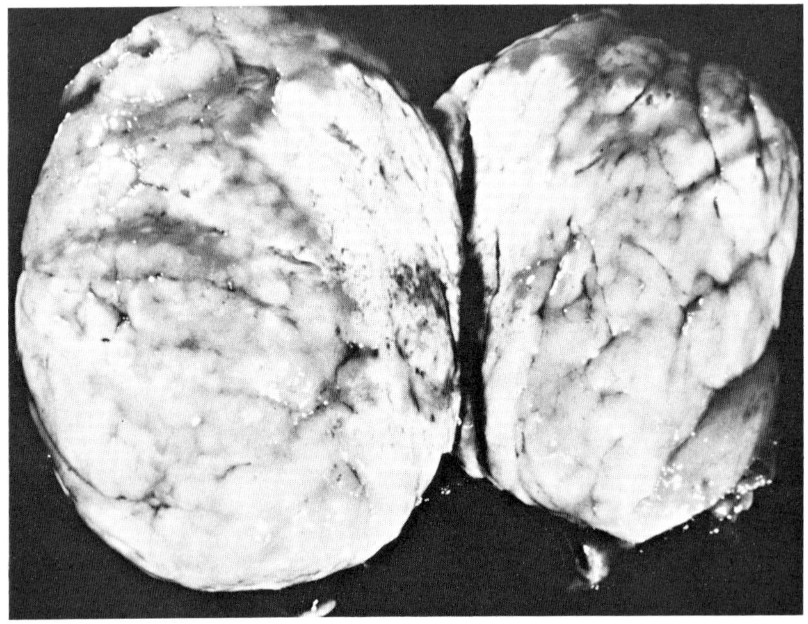

Figure 88
(Figures 88−90 from same patient)
ADRENAL CORTICAL ADENOMA
Section of a 47 g adrenal mass removed from a six and one-half year old girl with isosexual precocity shows bulging nodular appearance. There is no evidence of a residual adrenal. X1.5. (Courtesy of Dr. G.R. Dickersin, Boston, MA. Also from Case Records of the Massachusetts General Hospital. Case 23-1979. Adrenocortical adenoma with isosexual precocity. N. Engl. J. Med. 300:1322-1328, 1979.)

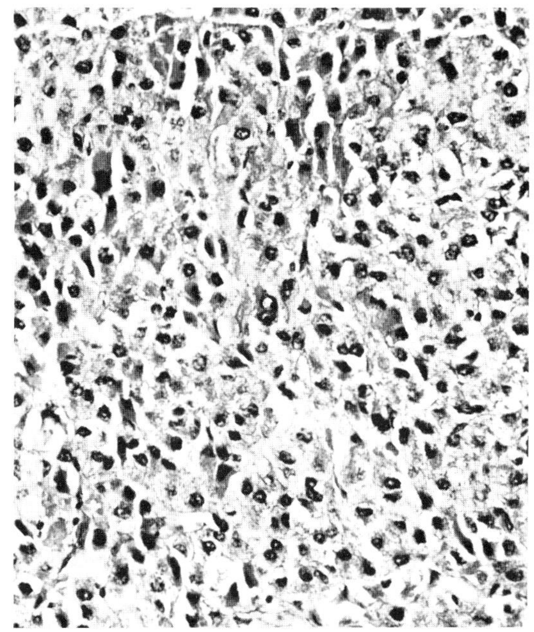

Figure 89
ADRENAL CORTICAL ADENOMA
Microscopic section of the tumor reveals pleomorphism
and hyperchromatism of adrenal tumor cells. In spite of the
ominous appearance, the patient was well five years later.
X256.

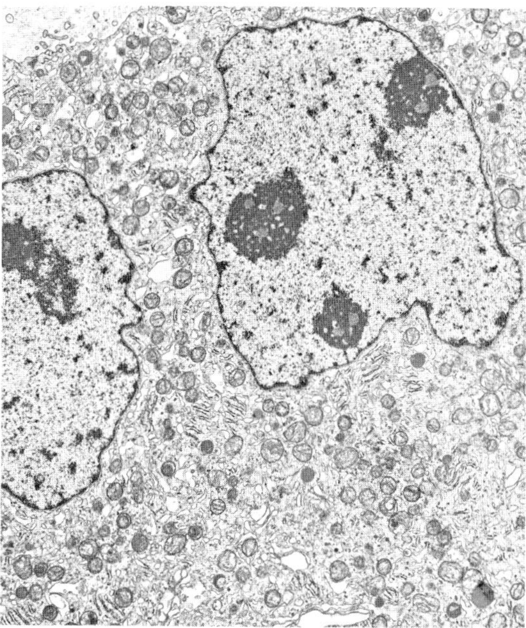

Figure 90
ADRENAL CORTICAL ADENOMA
Ultrastructure of this feminizing tumor reveals numerous
mitochondria and parallel arrays of rough endoplasmic
reticulum. This histologic and electron microscopic appearance of feminizing tumors does not differ from masculiniz-
ing ones. Uranyl acetate-lead citrate. X4080.

more variable than those producing either
Cushing's syndrome or primary aldosteronism. This discrepancy arises from the fact
that many of these tumors behave in an
aggressive fashion with local recurrence
and subsequent metastasis, even though
clinically and histologically benign. Careful
systematic appraisal of clinical and histologic characteristics may be necessary to
accurately predict the outcome in these
cases (see Adrenal Cortical Carcinoma).
Surgical intervention, with complete extirpation of the tumor and surrounding adrenal gland with the involved capsule, offers
the best means of curing these patients. In
the case of benign tumors, such therapy is
almost always curative. Rarely, benign
tumors producing the adrenogenital (or,
more rarely, Cushing's syndrome) may be

so large as to involve vital vascular structures making total removal impossible. In
these circumstances, the adrenolytic agent,
o'p'-DDD, may produce beneficial response.

DIFFERENTIAL DIAGNOSIS

The differential diagnosis of adrenal
cortical adenomas is a complicated one
encompassing on one hand, adrenal cortical
and metastatic carcinomas and, on the
other, pseudotumorous hyperplastic states
and incidental adrenocortical nodules. The
separation of adrenal cortical adenomas
from carcinomas, medullary neoplasms,
and other disease states is best performed
by using a variety of criteria, rather than
relying on a small number of purely
histologic ones.

Adrenal Nodule

These nodular collections of adrenal cortical cells may approach the size seen with adenomas producing a clinical syndrome (Neville). However, several gross and microscopic distinctions are present. The nodules may be multiple, are usually pale yellow, and tend to be irregular in outline on slab section (pl. III), often occupying the entire central portion of the gland. This is in contrast to the spherical, localized appearance of adenomas. Examination of the surrounding gland discloses no atrophy or hyperplasia, and compression of the gland by the nodule is unusual. Pleomorphism, especially of the hyperchromatic nuclear type, is very unusual in nodules. On light and electron microscopic examination, zona glomerulosa-type cells are absent from the nodules, a distinguishing point from adenomas causing primary hyperaldosteronism (Reidbord and Fisher; Mackay). Nodules may form cortisol in vitro, but not aldosterone. In contrast, aldosterone may be found in adenomas causing hyperaldosteronism (Vecsei et al.).

Adrenal Cortical Carcinoma

The distinction of a small well differentiated adrenal cortical carcinoma from an adenoma may be difficult. This subject is discussed in detail in the section on Adrenal Cortical Carcinoma.

Multinodular Hyperplasia

This condition differs from an adrenal adenoma in that multiple nodules are present; moreover, the intervening cortex is hyperplastic, not atrophic, and the condition is virtually always bilateral. This is in contrast to the unilateral occurrence of adenomas. Multinodular hyperplasia is distinguished from incidental adrenal nodules by the presence of a clinical syndrome (usually hypercortisolism) and by the hyperplastic character of the intervening cortex.

Pheochromocytoma

Some adrenal medullary tumors may superficially resemble an adrenal cortical adenoma. However, the characteristic gray brown gross appearance, with frequent occurrence of blood filled sinusoids, positive chromaffin reaction, and microscopic pattern of large or small alveolar (nesting) growth are usually sufficient to distinguish these tumors. Confirmatory tissue analysis for catecholamine content or histochemical studies are discussed in the section on Adrenal Medullary Tumors. Additional characteristics include the formalin-induced fluorescence (Falck) and specific granules on ultrastructural examination. At times, ACTH production by adrenal medullary tumors may induce adrenal cortical hyperplasia with clinical or biochemical evidence of hypercortisolism (Spark et al.).

Multiple Endocrine Neoplasia

Nodular adrenal glands have been reported in multiple endocrine, neoplasia, type I. In fact, the review of Ballard and associates on the multiple endocrine neoplasia syndrome type I (involvement of pituitary, pancreas, and parathyroid) reports abnormalities in the adrenals in 38 percent of 85 cases reported in the literature and in 4 of 16 affected members of the reported pedigree. However, none of these are solitary adenomas; most are noted at autopsy as adrenals with nodules and some are reported to be enlarged at surgical exploration. As noted in the review, "The frequent incidental finding of adrenal cortical adenomas in autopsy material raises the question of their particular significance in polyglandular adenomatosis." No patients had adrenocortical hyperfunction, but at autopsy one patient had pituitary basophil hyperplasia and adrenals weighing 18 g, with an appearance of diffuse hyperplasia and mild nodularity — probably representing Cushing's disease. There is a patient (Steiner et al.) reported with Cushing's disease and medullary carcinoma in the multiple endocrine neoplasia II syndrome (medullary carcinoma of the thyroid gland, pheochromocytoma, and parathyroid hyperplasia). Several of the reported patients with multiple endocrine neoplasia, type II, have had hypercortisolism, probably due to ACTH

production by the adrenal medullary neoplasm.

It is apparent that adrenal cortical adenomas and carcinomas as defined by autonomous function have not been described in the multiple endocrine neoplasia syndromes. Pituitary dependent Cushing's disease and hypercortisolism due to ectopic ACTH production by neoplasm are described, but are uncommon.

Metastatic Carcinoma

The cytologic characteristics of most carcinomas metastatic to the adrenal gland are sufficiently bizarre to suggest a malignancy of extracortical origin (see Metastatic Carcinoma). One notable exception is renal cell carcinoma (figs. 91–93), which may resemble an adrenal adenoma or nodular

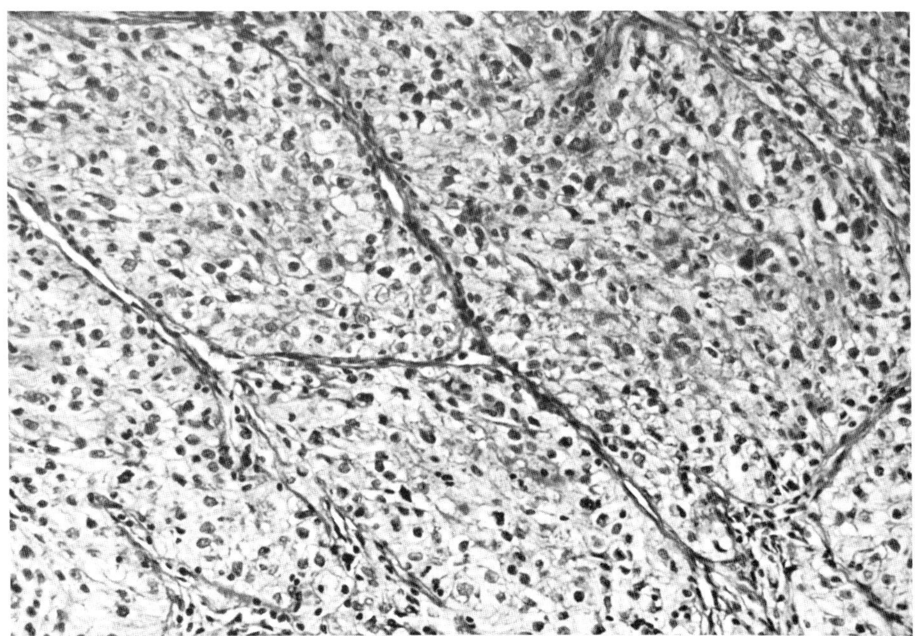

Figure 91
(Figure 91 and plate X-A from same patient)
RENAL CELL CARCINOMA
Microscopic appearance of renal cell carcinoma reveals a coarse nodularity with alveolar groups larger than in adrenal cortical adenoma. Renal cell carcinomas often have minimal pleomorphism compounding the differential diagnosis. X260. (Courtesy of Dr. G. Gray, New York, NY.)

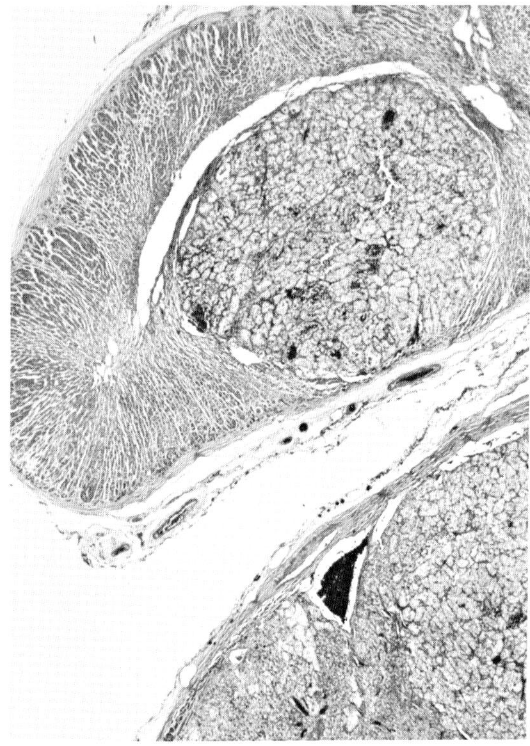

Figure 92
(Figures 92 and 93 from same patient)
RENAL CELL CARCINOMA
Nodular appearance of metastatic renal cell carcinoma is apparent in this low power view. (Courtesy of Royal Marsden Hospital, London, England.). X13.

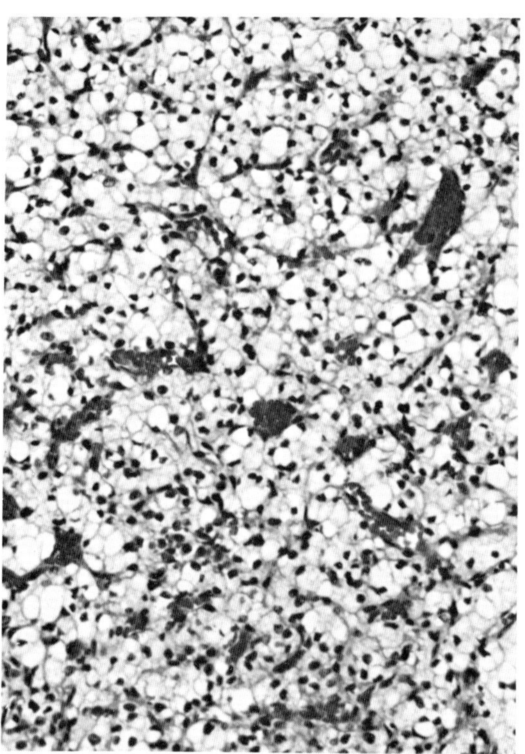

Figure 93
RENAL CELL CARCINOMA
Higher power view of figure 92 shows closer resemblance to adrenal cortical adenoma. X210.

hyperplasia superficially. However, the tendency toward a coarse alveolar growth pattern, the absence of an admixture of adrenal cortical cell types, and the sharp demarcation from the surrounding cortex are usually diagnostic (see p. 157). Other examples of secondary adrenal tumors are discussed in the section on Metastatic Carcinoma.

References

Adashi, E. Y., Rosenwaks, A., Lee, P. A., Jones, G. S., and Migeon, C. J. Endocrine features of an adrenal-like tumor of the ovary. J. Clin. Endocrinol. Metab. 48:241-245, 1979.

Akhtar, M., Gasalbez, T., and Young, I. Ultrastructural study of androgen-producing adrenocortical adenoma. Cancer 34:322-327, 1974.

Ballard, H. S., Frame, B., and Hartsock, R. J. Familial multiple endocrine adenomapeptic ulcer complex. Medicine 43:481-516, 1964.

Bhettay, E. and Bonnici, F. Pure oestrogen-secreting feminizing adrenocortical adenoma. Arch. Dis. Child. 52:241-243, 1977.

Blau, N., Miller, W. E., Miller, E. R., Jr., and Cervi-Skinner, S. J. Spontaneous remission of Cushing's syndrome in a patient with an adrenal adenoma. J. Clin. Endocrinol. Metab. 40:659-663, 1975.

Burr, I. M., Graham, T., Sullivan, J., Hartmann, W. H., and O'Neill, J. A testosterone-secreting tumour of the adrenal producing virilisation in a female infant. Lancet 2:643-644, 1973.

Caplan, R. H. and Virata, R. L. Functional black adenoma of the adrenal cortex. Am. J. Clin. Pathol. 62:97-103, 1974.

Case Records of the Massachusetts General Hospital. Case 23-1979. Adrenocortical adenoma with isosexual precocity. N. Engl. J. Med. 300:1322-1328, 1979.

Conn, J. W. and Hinerman, D. L. Spironolactone-induced inhibition of aldosterone biosynthesis in primary aldosteronism: morphological and functional studies. Metabolism 26:1293-1307, 1977.

Costin, G., Goebelsmann, U., and Kogut, M. D. Sexual precocity due to a testosterone-producing adrenal tumor. J. Clin. Endocrinol. Metab. 45:912-919, 1977.

Dahms, W. T., Gray, G., Vrana, M., and New, M. I. Adrenocortical adenoma and ganglioneuroblastoma in a child. Am. J. Dis. Child. 125:608-611, 1973.

Eto, T., Kumamoto, K., Kawasaki, T., Omae, T., Masaki, Z., and Yamamoto, T. Ultrastructural types of cell in adrenal cortical adenoma with primary aldosteronism. J. Pathol. 128:1-6, 1979.

Falck, B. and Owman, C. A detailed methodological description of the fluorescence method for the cellular demonstration of biogenic monoamines. Acta Univ. Lund. Section 2, No. 7:1-23, 1965.

Favre, L. Jacot-des-Combes', E., Morel, P., Hauser, H., Riondel, A-M., et al. Primary aldosteronism with bilateral adrenal adenomas. Virchows Arch. [Pathol. Anat.] 388:229-236, 1980.

Fidler, W. J. Ovarian thecal metaplasia in adrenal glands. Am. J. Clin. Pathol. 67:318-323, 1977.

Fraumeni, J. F. and Miller, R. W. Adrenocortical neoplasms with hemihypertrophy, brain tumors, and other disorders. J. Pediatr. 70:129-138, 1967.

Garret, R. and Ames, R. P. Black-pigmented adenoma of the adrenal gland. Arch. Pathol. 95:349-353, 1973.

Gorgas, K., Böck, P., and Wuketich, S. Fine structure of a virilizing adrenocortical adenoma. Beitr. Pathol. 159:371-397, 1976.

Hamwi, G. J., Gwinup, G., Mostow, J. H., and Besch, P. K. Activation of testicular adrenal rest tissue by prolonged excessive ACTH production. J. Clin. Endocrinol. Metab. 23:861-869, 1963.

Hough, A. J., Hollifield, J. W., Page, D. L., and Hartmann, W. H. Prognostic factors in adrenal cortical tumors. Am. J. Clin. Pathol. 72:390-399, 1979.

Howard, C. P., Takahashi, H., and Hayles, A. B. Feminizing adrenal adenoma in a boy. Mayo Clin. Proc. 52:254-357, 1977.

Hutter, A. M., Jr., and Kayhoe, D. E. Adrenal cortical carcinoma. Am. J. Med. 41:572-580, 1966.

Josse, R. G., Bear, R., Kovacs, K., and Higgins, H. P. Cushing's syndrome due to unilateral nodular adrenal hyperplasia: a new pathophysiological entity? Acta Endocrinol. 93:495-504, 1980.

Kable, W. T. and Yussman, M. A. Testosterone-secreting adrenal adenoma. Fertil. Steril. 32:610-611, 1979.

Kovacs, K., Horvath, E., and Feldman, P. S. Pigmented adenoma of adrenal cortex associated with Cushing's syndrome. Urology 7:641-645, 1976.

Lecky, J. W., Wolfman, N. T., and Modic, C. W. Current concepts of adrenal angiography. Radiol. Clin. North Am. 14:309-352, 1976.

Liddle, G. W. Cushing's syndrome. Ann. N.Y. Acad. Sci. 297:594-602, 1977.

Macadam, R. F. Black adenoma of the human adrenal cortex. Cancer 27:116-119, 1971.

Mackay, A. Atlas of Human Adrenal Cortex Ultrastructure. In: Functional Pathology of the Human Adrenal Gland. Symington, T. (Ed.). Baltimore: The Williams & Wilkins Company, 1969.

Mathison, D. A. and Waterhouse, C. A. Cushing's syndrome with hypertensive crisis and mixed adrenal cortical adenoma-pheochromocytoma (corticomedullary adenoma). Am. J. Med. 47:635-641, 1969.

Neville, A. M. The nodular adrenal. Invest. Cell Pathol. 1:99-111, 1978.

——— and Mackay, A. M. The Structure of the Human Adrenal Cortex in Health and Disease, pp. 361-395. In: Clinics in Endocrinology and Metabolism., Vol. 1, No. 2. London, Philadelphia, Toronto: W. B. Saunders Company, 1972.

——— and O'Hare, M. J. Aspects of Structure, Function, and Pathology, pp. 1-65. In: The Adrenal Gland. James, V. H. T. (Ed.). New York: Raven Press, 1979.

——— and Symington, T. The pathology of the adrenal gland in Cushing's syndrome. J. Pathol. 93:19-35, 1967.

Orth, D. N. and Liddle, G. W. Results of treatment in 108 patients with Cushing's syndrome. N. Engl. J. Med. 285:243-247, 1971.

Reidbord, H. and Fisher, E. R. Aldosteronoma and nonfunctioning adrenal cortical adenoma. Arch. Pathol. 88:155-161, 1969.

Sasano, N., Ojima, M., and Masuda, T. Endocrinologic pathology of functioning adrenocortical tumors. Pathol. Annu. 15:105-142, 1980.

Sebold, J. E., Cohen, E. L., Beierwaltes, W. H. et al. Adrenal Imaging with [131]I-19-iodocholesterol in the diagnostic evaluation of patients with aldosteronism. J. Clin. Endocrinol. Metab. 42:41-51, 1976.

Shrago, S. S., Waisman, J., and Cooper, P. H. Spironolactone bodies in an adrenal adenoma. Arch. Pathol. 99:416-420, 1975.

Sienkowski, I., Watkins, R. M., and Anderson, V. Primary tumorous aldosteronism due to a black adrenal adenoma: a light and electron microscopic study. J. Clin. Pathol. 37:143-149, 1984.

Spark, R. F., Connolly, P. B., Gluckin, D. S., et al. ACTH secretion from a functioning pheochromocytoma. N. Engl. J. Med. 301:416-418, 1979.

Steiner, A. L., Goodman, A. D., and Powers, S. R. Study of a kindred with pheochromocytoma, medullary thyroid carcinoma, hyperparathyroidism, and Cushing's disease: multiple endocrine neoplasia, type 2. Medicine 47:371-409, 1968.

Strauch, G. O. and Vinnick, L. Persistent Cushing's syndrome apparently cured by ectopic adrenalectomy. J.A.M.A. 221:183-184, 1972.

Symington, T. Functional Pathology of the Human Adrenal Gland. Baltimore: The Williams & Wilkins Company, 1969.

Tannenbaum, M. Ultrastructural pathology of the adrenal cortex. Pathol. Ann. 8:109-156, 1973.

Uehling, D. T. Adrenal rest tumors of the testis: a case report of fertility following treatment. Fertil. Steril. 29:583-584, 1978.

Vecsei, P., Purjesz, I., and Wolff, H. P. Studies on the biosynthesis of aldosterone in solitary adenoma and in nodular hyperplasia of the adrenal cortex in patients exhibiting Conn's syndrome. Acta Endocrinol. 62:391-398, 1969.

Visser, H. K. A. The adrenal cortex in childhood. Arch. Dis. Child. 41:113-136, 1966.

————, Boeijinga, J. K., and Meer, C. V. D. A functioning black adenoma of the adrenal cortex: a clinico-pathological entity. J. Clin. Pathol. 27:955-959, 1974.

Werk, E. E., Jr., Sholiton, L. J., and Kalejs, L. Testosterone-secreting adrenal adenoma under gonadotropin control. N. Engl. J. Med. 289:767-770, 1973.

Williams, E. D., Siebenmann, R. E., and Sobin, L. H. Histological typing of endocrine tumours. International Histological Classification of Tumours, No. 23. Geneva: World Health Organization, 1980.

Zaniewski, M. and Sheeler, L. R. Cushing's syndrome associated with functional black adenoma of the adrenal cortex. South. Med. J. 73:1410-1412, 1980.

ADRENAL CORTICAL CARCINOMA

SYNONYMS AND RELATED TERMS: Adrenal adenocarcinoma; adrenocortical carcinoma; adrenal carcinoma; primary adrenal carcinoma.

Definition. A malignant tumor of adrenal cortical cells demonstrating various degrees of histologic and biochemical differentiation.

Incidence. Primary malignant tumors of the adrenal cortex are rare neoplasms. They comprise from less than 0.05 percent (Ibanez; Macfarlane) to approximately 0.2 percent (Hutter and Kayhoe) of all malignancies, with an incidence of about two per million in the general population (DHEW). Adrenal cortical carcinomas occur worldwide. Although almost all published series would indicate a two to one predilection for females, tumor registry reports from a variety of sources (Hutter and Kayhoe) show an equal or greater frequency in males. This apparent contradiction may be due to the fact that many of the endocrinologic manifestations are more apparent in females. Comparatively few large series of "nonfunctioning" or endocrinologically silent adrenal cortical tumors have been reported (Lewinsky et al.; Shons and Gamble; Ibanez). In this group of "nonfunctioning" tumors, males outnumber females considerably.

There is no consistent predilection for either right or left adrenal, although bilaterality and ectopic origin are uncommon. There is, however, a bimodal distribution with respect to age (fig. 94), the two periods of peak incidence occurring in childhood and in late middle life (Lewinsky et al.). The great majority of childhood cases occur before the age of five years (Benaily et al.). Congenital adrenal hyperplasia, which may be mistaken for primary adrenocortical carcinoma due to the large size of the adrenals, apparently plays no role in the development of juvenile adrenocortical carcinoma (Visser; see p. 72). However, juvenile adrenal cortical carcinomas have been described sporadically (Artigas et al.) and in association with congenital hemihypertrophy (Miller). Adrenocortical carcinoma is a part of a complex hereditary cancer syndrome with sarcomas, breast cancer, and lung cancer (Lynch et al.).

Clinical Diagnosis. Adrenal cortical carcinomas may attain a large size prior to initial presentation. This is especially true in the group of tumors (20 to 40 percent of the total) which produce no apparent endocrine syndrome (Lewinsky et al.). Thus, a palpable abdominal mass, or pain referrable to it, are common presenting complaints (Hutter and Kayhoe; Didolkar et al.). Some adrenal cortical carcinomas produce a systemic febrile reaction, connoting a poor prognosis (Cassan et al.).

The majority of adrenal cortical carcinomas, however, present with one of several endocrine abnormalities due to uncontrolled secretion of various hydroxycorticosteroids or their precursor substances. This phenomenon usually leads to a clinical picture of Cushing's syndrome, with elevated corticosteroid levels unsuppressible by high dose dexamethasone (Liddle). Plasma ACTH is usually undetectable. In contrast to the relatively "pure" Cushing's syndrome produced by adrenal cortical adenomas, that resulting from an adrenal cortical carcinoma is often mixed with clinical virilism and may be associated with a picture of mineralocorticoid excess as well (Symington). The greater production of androgens

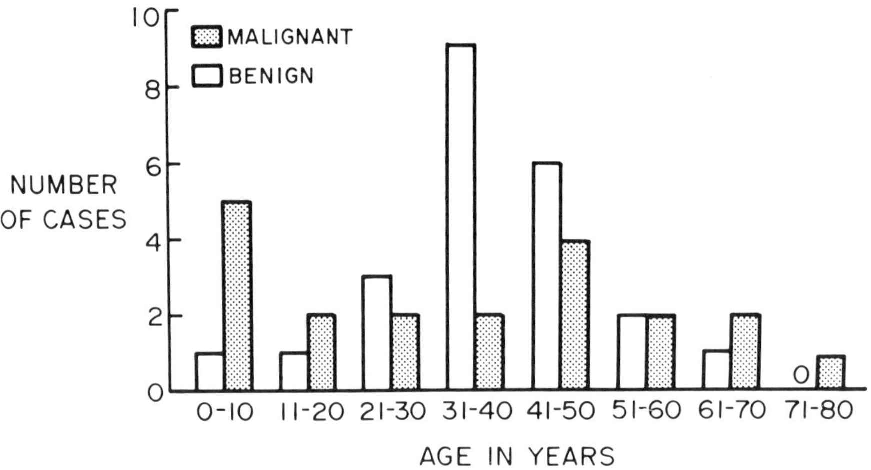

Figure 94
ADRENAL CORTICAL CARCINOMA
Histogram demonstrates age incidence of adrenal neoplasms. Increased incidence of carcinoma
is present in childhood. (From Hough, A.J., Hollifield, J.W., Page, D.L., and Hartmann, W.H.
Prognostic factors in adrenal cortical tumors. Am. J. Clin. Pathol. 72:390-399, 1979.)

in adrenal cortical carcinoma is often associated with markedly elevated urinary 17-ketosteroid levels, a finding less common in adrenal adenomas (Schteingart et al.). Some adrenal cortical carcinomas are relatively deficient in 11-β-hydroxylase (O'Hare et al.) and consequently produce large amounts of 11-deoxycorticosteroids and their metabolites, many of which are potent virilizing agents (Neville and O'Hare).

Feminization, in contrast to virilism, is an extremely uncommon presenting symptom (Symington). However, the few feminizing tumors reported were usually malignant in outcome. The clinical features of primary hyperaldosteronism (hyporeninemic hyperaldosteronism), although common with adrenal tumors, is rarely associated with adrenal cortical malignancy (Alterman et al.). When hyperaldosteronism is present with adrenal carcinoma, other steroids are usually increased as well (Telner; Arteaga et al.). Adrenal carcinomas may demonstrate excessive mineralocorticoid activity

with production of deoxycorticosterone (Kelly et al.; Powell-Jackson et al.).

In contrast to many adrenal adenomas, most adrenal carcinomas are poorly responsive to ACTH in vivo, as manifested by failure to increase steroidogenesis in response to ACTH administration (Symington; Harrison et al.). Due to the anabolic actions of various corticoid hormones (particularly androgens), weight loss with adrenal carcinoma is not a common presenting complaint. However, it is extremely ominous when present (Hutter and Kayhoe; Hajjar et al.).

Even small (c. 100 g) adrenal carcinomas may be localized by selective arteriography and ultrasound technics (fig. 95). Larger tumors are usually apparent on intravenous pyelograms (fig. 96) or on plain films of the abdomen (fig. 97).

Because most adrenal cortical carcinomas produce endocrine manifestations (predominantly mixed Cushing's-virilism

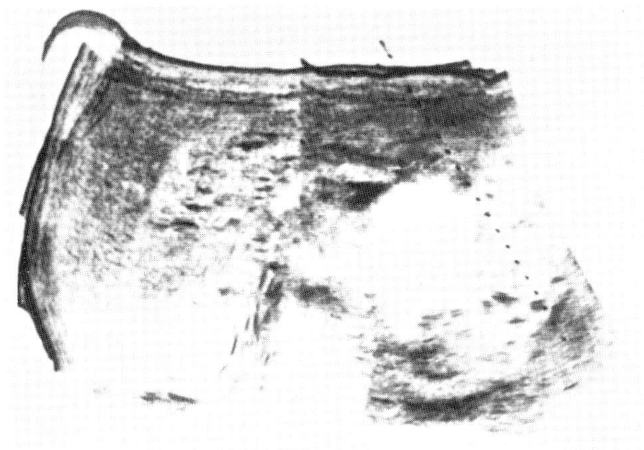

Figure 95
(Figures 95 and 96 from same patient)
ADRENAL CORTICAL CARCINOMA
An ultrasound study demonstrates a large adrenal carcinoma seen to the
left of dotted line as a solid mass. A portion of the kidney with cysts is seen
to the right of the adrenal mass. (See plate VIII-A, B.)

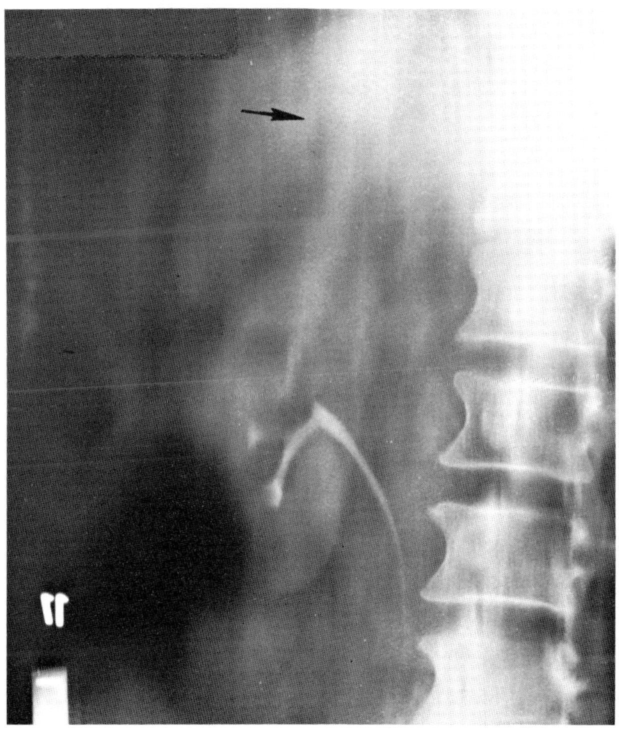

Figure 96
ADRENAL CORTICAL CARCINOMA
An intravenous pyelogram shows a large suprarenal mass (arrow)
greater in size than the kidney.

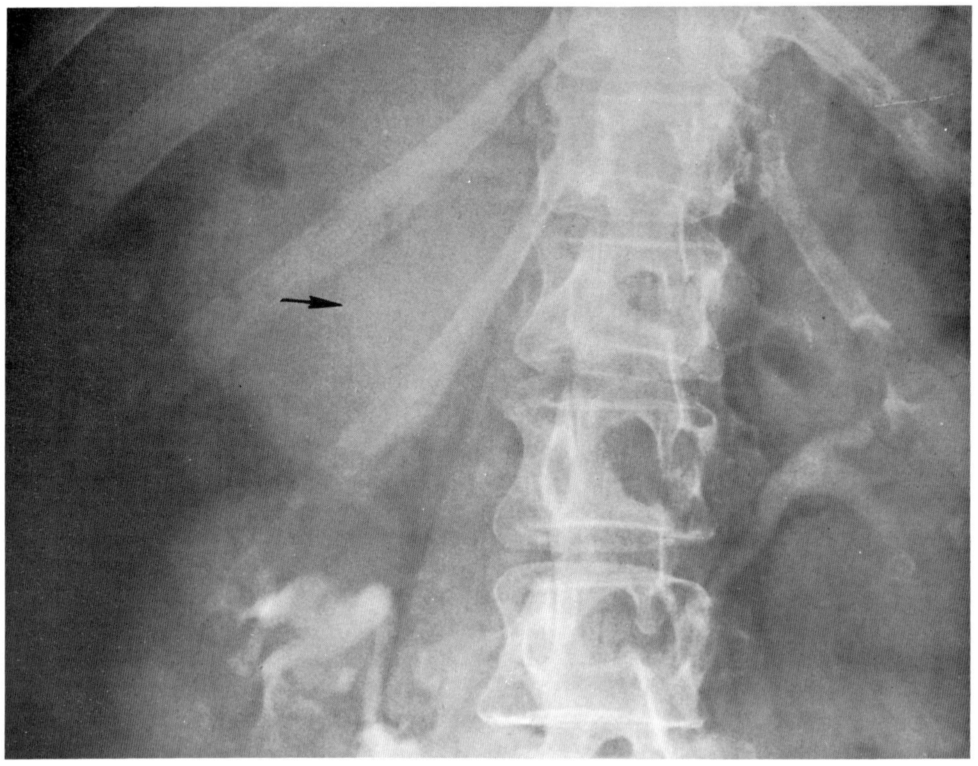

Figure 97
(Figures 97 and 98 from same patient)
ADRENAL CORTICAL CARCINOMA
Plain film of abdomen demonstrates a large suprarenal mass (arrow) above the kidney. (Courtesy of Dr. G.A.K. Missen, London, England.)

syndrome), attain considerable size (greater than 100 g), and demonstrate no responsiveness to ACTH, the differentiation from Cushing's syndrome due to adrenal adenoma is often apparent on clinical and biochemical grounds. However, a clear determination of malignancy may be difficult and careful application of biochemical and pathologic data will be necessary. Adrenal adenomas, especially those associated with virilism (Neville and O'Hare, Akhtar et al.) may be large, and there is considerable overlap between benign and malignant variants with respect to weight. Thus, histologic confirmation of malignancy is necessary.

Gross. Adrenal cortical carcinomas vary in size from less than 100 to greater than 5000 g. Malignant adrenal cortical lesions weighing less than 100 g are rare. Most are encapsulated, soft fleshy masses with an overall pink, gray, brown, or yellow coloration (pls. VII and VIII). Areas of hemorrhage and necrosis (fig. 98) and/or coarse trabeculation (fig. 99) are often present and are presumptive signs of malignancy. Some very large tumors are cystic and may be easily ruptured at time of operative manipulation. Invasion and fixation to adjacent structures are common (figs. 99, 100).

Although origin or growth beneath the renal capsule is uncommon (pl. VII-A),

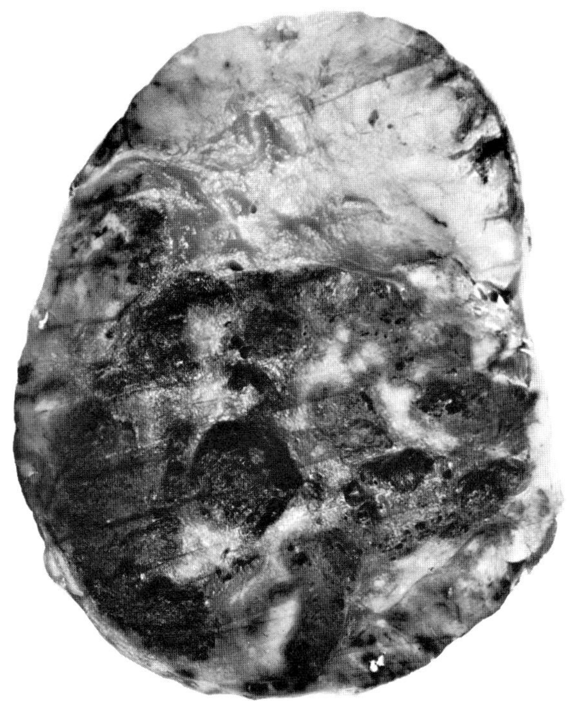

Figure 98
ADRENAL CORTICAL CARCINOMA
Note dull, dark areas of necrosis in this adrenal cortical carcinoma from a 64 year old
woman with hypertension ameliorated by removal of tumor. Actual size. (Courtesy of Dr.
G.A.K. Missen, D.M., London, England).

adrenal cortical tumors with this gross appearance may mimic renal cell carcinoma. Gross evidence of vascular invasion is present in a minority of cases (Symington), a point of distinction from renal cell carcinoma. Careful dissection is usually required to identify the remnant of the adrenal, if one is present at all.

Microscopic. Adrenal cortical carcinomas vary greatly in histologic appearance. Such variation occurs not only among different tumors producing similar syndromes, but also among different areas of the same tumor. Tumors may reproduce the alveolar or trabecular pattern of the normal adrenal (fig. 101) or show sheetlike or diffuse growth instead (fig. 102). A fine fibrovascular stroma separates the alveolar groups in many tumors. Cells may be lipid rich or poor, and malignant tumors usually contain admixtures of cortical cells of various descriptions. Abrupt transition from well to poorly differentiated areas is common (fig. 103). Although many benign adrenal cortical tumors contain cells with enlarged swollen nuclei (Schteingart et al.; Symington) and distorted cytoplasm (fig. 66), the presence of nuclear hyperchromatism (fig. 104), or vesicular nuclei with prominent nuclear membranes and enlarged nucleoli (fig. 105) constitutes presumptive evidence of malignancy (Tang and Gray;

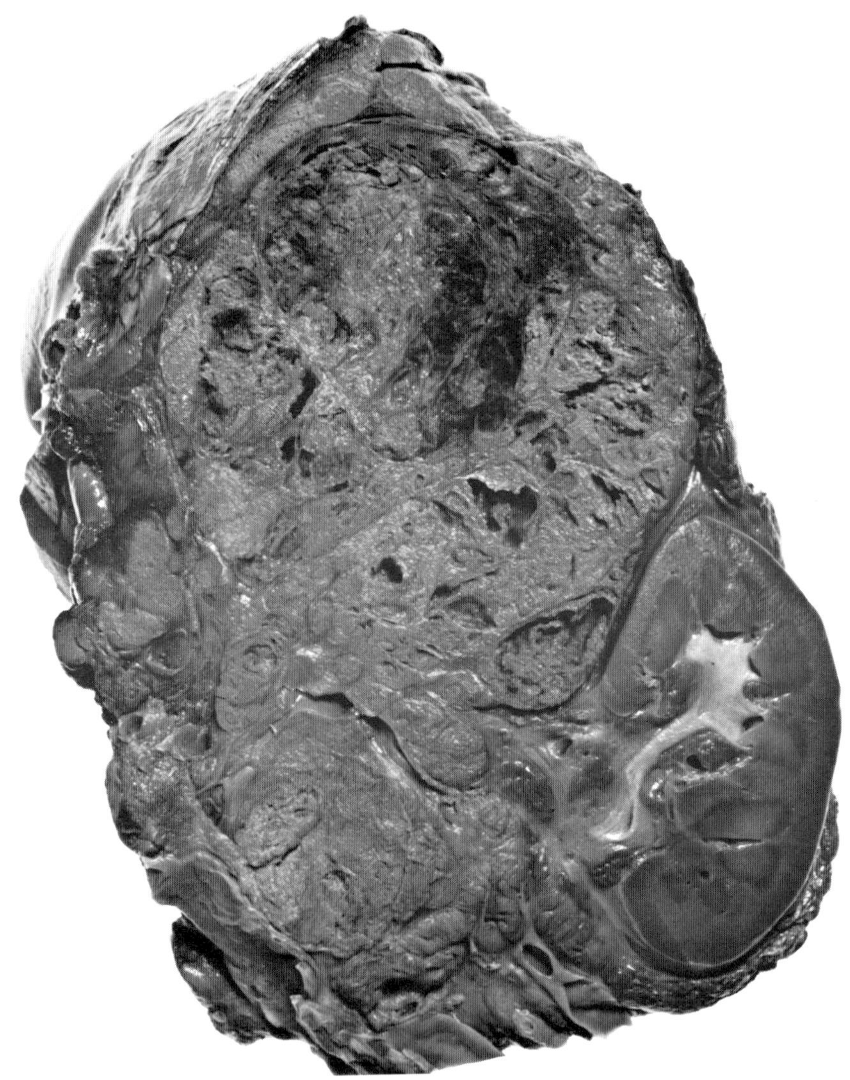

Figure 99
ADRENAL CORTICAL CARCINOMA
Invasion of surrounding soft tissues, with relative sparing of kidney is seen in this adrenal cortical carcinoma from a 51 year old woman with 11 years' history of deepening voice and beard development. X0.5. (Courtesy Mr. J.D. Maynard, M.S., Curator, Gordon Museum, Guy's Hospital, London, England.)

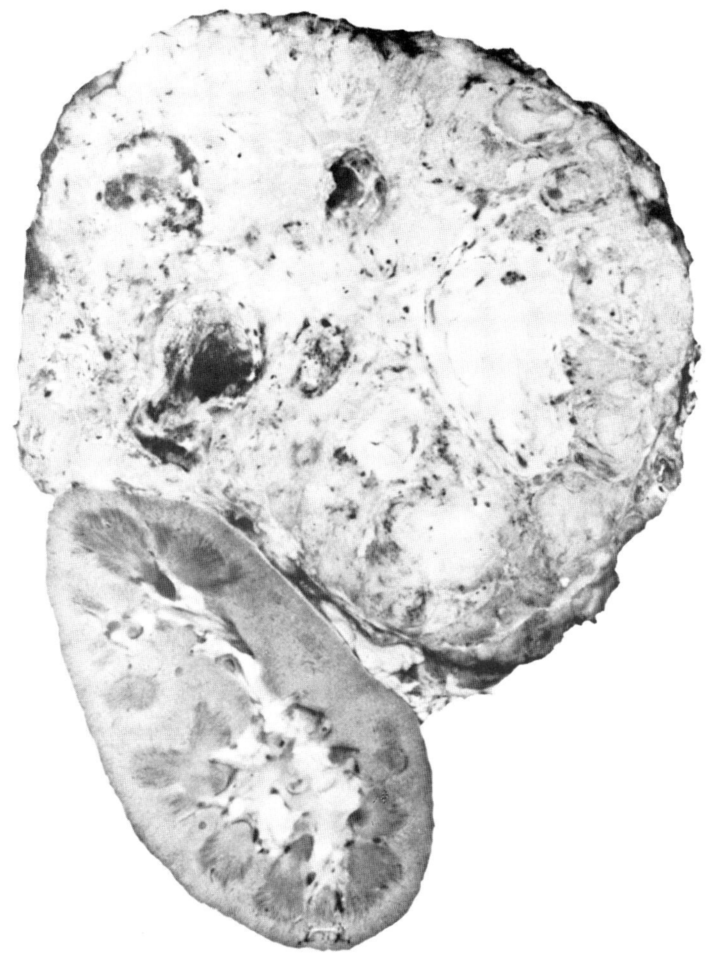

Figure 100
ADRENAL CORTICAL CARCINOMA
Adrenal cortical carcinoma in a 62 year old man is apparently well circumscribed in this cross section, but invasion of vena cava and widespread metastases in lung and liver were noted. There was no apparent hormonal function. X0.6. (Courtesy of Department of Pathology, Radcliffe Infirmary, Oxford, England.)

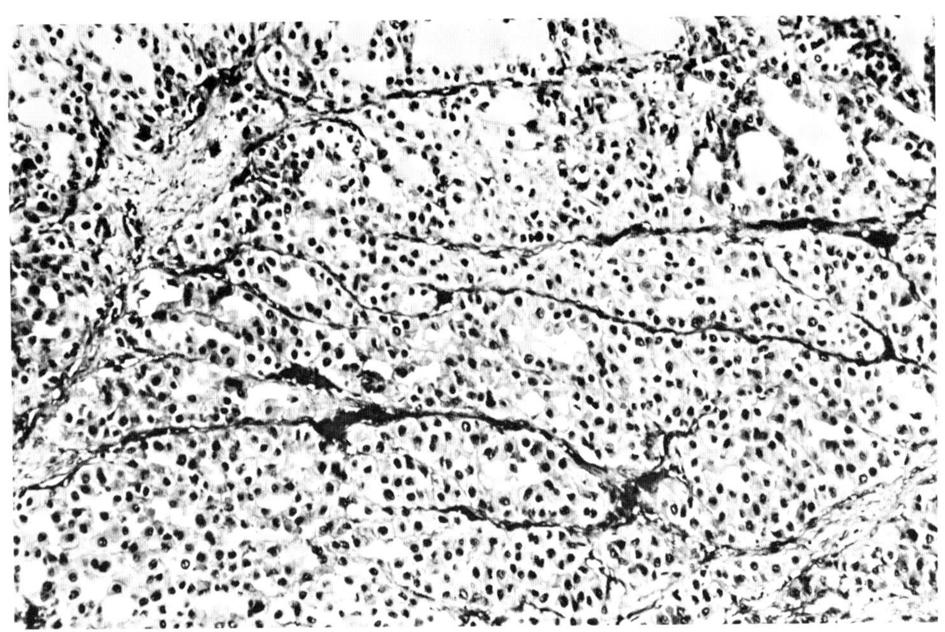

Figure 101
(Figures 101 and 108 from same patient)
ADRENAL CORTICAL CARCINOMA
The virilizing adrenal cortical carcinoma demonstrates a trabecular pattern of growth. Patient was a 38 year old woman who died with metastatic disease three years after operation. X120.

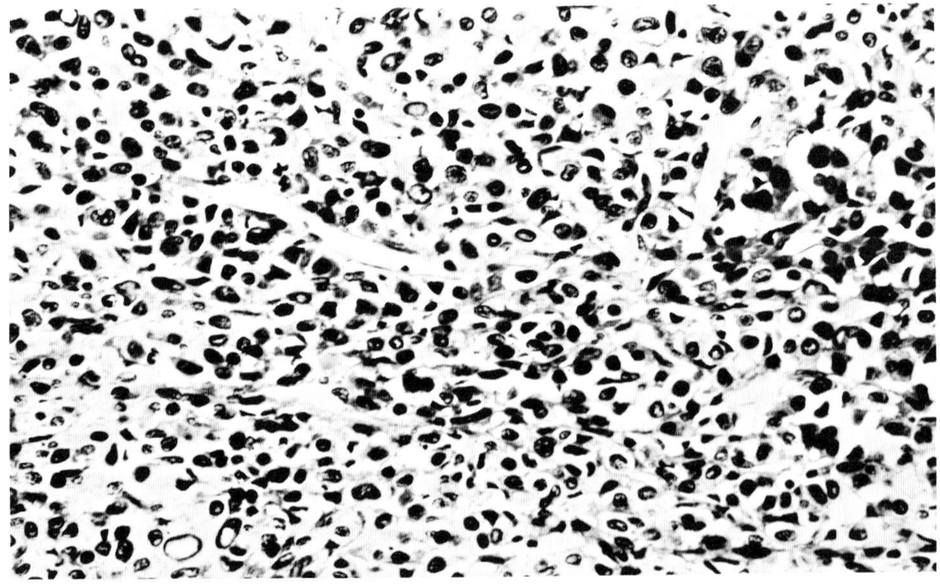

Figure 102
ADRENAL CORTICAL CARCINOMA
Another common histologic pattern is that of diffuse growth as in this adrenal cortical carcinoma. Patient was a 12 year old girl who died with metastatic disease nine months after operation. The patient suffered from a mixed Cushing's-virilism syndrome. X140.

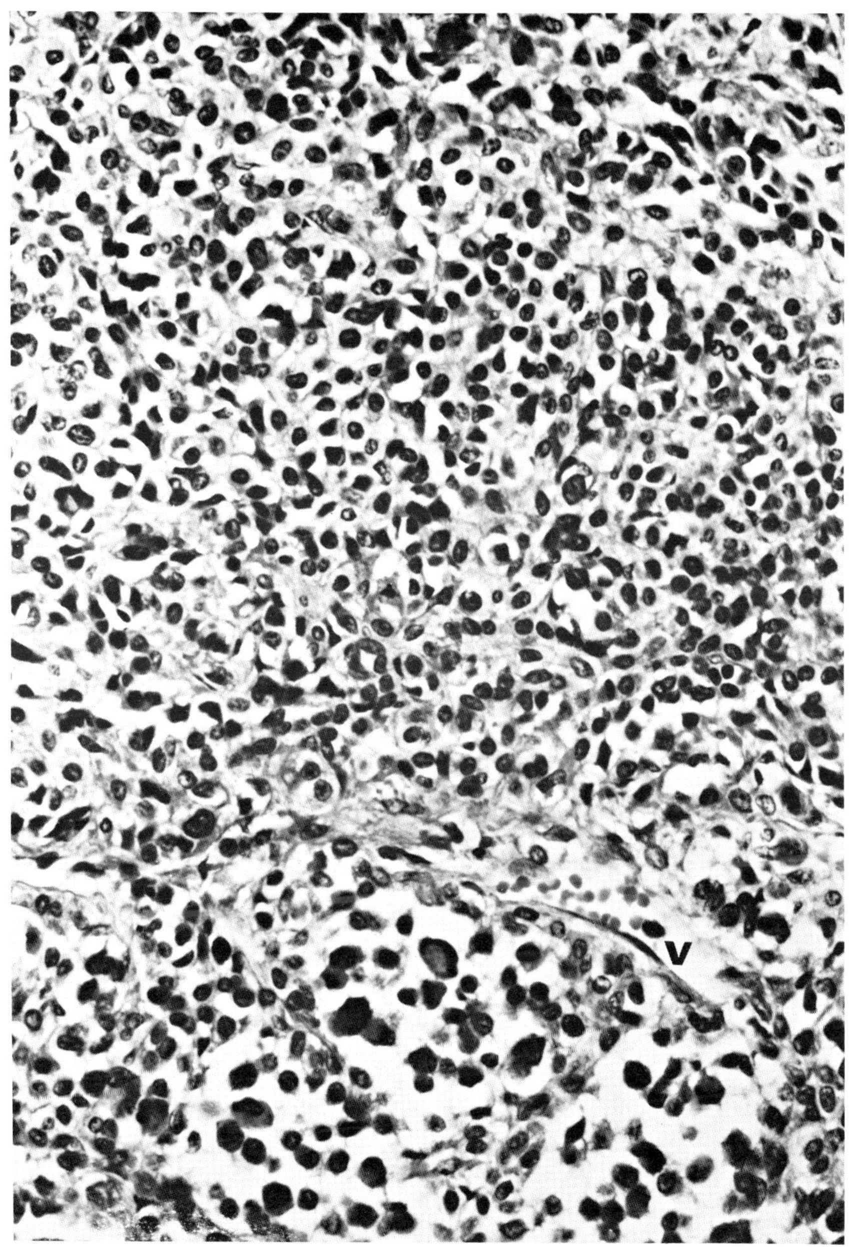

Figure 103
ADRENAL CORTICAL CARCINOMA
Adrenal cortical carcinoma demonstrates well differentiated trabecular pattern (above)
and poorly differentiated area (below). Note subtle abutment of tumor cells on thin walled
vascular space (V). Mixed Cushing's-virilism syndrome was present. X400.

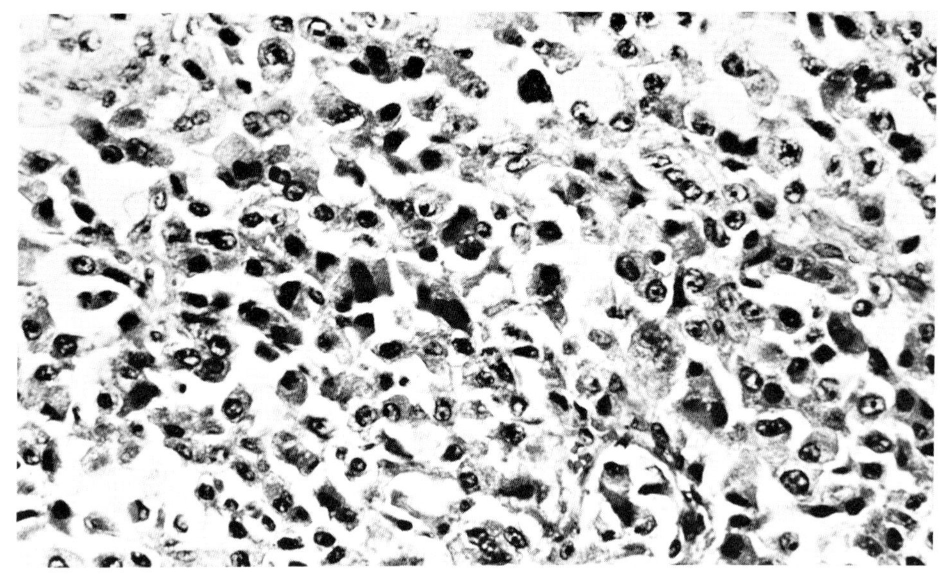

Figure 104
ADRENAL CORTICAL CARCINOMA
Marked nuclear pleomorphism is present in a 1500 g tumor occurring in a 65 year old man. This carcinoma produced no definite clinical syndrome. X400.

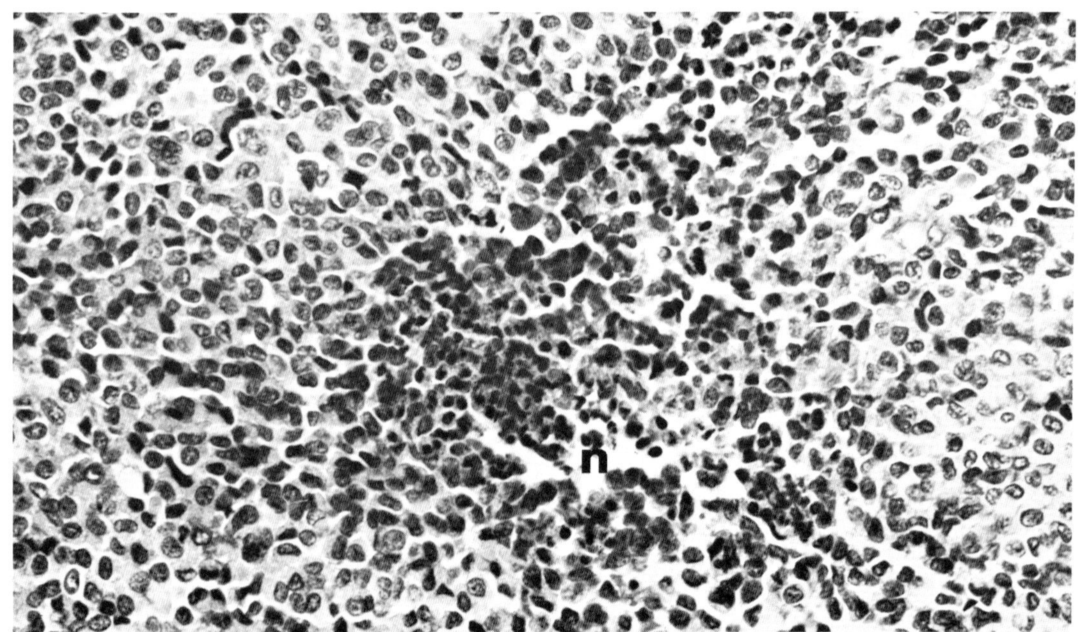

Figure 105
(Figures 105 and 106 from same patient)
ADRENAL CORTICAL CARCINOMA
Vesicular, deceptively uniform nuclei characterize an 1800 g adrenal cortical carcinoma. Patient was an 11 year old girl with a mixed Cushing's-virilism syndrome. Note focal necrosis (n). Metastases were present at initial exploration. X400.

Symington; Neville and O'Hare). These nuclear changes are often present, even though the cells themselves have a deceptively uniform appearance on low power examination (fig. 101). It is to be emphasized that the histologic appearance of these tumors may vary greatly from region to region, necessitating multiple blocks for adequate histologic sampling, and that tumors with minimal pleomorphism may metastasize.

Marked nuclear and cytoplasmic aberration is more frequent in large tumors (greater than 500 g). Mitotic activity (fig. 106) and vascular invasion (figs. 107, 108) are present in a minority of adrenal cortical carcinomas. Their presence, however, is indicative of malignancy. The presence of

confluent (rather than individual cellular) necrosis is seen in most adrenal cortical carcinomas (Symington), and a careful search should be made for this finding (fig. 109). Although individual cell necrosis may be seen in benign adrenal cortical tumors, areas of confluent cellular necrosis two high power fields or greater in diameter (fig. 110) are associated with subsequent metastasis in 80 percent of cases so identified (Hough et al.). Likewise, the finding of broad fibrous bands traversing the tumor (fig. 111) is associated with subsequent metastatic spread in a high percentage of cases (Schteingart et al.). Capsular invasion is a less valuable sign of malignant potential, due in part to the tendency of normal adrenal tissue to be found in extra-

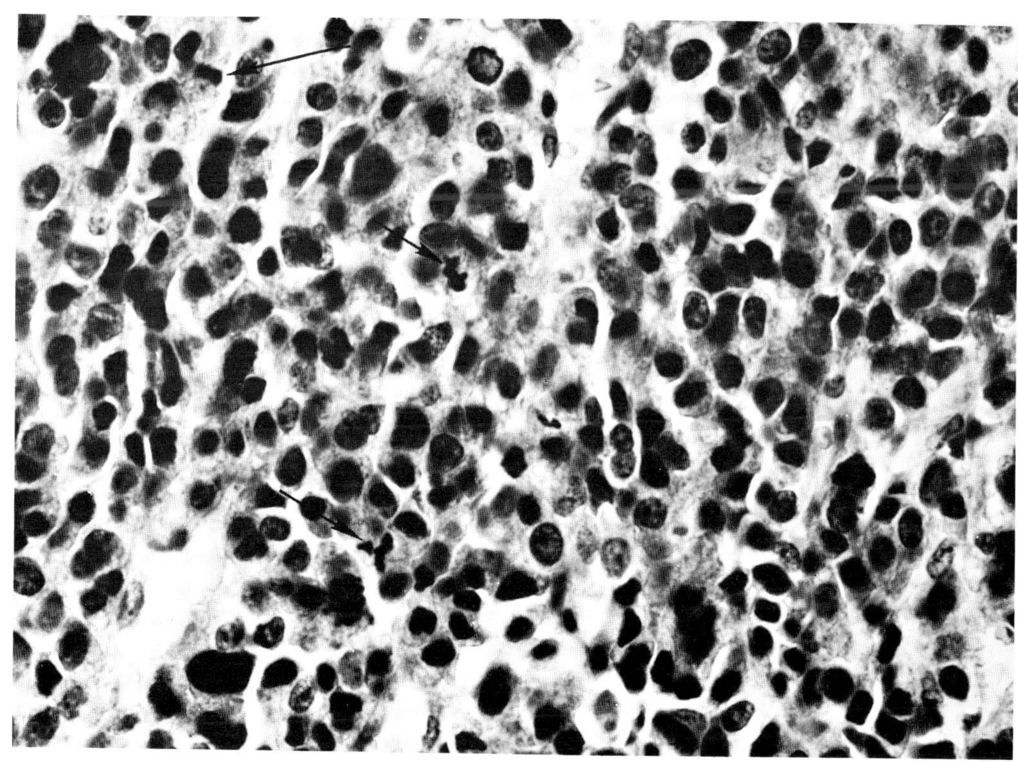

Figure 106
ADRENAL CORTICAL CARCINOMA
Numerous mitoses (arrows) are present in this section from case shown in figure 105. X650.

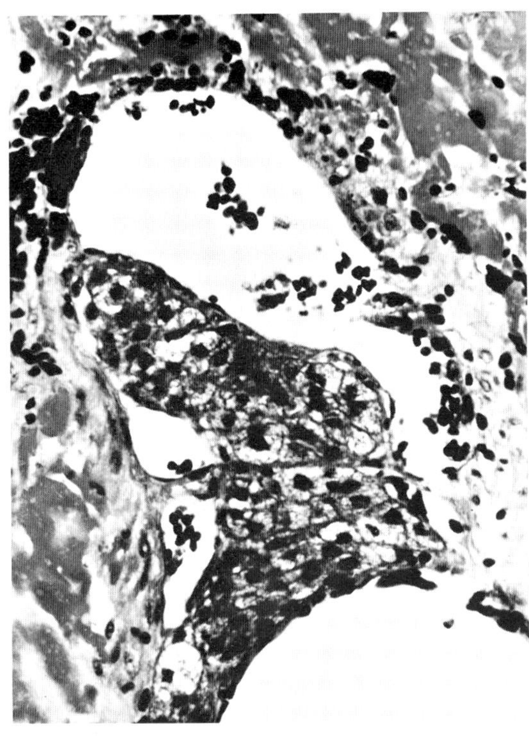

Figure 107
ADRENAL CORTICAL CARCINOMA
Vascular invasion is present in a 108 g adrenal cortical carcinoma occurring in a 38 year old woman with mixed Cushing's-virilism syndrome. Metastases were noted at original exploration. X260.

Figure 108
(Figures 101 and 108 from same patient)
ADRENAL CORTICAL CARCINOMA
Piecemeal, single cell vascular invasion (arrow) is pictured in a well differentiated 39 g virilizing adrenal cortical carcinoma. Tumor had invaded the wall of the vena cava and metastasized three years later. X400.

capsular locations. The consensus of available opinion on microscopic criteria of malignancy is summarized in Table 6. The usefulness of these features in determining malignant behavior is supported by Weiss.

Attempts to correlate histology with functioning status in adrenal cortical carcinomas (Birke et al.) have been generally disappointing (Symington; Lewinsky et al.). Although tumors producing the adrenogenital syndrome usually are composed almost exclusively of compact, reticularis-like cells (fig. 112), the converse is not true. Carcinomas producing the Cushing's syndrome (either pure or mixed with virilism) usually are composed of mixtures of clear fasciculata-like and compact reticularis-like cells. In general, the tumors producing the adrenogenital syndrome show less pleomorphism and other characteristics of malignancy (Table 7) than do those tumors of similar size producing Cushing's syndrome (Neville and O'Hare). Tumors producing feminization histologically resemble those producing virilism (Symington), but are almost always aggressive neoplasms, especially in adult males (Gabrilove et al.). Conversion of virilization to feminization has been reported with adrenal cortical carcinoma (Halmi and Lascari).

Table 6

SIGNIFICANT HISTOLOGIC CRITERIA IN ADRENAL CORTICAL TUMORS

		PATHOLOGIC DIAGNOSIS			CLINICAL RESULT		
Criterion	Definition	Benign N=20	Malignant N=17	Indeterminate N=4	Metastatic Tumors N=14	Nonmetastatic Tumors N=27	P Value*
Diffuse growth pattern	Growth of cells in sheets without organization into trabeculae or alveolae	0	7	1	7(2.7)***	1(5.3)	$<$.001
Vascular invasion	Presence of tumor cells with lumina of blood vessels	0	8	0	7(2.7)	1(5.3)	$<$.001
Tumor cell necrosis	Absent or focal if isolated areas 1 HPF** in diameter present; widespread if areas $>$ 2 HPF in diameter present	0	14	1	12(5.1)	3(9.9)	$<$.0001
Broad fibrous bands	Fibrous connective tissue septae greater than 1 HPF in diameter	1	8	1	9(3.4)	1(6.6)	$<$.0001
Capsular invasion	Nests of tumor cells present in capsule	2	10	2	8(4.8)	6(9.2)	$<$.03
Mitotic Index	Number of mitoses $>$ 1 HPF	0	8	0	6(2.7)	2(5.3)	$<$.02
Pleomorphism	Hyperchromatic nuclei with high nuclear-cytoplasmic ratio, marked variation in nuclear characteristics; tumor giant cells have hyperchromatic nuclei	3	15	4	13(7.5)	9(14.5)	$<$.001

Adapted from Hough, et al.

*F sher's exact test for significance of criterion comparing metastatic vs. nonmetastatic groups.

**High power field

***Observed (Expected from a series of 41 adrenal neoplasms)

Table 7

FACTORS INDICATING MALIGNANCY IN ADRENAL CORTICAL TUMORS

HIGHLY RELIABLE

Common: Tumor necrosis, tumor weight >100 g, broad fibrous bands, diffuse growth
pattern
Less Common: Vascular invasion, mitotic activity
Uncommon: Weight loss, feminization syndrome

MODERATELY RELIABLE

Virilism, mixed Cushing's/virilism syndrome, or no endocrine syndrome, marked nuclear
pleomorphism

SOMEWHAT RELIABLE

Markedly elevated urine 17-ketosteroids, negative clinical ACTH stimulation test, capsular invasion

UNRELIABLE

Tumor giant cells, cytoplasmic size variation, ratio between compact and clear cells

RECENTLY DEVELOPED TESTS

Elevated plasma 11-deoxysteroid and Δ-5 pregnenolone levels, absent ACTH response or elevated
11-deoxysteroid production in tissue culture

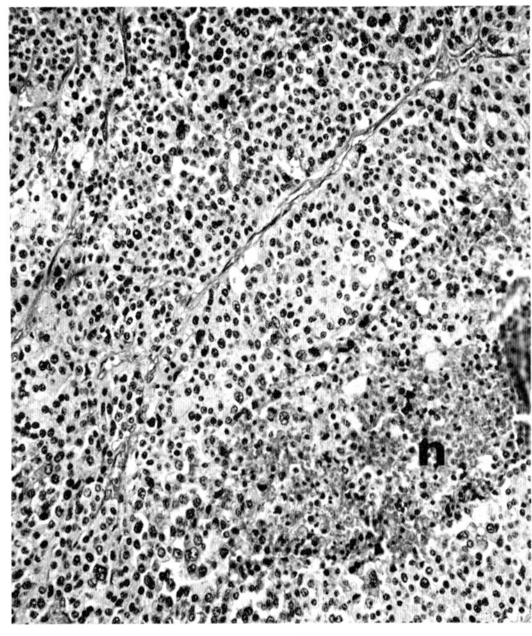

Figure 109
ADRENAL CORTICAL CARCINOMA
Focal necrosis (n) is noted in an adrenal cortical carci-
noma manifesting a trabecular pattern of growth. X120.

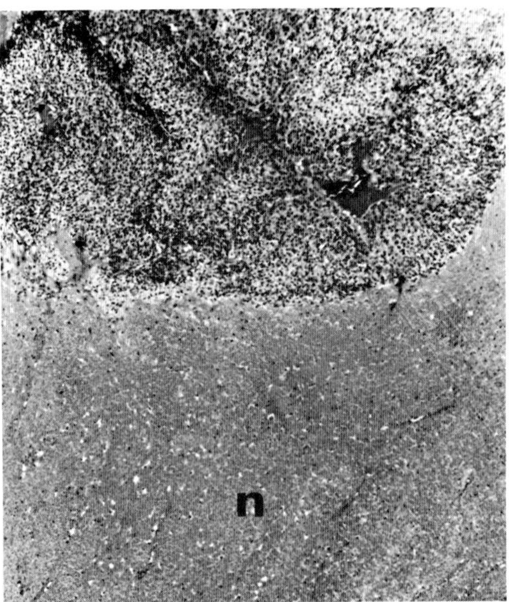

Figure 110
ADRENAL CORTICAL CARCINOMA
Confluent widespread necrosis (n) is a characteristic in
this 45 g adrenal cortical carcinoma which metastasized one
year after initial operation. X50.

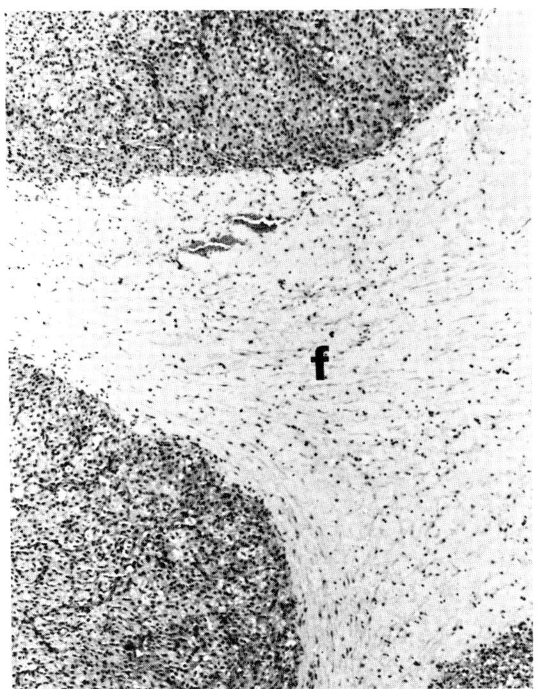

Figure 111
ADRENAL CORTICAL CARCINOMA
Broad fibrous band (f) traverses a virilizing adrenal cortical carcinoma. Such bands are probably the sequelae of necrosis. X50.

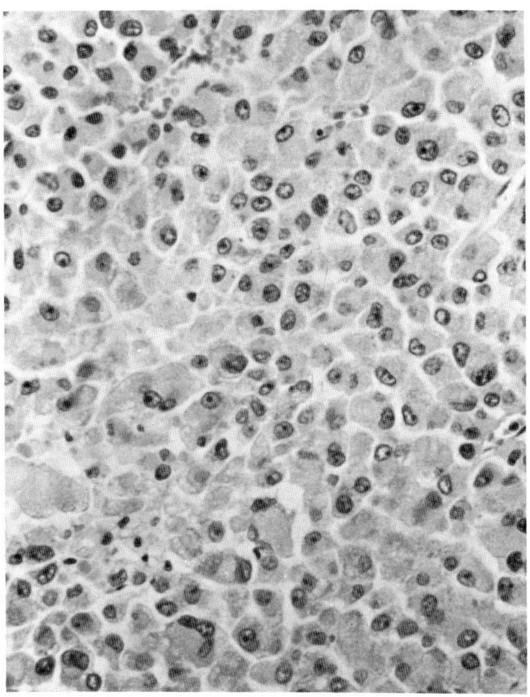

Figure 112
ADRENAL CORTICAL CARCINOMA
Compact, lipid poor cells with vesicular nuclei are seen in a virilizing adrenal cortical carcinoma. Such cells, although characteristic of androgen-producing tumors, may also be seen in tumors producing Cushing's syndrome. X160.

Although primary aldosteronism in association with malignant adrenal cortical tumors is rare (Åberg et al.), the neoplasms may have a characteristic appearance (figs. 113, 114) marked by trabeculae and thick walled vascular sinusoids. Carcinomas producing this syndrome are composed of hybrid fasciculata — glomerulosa cells differing histologically little from those seen in adrenal adenomas producing Conn's syndrome (Neville and O'Hare). So-called nonfunctioning adrenal cortical carcinomas do not differ reproducibly from those producing an endocrine syndrome (Lewinsky et al.). Although they are usually sheetlike (fig. 101) rather than trabecular (fig. 102) in appearance, no reproducible differential characteristics are present.

Ultrastructural Pathology. The cytologic aberrations observed in adrenal cortical carcinomas with routine histologic technics are reflected at the ultrastructural level. There is an extensive literature on this subject (Tannenbaum; Mackay; Neville and O'Hare; Mitschke et al.; Valente et al.). Electron microscopy of these tumors reveals progressive differences from normal, such as increased numbers of mitochondria, giant deformed mitochondria, and marked variation in content of organelles among neighboring individual cells (fig. 115). One of the most characteristic findings (Tannenbaum) has been disruption and dissolution of the basement membrane material normally surrounding the alveolar groups of adrenal cells. This may be the ultrastruc-

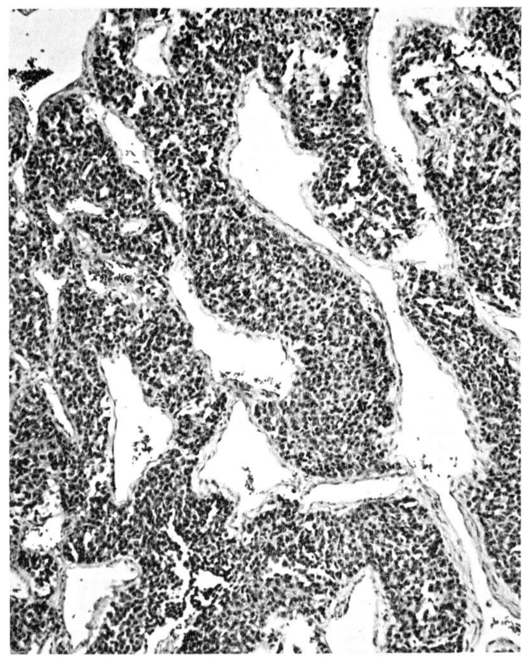

Figure 113
(Figures 113 and 114 from same patient)
ADRENAL CORTICAL CARCINOMA
Characteristic anastomosing, thick walled, vascular sinusoids are surrounded by uniform but dysplastic cells in an adrenal cortical carcinoma producing primary aldosteronism. Not all malignant tumors with aldosteronism have this appearance. X50. (Courtesy of Dr. A.M. Neville, London, England).

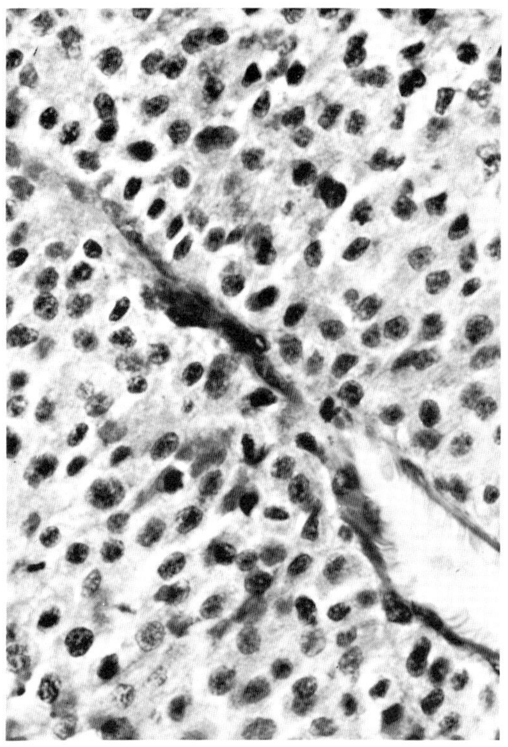

Figure 114
ADRENAL CORTICAL CARCINOMA
Nuclei are relatively uniform, but vesicular and hyperchromatic with occasional mitoses in the case shown in figure 113. X400. (Courtesy of Dr. A.M. Neville, London, England.)

tural counterpart of the loss of trabecular structure associated with more poorly differentiated adrenal cortical carcinomas. Electron microscopic study is particularly valuable in establishing adrenal cortical features in apparently nonfunctioning carcinomas, such as the case of Tang and colleagues, which had myxoid histologic features.

Tumors producing the adrenogenital syndrome are often composed of cells resembling the zona reticularis of the normal adrenal gland. These carcinomas demonstrate lipid-poor cytoplasm with abundant lysosomes and smooth endoplasmic reticulum (Tannenbaum; Valente et al.; Gorgas et al.). However, the rough endoplasmic retic-

ulum is apparently in parallel rows, as is usually seen in carcinomas associated with Cushing's syndrome. In addition, these tumors, as well as many producing Cushing's syndrome, possess an abnormally large number of microvilli. However, ultrastructural details are not significantly reproducible to allow a distinction between carcinomas producing various syndromes.

Adrenal cortical carcinomas producing no endocrine syndrome may be poorly differentiated. However, this is often not the case, since the failure to produce a syndrome may be a manifestation of absence of one or more enzymes in the steroid synthetic pathway, rather than a morphologic change in cytoplasmic organelles.

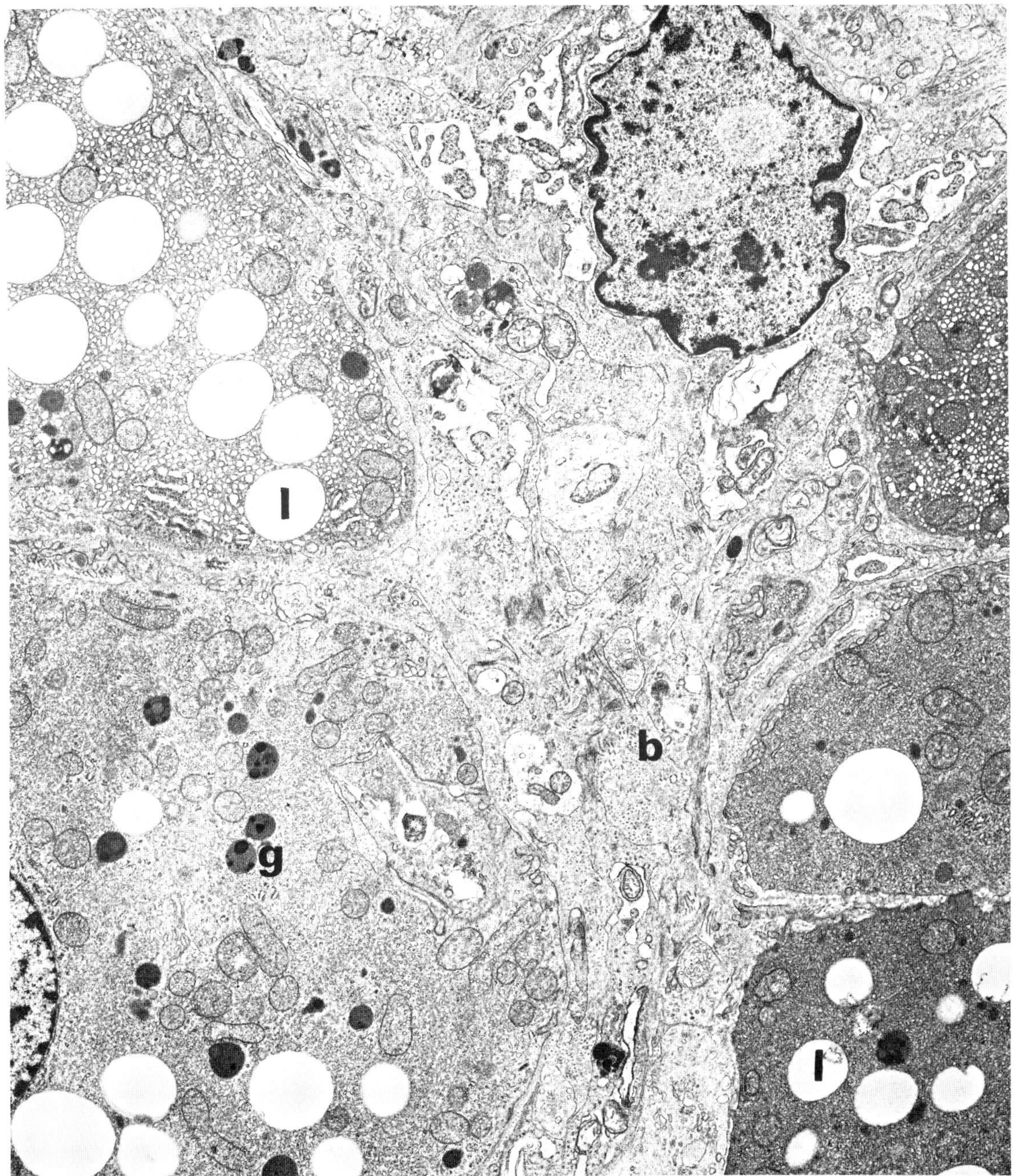

Figure 115
ADRENAL CORTICAL CARCINOMA
Pleomorphism of adrenal cortical carcinoma cells is shown in this electron micrograph of a well differentiated adrenal cortical carcinoma weighing 200 g. Patient did not have Cushing's syndrome and was free of disease five years later. Note marked variation in appearance of individual cells and deposition of excess basement membrane material (b). Some cells contain abundant lipid (l) and scattered lipofuscin granules (g). Mitochondria are of the ovoid tubulovesicular type. Uranyl acetate-lead citrate. X7000.

ECTOPIC ADRENAL
CORTICAL CARCINOMA

The majority of adrenal cortical carcinomas produce characteristic clinical and pathologic findings. There exists a group of tumors which are more difficult to categorize as adrenal cortical neoplasms. These tumors are unusual in arising from ectopic adrenal cortical tissue within the kidney (pl. VII), liver (fig. 116), or in para-aortic region (figs. 117–119). More rarely, ectopic adrenal tumors have been described in the gonads. These tumors may or may not produce an endocrine syndrome. Preoperative measurement of plasma and urine steroids, including precursor substances such as Δ-5-pregnenolone (McKenna et al.) may be useful in the accurate diagnosis of these lesions when an endocrine syndrome is not apparent. When Cushing's syndrome is produced by these ectopic tumors, the adrenal glands will be atrophic.

These tumors often have microscopic features similar to adrenal cortical carcinomas arising within the substance of the adrenal glands (fig. 118). In the absence of adequate preoperative biochemical analyses of serum and urine, electron microscopy is vital in establishing the steroid secreting nature of these neoplasms (fig. 119). However, Leydig cell tumors can

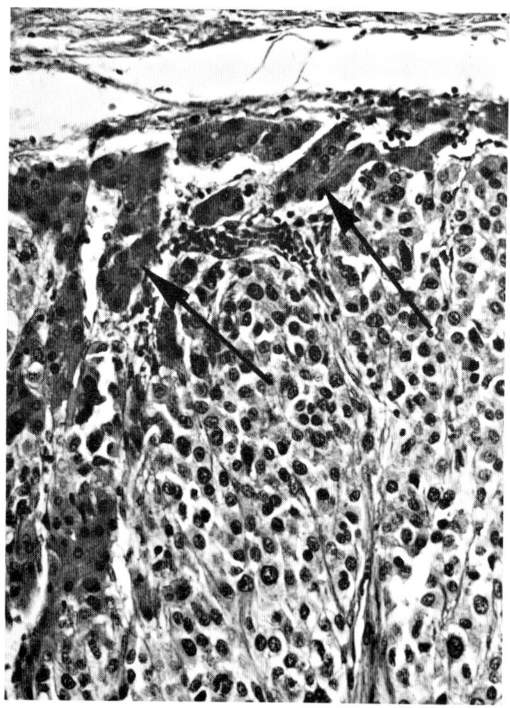

Figure 116
ADRENAL CORTICAL CARCINOMA
This ectopic adrenal cortical carcinoma originated beneath capsule of liver. Patient was a virilized 23 year old woman. Residual hepatic cells (arrows) are present. X80. (Courtesy of Dr. A. Stanek, New York, NY.).

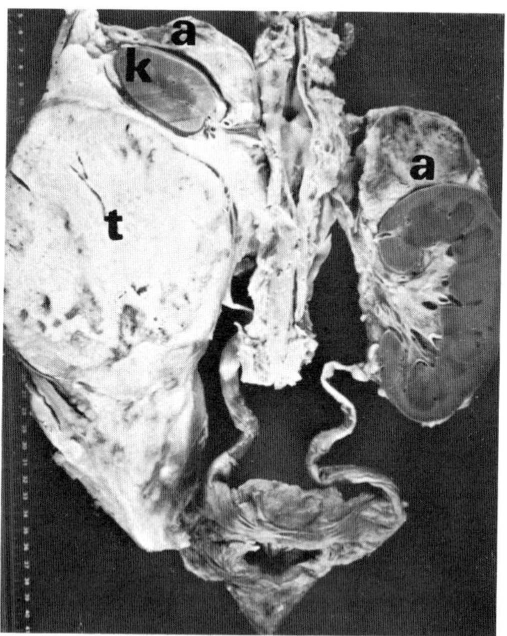

Figure 117
(Figures 117–119 from same patient)
ADRENAL CORTICAL CARCINOMA
This case is that of a 48 year old man without endocrine symptomatology, but with elevated urinary 17-ketosteroids. Massive tumor (t) occupies the left retroperitoneum, displacing the kidney (k) rostrally. Tumor is present in both adrenal glands (a). Other possible primary sites, such as lung, pancreas, and liver were negative.

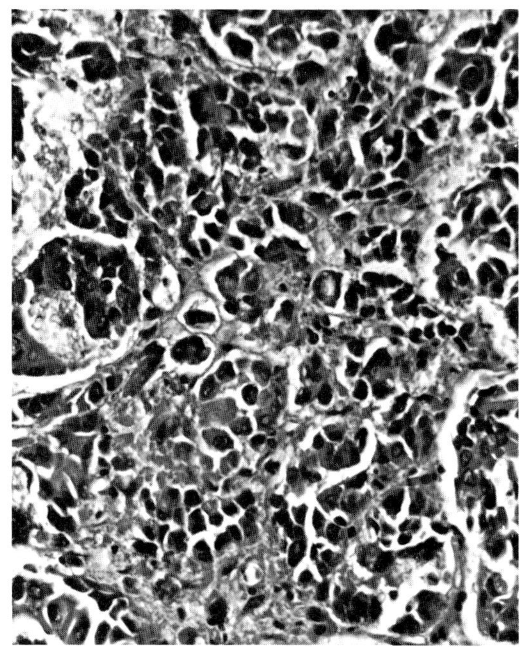

Figure 118
ADRENAL CORTICAL CARCINOMA
Microscopic appearance demonstrates poorly differenti-
ated polygonal cells arranged in nests and alveolar groups.
An origin in a pararenal adrenocortical nest was considered
a strong possibility. X300.

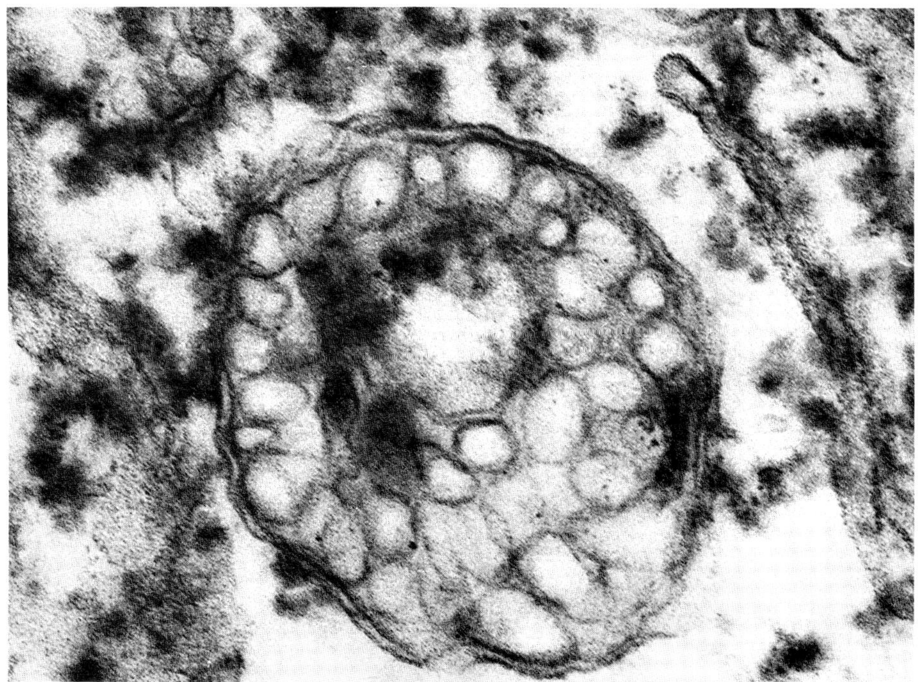

Figure 119
ADRENAL CORTICAL CARCINOMA
Electron micrograph reveals a tubulovesicular mitochondrion of the type associated with steroid
secreting cells, supporting the interpretation that this was an ectopic adrenal cortical carcinoma.
Uranyl acetate-lead citrate. X116,400.

closely resemble adrenal cortical tumors ultrastructurally, especially if Reinke crystalloids are not present in the former.

Natural History, Prognostic Factors. Although the difference between the natural history of benign and malignant adrenal cortical tumors is obvious, it is not always easy to separate one from another at the time of diagnosis (Symington; Neville and O'Hare). No single criterion will reliably separate all metastasizing from nonmetastasizing cases (Schteingart et al.). However, a combination of clinical and morphologic data will leave very few cases in which a decision cannot be made (Symington). Nonparametric analysis of clinical and morphologic data (Hough et al.) is an example of combining prognostic factors to produce a sharp separation between benign and malignant groups.

Other authors have found tumor mass an extremely important discriminant (Tang and Gray; Symington). Based on the studies available, it is apparent that tumor mass, type of endocrine syndrome produced, confluent tumor necrosis, and/or broad fibrous bands traversing the tumor, and weight loss are very important clinical and morphologic criteria in assessing prognosis. These criteria, as well as others, may be separated into groups depending upon the frequency with which they occur in adrenal cortical carcinomas (Table 7). Although vascular invasion and appreciable numbers of mitoses are seen in a minority of adrenal cortical carcinomas, their presence is indicative of an unfavorable prognosis. In addition, some authors (Lewinsky et al.) regard all large "nonfunctioning" tumors as potentially, if not actually, malignant.

At the present time, it appears that the responses of human adrenal cortical tumor cells in tissue culture may prove a valuable adjunct to more customary morphologic diagnosis (Neville and O'Hare; O'Hare et al.). Cells from functioning malignant adrenal cortical tumors produce abnormal amounts of androgens and 11-deoxysteroids and show a blunted functional response to ACTH, as compared with benign ones (O'Hare et al.). This difference is present even in small (< 100 g) well differentiated carcinomas which subsequently metastasized.

Metastatic Spread. Adrenal cortical carcinomas are among the most lethal of all neoplasms. Ultimate mortality ranges from 67 to 94 percent for various series reported (Hutter and Kayhoe; Harrison et al; Hajjar et al.; Huvos et al.; King and Lack). Metastatic spread may take one or both of two forms: a pronounced tendency toward local recurrence in the retroperitoneum with local nodal metastases, or hematogenous spread (fig. 120). The former phenomenon may be obvious at initial presentation, rendering the distinction among adrenal cortical, renal cell, and metastatic pulmonary carcinoma difficult (pl. IX).

Most patients develop metastases within two years from initial presentation. Death within one year after the development of metastases is usual (Hutter and Kayhoe; Sullivan et al.). In most instances, the histology of the metastatic lesions resembles that of the primary lesion, as does the endocrine syndrome which may reappear with the emergence of metastases. Although death from nonendocrine-related sequelae of metastatic spread is common (Hajjar et al.), some patients may succumb to uncontrollable Cushing's syndrome induced by metastases (Hutter and Kayhoe).

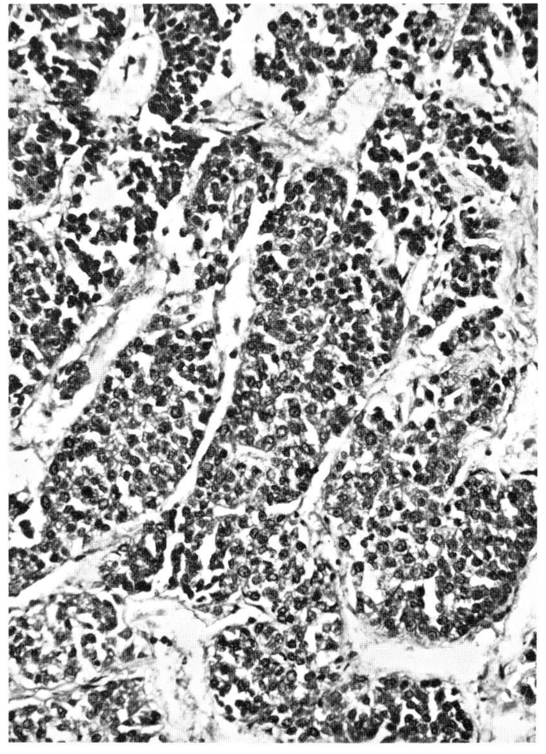

Figure 120
ADRENAL CORTICAL CARCINOMA
Histologic appearance of adrenal cortical carcinoma metastatic to lung reveals a plexiform trabecular pattern of growth. Such tumors may be confused with primary carcinoma of this site. X160.

At least one-fourth of patients with adrenal cortical carcinoma present with obvious metastases. Liver, lung, and lymph nodes are the common sites for distant spread (fig. 121). A staging system incorporating size, evidence of local invasion, and distant metastases (Sullivan et al.) demonstrates a correlation with length of survival. However, the difficulty of separating small adrenal cortical carcinomas from adenomas may be reflected in any such system. Local spread to the abdomen occurs in a high percentage of cases and reflects a very poor prognosis. Brain metastases are distinctly uncommon (Hutter and Kayhoe; Lipsett et al.), in contrast with the natural history of renal cell carcinoma with which metastatic adrenal cortical carcinoma may be confused. A recent review of the literature (Friedland and Whetsell) revealed only two histologically proven examples of intracerebral metastases in 243 cases of adrenal cortical carcinoma. Bone metastases are likewise relatively uncommon, although most large series contain several documented examples of this phenomenon (fig. 122). Subcutaneous metastases are also seen (fig. 123), but much less commonly than with renal cell carcinoma. It is also not uncommon for adrenal cortical carcinoma to present with distant metastases in unusual sites, such as mediastinal or cervical lymph nodes. Electron microscopy may be quite useful in this situation.

Response to Therapy. Surgery is the primary mode of treatment in this disease (Hajjar et al.; Ibanez; Lewinsky et al.). However, survival is poor in most large series reported (Javadpour et al.). Larger tumors frequently require radical resection of kidney and portions of adjacent viscera, such as liver, spleen, and pancreas (Scott et al.; Hajjar et al.). In many instances, complete resection of the primary may be impossible. This is often the case in "nonfunctioning" variants which are often quite large at initial presentation (Lewinsky et al.). In most large series, males survive significantly less frequently than females (Hajjar et al.; Hoffman and Mattox; Hutter and Kayhoe).

Although many patients receive radiotherapy for residual tumor, there is no statistical evidence for prolonged survival over surgery alone (Hajjar et al.; Hutter and Kayhoe). However, external radiation in high doses may be beneficial for isolated patients, especially those with osseous metastases (Lewinsky et al.).

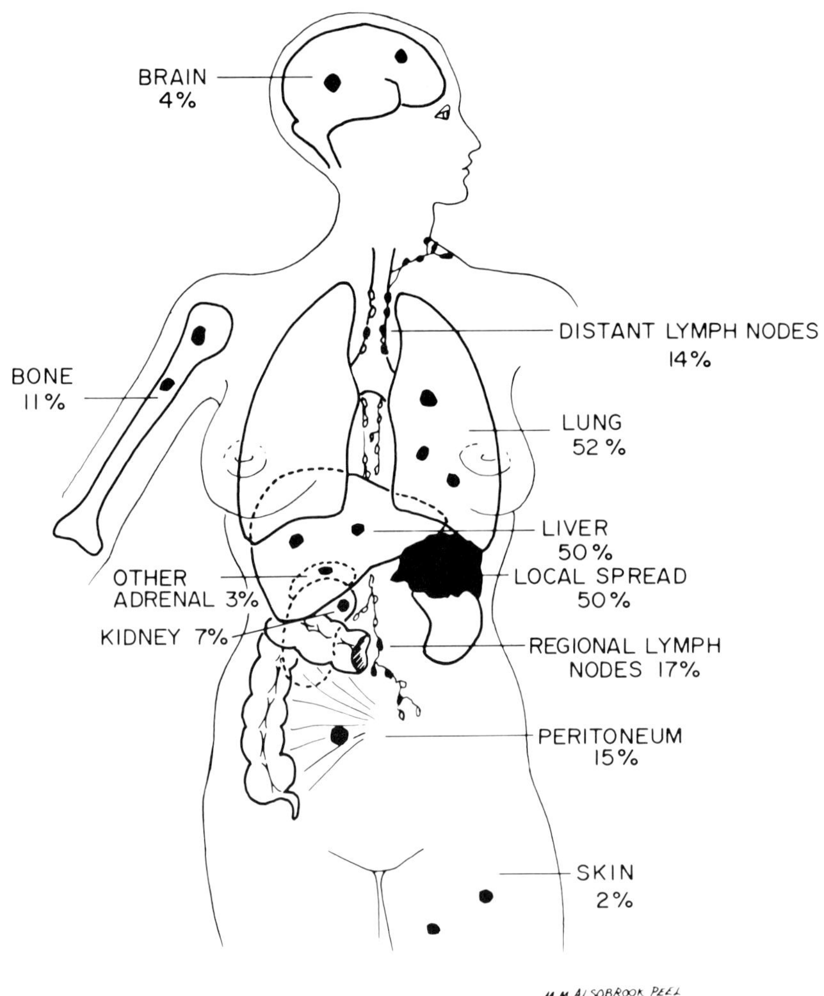

Figure 121
ADRENAL CORTICAL CARCINOMA
This schematic diagram depicts the anatomic distribution of the lesions from 262 cases of metastatic adrenal cortical carcinoma collected from the literature references cited in this chapter. Note that spread to the kidney, opposite adrenal, brain, and skin are uncommon.

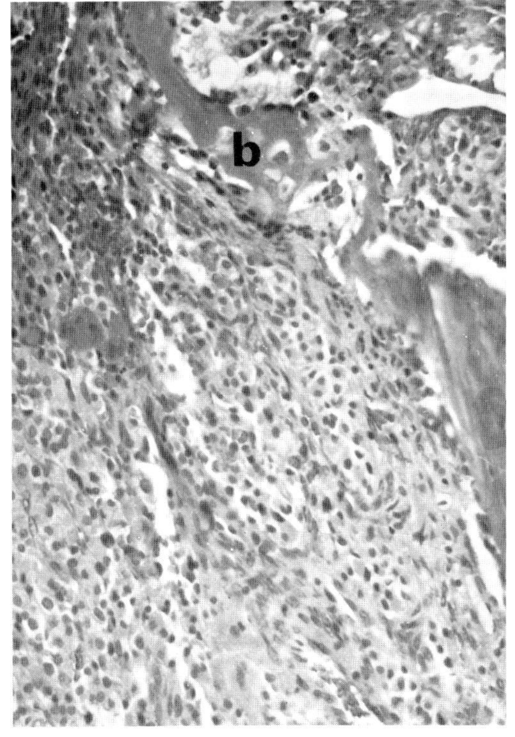

Figure 122
ADRENAL CORTICAL CARCINOMA
This adrenal cortical carcinoma presented with a metastasis to the humerus. Considerable new bone formation (b) is present. Cushing's syndrome was present. Note poorly differentiated nature of tumor deposit. The patient subsequently developed widespread metastases. X160.

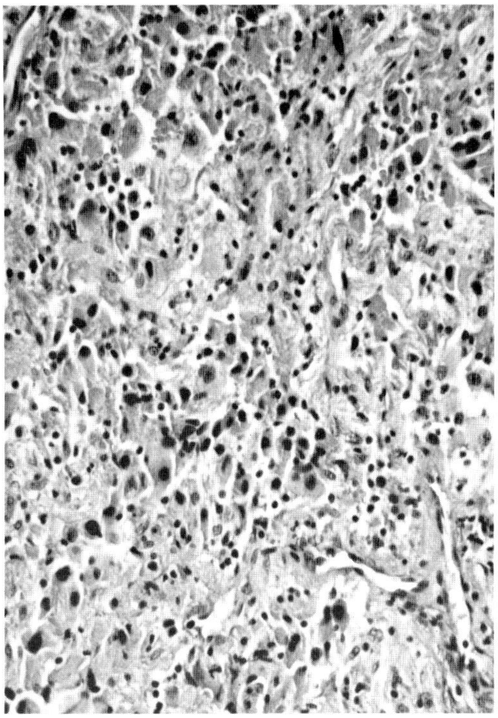

Figure 123
ADRENAL CORTICAL CARCINOMA
This poorly differentiated adrenal cortical carcinoma presented with widespread metastatic involvement, including this lesion in the subcutaneous tissue of the forearm. Mixed Cushing's-virilism syndrome was present. Note the pleomorphic cells with abundant cytoplasm infiltrating among collagen fibers. Such tumors may be misinterpreted as lung or renal carcinomas. X160.

Chemotherapy with 1,1,dichloro-2-(o-chlorophenyl)-2-(p-chlorophenyl)-ethane or o'p'DDD (Hutter and Kayhoe) is useful in alleviating the symptoms of hypercortisolism (Orth and Liddle) which accompany the majority of recurrent and metastatic adrenal cortical carcinomas (Hajjar et al.). In a small percentage of patients, the lysis of cortical tumor cells induced by o'p'DDD not only alleviates symptoms, but induces objective remission of tumor growth (Ostuni and Roginsky; Becker and Schumacher). Experience with other chemotherapeutic agents has shown no apparent increment in benefits over those provided by o'p'DDD alone.

DIFFERENTIAL DIAGNOSIS

General Approach. The customary case of adrenal cortical carcinoma, producing Cushing's syndrome or some variant thereof and adequately evaluated biochemically preoperatively, is not often confused with other malignant tumors. There are, however, many examples of adrenal cortical carcinoma where clinical confirmation of

PLATE VII
ADRENAL CORTICAL CARCINOMA

A. Adrenal cortical carcinomas vary considerably in gross appearance. This tumor was 15 cm in diameter and originated beneath the renal capsule. The patient was a woman with mild hypercortisolism and elevation of many cortisol precursors and their metabolites, including pregnenolone. Note extensive necrosis within the tumor. X.5. (Courtesy of Dr. L. Graham, Nashville, TN.)

B. This case is of a 33 year old man with a 250 g nonfunctioning adrenal cortical carcinoma closely adherent to, but not invading, the right kidney. The tumor is composed of cysts filled with necrotic tumor and separated from one another by broad fibrous bands. Viable tumor is present at the expanding margins of the tumor. The tumor presented with a cerebral metastasis. X.06.

C. Cross section of a 357 g adrenal cortical carcinoma reveals multiple foci of necrosis, denoted by pale chalk white areas. The patient was a 57 year old woman with Cushing's syndrome and hepatic metastases. X.5.

PLATE VII

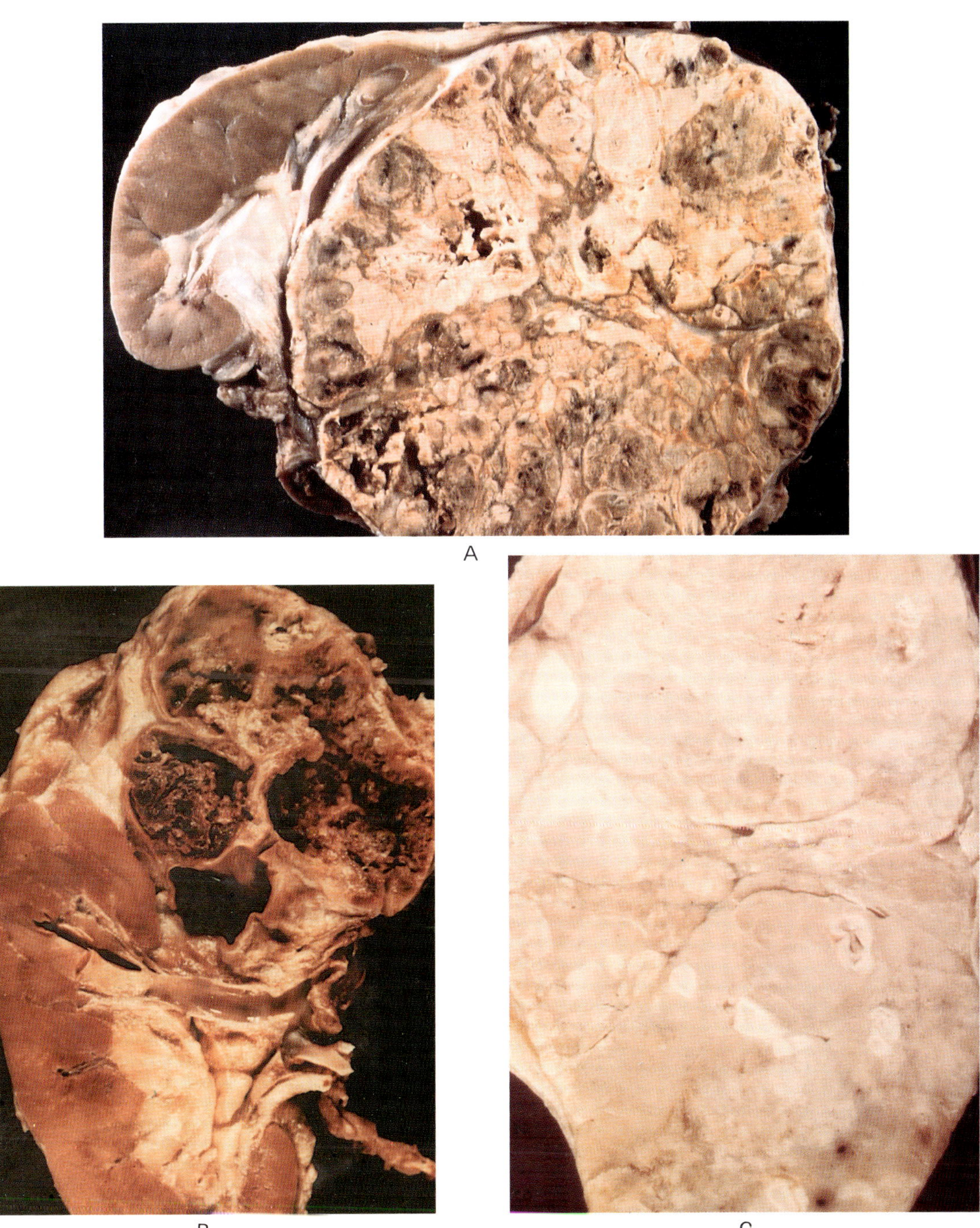

A

B

C

PLATE VIII
ADRENAL CORTICAL CARCINOMA

(Plate VIII-A and B from same patient)

A. This 380 g adrenal cortical carcinoma occurred in a middle-aged man without endocrine symptomatology. No metastases were present at initial exploration, but the patient died with metastatic disease within a year. X.6.

B. A macrosection demonstrates massive necrosis of the tumor, with viable tissue confined to the outer zone. X0.6.

C. Characteristic broad fibrous band (f) is seen in this adrenal cortical carcinoma occurring in a virilized 41 year old woman. X120.

D. Hyperchromatic distorted nuclei characterize this 1800 g adrenal cortical carcinoma removed from a 16 year old boy with elevated urine 17-ketosteroids, but no evidence of feminization. X160. (Courtesy of Dr. S. Orr, Charlotte, NC.)

PLATE VIII

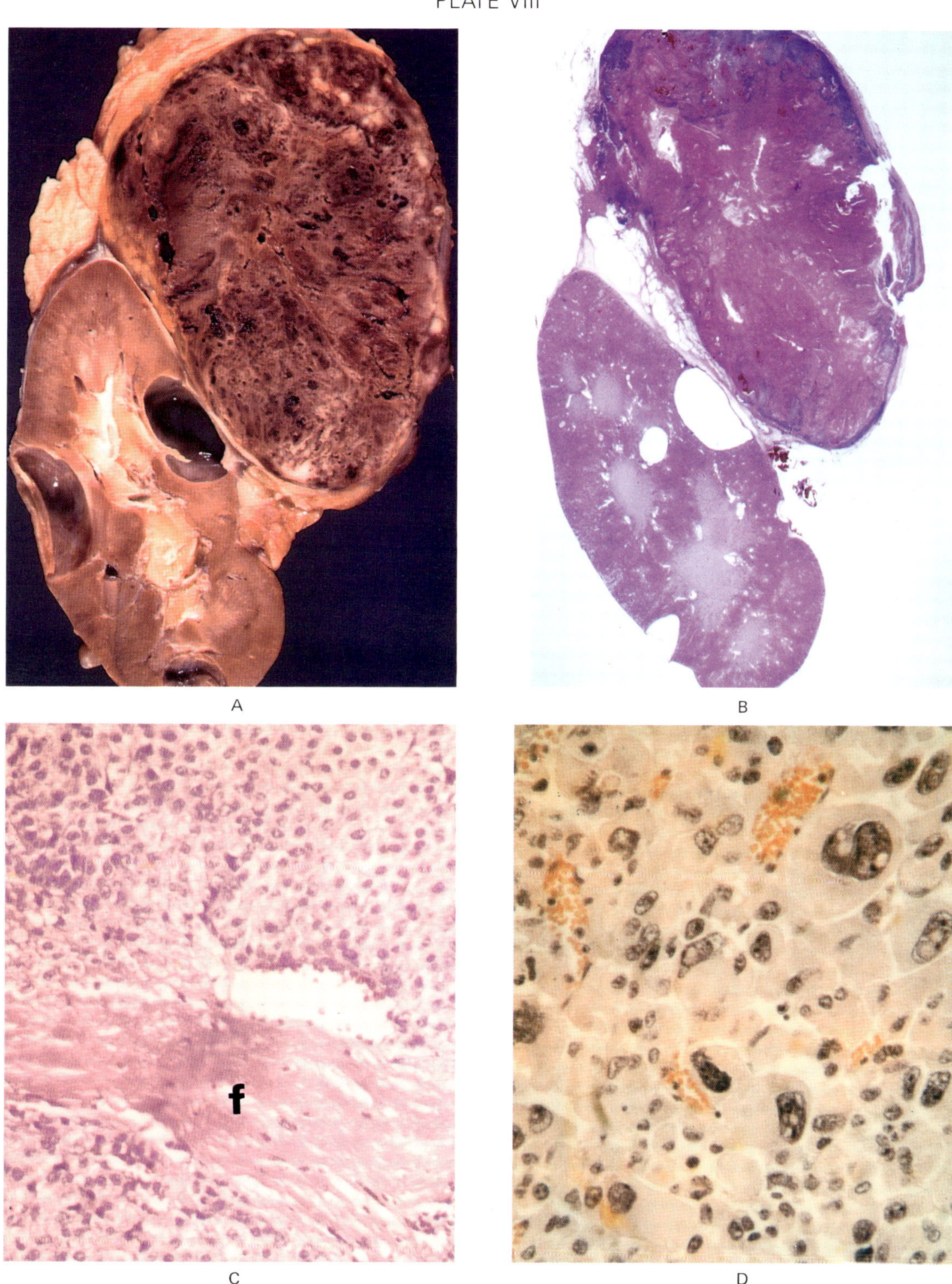

PLATE IX
DIFFERENTIAL DIAGNOSIS OF ADRENAL CORTICAL CARCINOMA

A. A poorly differentiated adrenal cortical carcinoma demonstrates diffuse growth pattern with uniform, but hyperchromatic, nuclei. The patient presented with subcutaneous metastases and extensive retroperitoneal involvement. Cushing's syndrome was present. X160.

B. An islet cell carcinoma demonstrates a ribbon-like growth pattern with uniform appearing nuclei. The patient presented with retroperitoneal spread of tumor. There was no clinical evidence of function. X160.

C. A large cell undifferentiated carcinoma of the lung demonstrates marked nuclear dysplasia with abundant cytoplasm. The patient presented with extensive metastases to abdomen and retroperitoneum. X160.

D. A hepatocellular carcinoma contains bile and shows evidence of tubular differentiation. Such discriminating features often are not present. This tumor also presented with extensive abdominal spread. X160.

PLATE IX

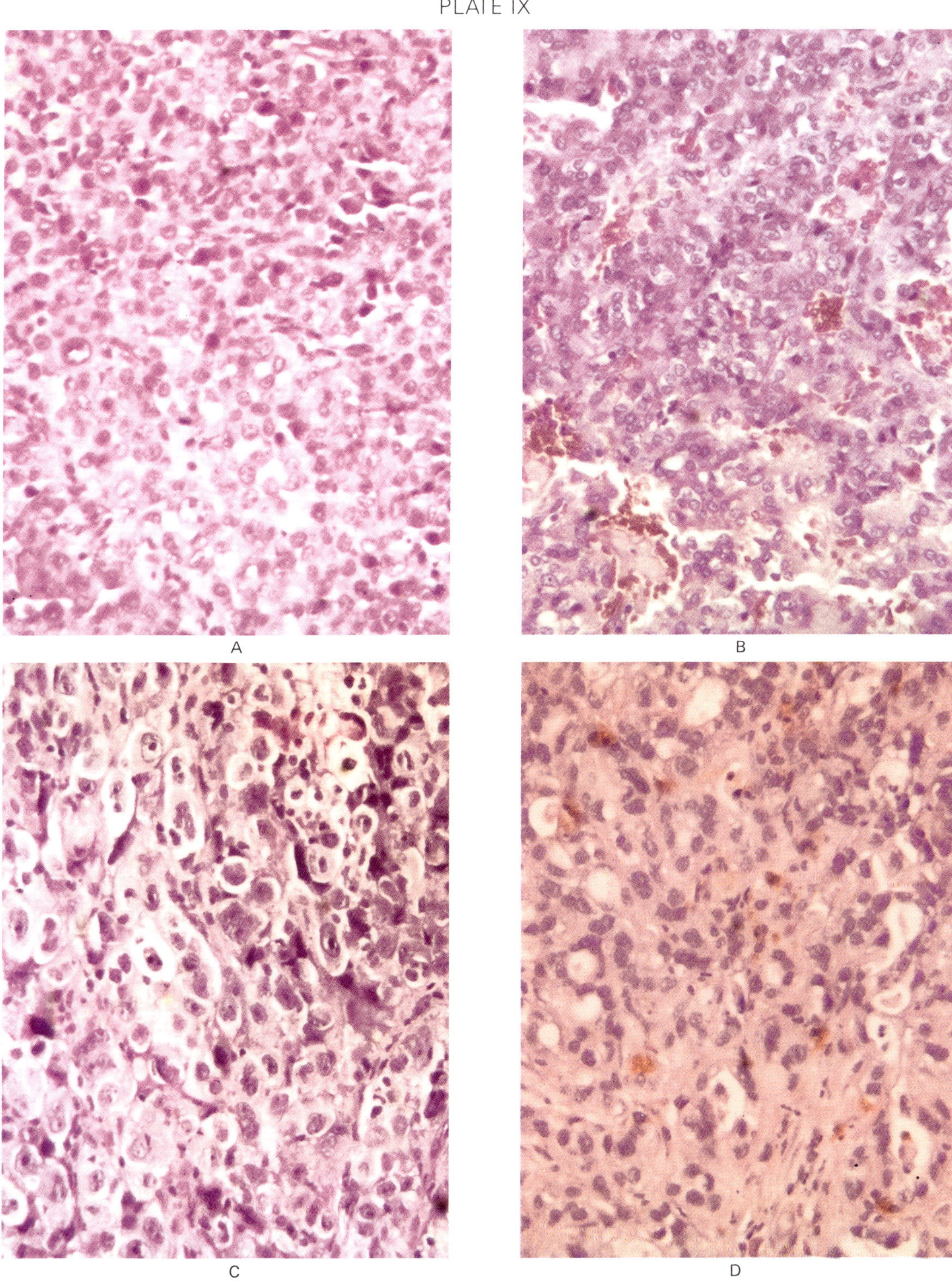

A

B

C

D

steroid secretion and primary site are lacking. These tumors may be confused with others made up to some degree of polygonal cells with eosinophilic cytoplasm and manifesting a tendency toward a trabecular arrangement (pl. IX). In many cases, this confusion is not due to limitations of the microscopist, but, instead, to those of light microscopy itself. In these cases, electron microscopy may be invaluable in establishing a diagnosis. This is especially true when the tumor available for study is from a metastatic site. In this situation, the characteristic mitochondria, parallel stacks of rough (fig. 115) and abundant smooth endoplasmic reticulum (Tannenbaum; Mackay) of adrenal cortical neoplasms seen with electron microscopy may be the only sure means of arriving at a distinction.

Renal Adenocarcinoma

Several important morphologic distinctions exist between malignancies of adrenal cortical and renal tubular origin. These differences are more apparent on ultrastructural observation (Tannenbaum). However, they are usually sufficiently marked at the gross and light microscopic levels to allow differentiation. Renal adenocarcinomas characteristically expand and distort the renal calyces, displacing rather than distorting the adrenal gland. More rarely, direct invasion of the adrenal gland may occur. Conversely, adrenal cortical carcinomas usually displace rather than distort the kidneys (figs. 98, 99). The extremely rare occurrence of adrenal cortical tumors primary beneath the renal capsule (pl. VII) usually requires electron microscopy for definitive diagnosis of the steroidogenic potential of the tumor, especially if no clinical syndrome is apparent. A careful search

for the ipsilateral adrenal is, of course, helpful both at surgery and in the operative specimen. Adrenal cortical carcinomas, regardless of site of origin, characteristically demonstrate more nuclear pleomorphism and mitoses than tumors of renal origin (Bennington and Beckwith), while renal carcinomas often have a nodularity readily apparent on low power microscopic examination (fig. 124) and usually contain glycogen demonstrable by histochemistry or electron microscopy.

Islet Cell Carcinoma

The biochemical and anatomic differences among islet cells and adrenal cortical malignancies are usually sufficient to facilitate their separation. Occasionally, adrenal cortical tumors, either benign or malignant, may arise within the pancreas (fig. 83). These neoplasms may closely resemble islet cell tumors (pl. IX) on light microscopic examination, even though Cushing's syndrome is present clinically. In the absence of a definite clinical syndrome, electron microscopy or immunocytochemistry may be needed, since many islet cell tumors cannot be characterized by conventional histochemistry alone. In addition, islet cell tumors rarely may produce ACTH (Azzopardi and Williams), resulting in Cushing's syndrome due to bilateral adrenal hyperplasia. The distinction is aided if some adrenal tissue is available for study, since atrophy will be obvious if the Cushing's syndrome is due to production of cortisol by an ectopic adrenal neoplasm. Regardless of the syndrome produced by an islet cell tumor, the ultrastructural appearance of characteristic secretory granules will serve to distinguish these lesions from those of ectopic adrenal cortical origin.

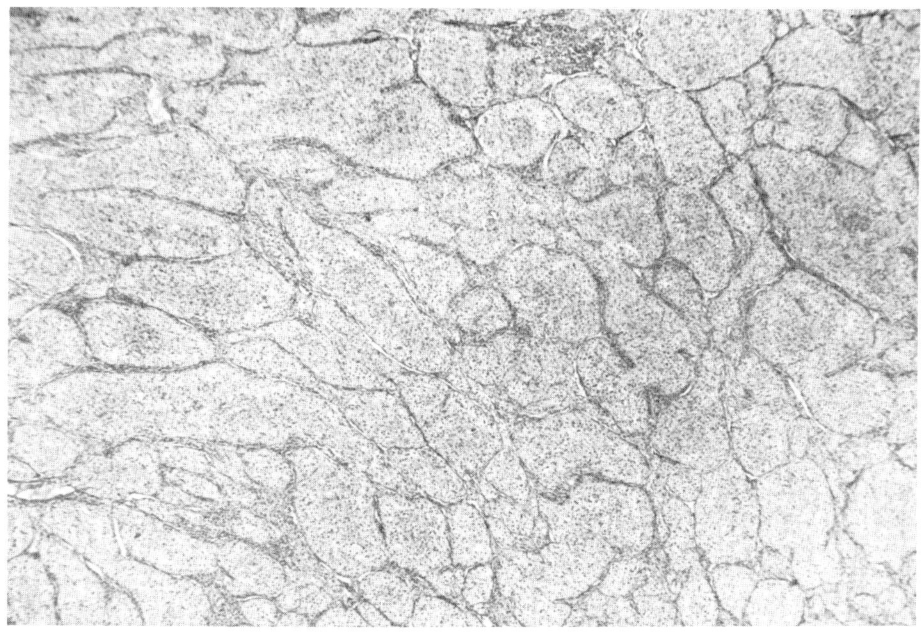

Figure 124
RENAL CELL CARCINOMA
This photomicrograph of a renal cell carcinoma depicts the nodular growth pattern commonly seen in these tumors. Pleomorphism of nuclei is usually less apparent than in adrenal cortical carcinoma. X40.

Hepatocellular Carcinoma

This group of tumors more rarely metastasize outside the abdomen than adrenal cortical carcinomas. The obvious hepatocellular carcinoma confined to the liver and manifesting bile production (pl. IX) is seldom confused with an adrenal cortical carcinoma. However, more poorly differentiated hepatocellular carcinomas may invade or metastasize to an adrenal gland. This situation is complicated by the rare occurrence of primary adrenal cortical tumors within the substance of the liver. Many of these tumors produce endocrine syndromes, usually involving some degree of virilism. More commonly, an adrenal cortical carcinoma will attain massive proportions, with invasion of hepatic parenchyma. In the absence of adequate preoperative studies, electron microscopy may be needed to distinguish between the tumors in this circumstance.

Bronchogenic Carcinoma

The possibility of confusing a poorly differentiated bronchogenic carcinoma with an adrenal cortical carcinoma is not confined to metastatic sites (pl. IX), but also occurs in the adrenal gland proper (see Metastatic Carcinoma of the Adrenal Gland). In the absence of histochemical markers such as mucin or keratin, large cell undifferentiated and poorly differentiated pulmonary adenocarcinomas closely simulate the histology of adrenal cortical carcinoma. This resemblance includes a tendency toward alveolar growth and extreme pleomorphism. Fortunately, most poorly differentiated pulmonary carcinomas of this type contain tonofilaments, vacuoles, and desmosomes, features not ordinarily seen in adrenal neoplasms. Although small cell undifferentiated pulmonary carcinoma is seldom confused histologically with primary adrenal cortical carcinoma, the clinical presentation may be similar, since hypercortisolism due to the ectopic ACTH syndrome is often present in this group of tumors (Strott et al.; Rees and Ratcliffe; Meador et al.).

Pheochromocytoma and Paraganglioma

Under usual circumstances, the distinction between adrenal tumors of cortical and medullary origin is readily made. In certain instances, however, absence of a distinct hypertensive syndrome or of differential histologic features may make the anatomic diagnosis more difficult (see Pheochromocytoma). More rarely, clinical or biochemical evidence of excessive steroid secretion may accompany medullary tumors. Although some authors have described compound corticomedullary neoplasms, our experience does not substantiate the existence of these tumors. The possibility that Cushing's syndrome is resulting from corticotrophic substances released by the medullary tumor is more likely. In practice, such cases can present with extreme contralateral adrenal hyperplasia and grossly elevated urinary steroid excretion. The characteristic histochemical and ultrastructural findings in medullary tumors will resolve the dilemma.

Alveolar Soft Part Sarcoma

The endocrine and alveolar pattern of the alveolar soft part sarcoma is well known to mimic renal adenocarcinoma (Shipkey et al.) and thus enters into the differential diagnosis of adrenal cortical neoplasms (fig. 125). Although usually presenting in soft tissues of the extremities, the alveolar soft part sarcoma may present in the retroperitoneum. Most alveolar soft part sarcomas will demonstrate rodlike cytoplasmic inclusions, positive with PAS stain after diastase digestion (fig. 126). Electron microscopy reveals suggestions of smooth muscle differentiation, as well as a distinctive periodicity to the membrane bound, cytoplasmic, crystalline granules (DeSchryver-Kecskemeti et al.). Secretory-like granules with crystalline arrays may also be seen (Welsh et al.).

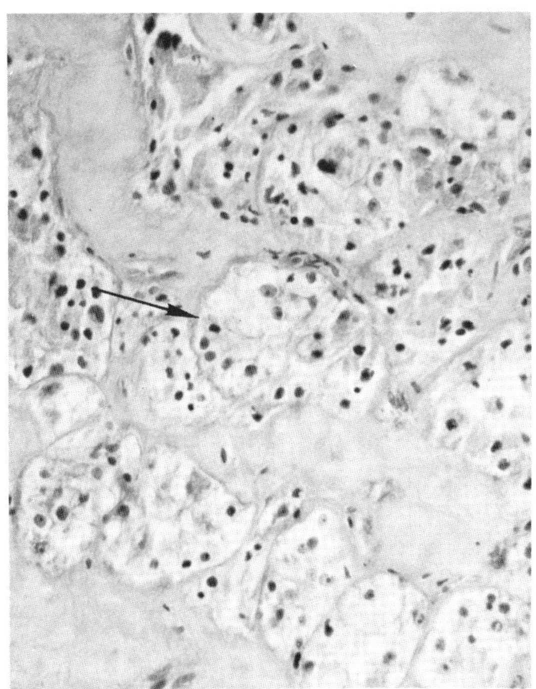

Figure 125
(Figures 125 and 126 from same patient)
ALVEOLAR SOFT PART SARCOMA
A large mass involving the retroperitoneum was present in a young adult man. The histology shows nests of clear cells surrounded by an apparent basement membrane (arrow). Such a microscopic appearance might be interpreted as consistent with either renal or adrenal cortical carcinoma. X160.

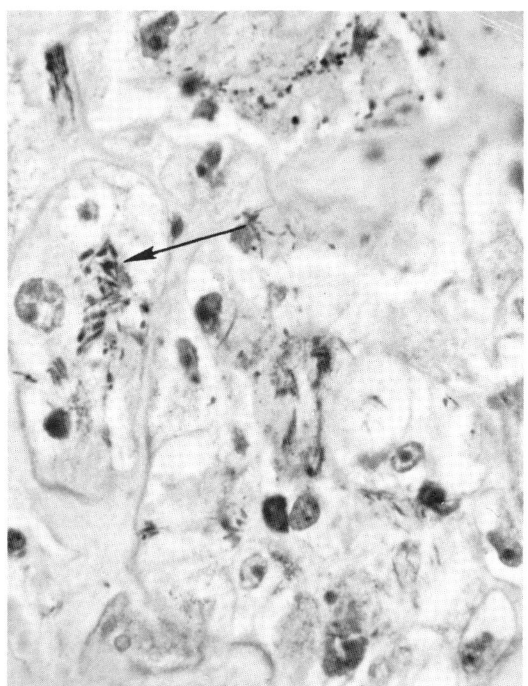

Figure 126
ALVEOLAR SOFT PART SARCOMA
A periodic acid-Schiff stain reveals rodlike inclusions (arrow) characteristic of an alveolar soft part sarcoma, in this case primary in the retroperitoneum. PAS-hematoxylin. X400.

References

Åberg, H., Johansson, H., Morlin, C., and El-Sherief, A. Malignant aldosteronoma. Acta Chir. Scand. 147:735-737, 1981.

Akhtar, M. Gosalbez, T., and Young, I. Ultrastructural study of androgen-producing adrenocortical adenoma. Cancer 34:322-327, 1974.

Alterman, S. L., Dominguez, C. Lopez-Gomez, A., and Lieber, A. L. Primary adrenocortical carcinoma causing aldosteronism. Cancer 24:602-609, 1969.

Arteaga, E., Biglieri, E. G., Kater, C. E., Lopez, J. M., and Schambelan, M. Aldosterone-producing adrenocortical carcinoma. Ann. Intern. Med. 101:316-321, 1984.

Artigas, J. L. R., Niclewicz, E. D., Silva, A. deP. G., Ribas, D. B, and Athayde, S. L. Congenital adrenal cortical carcinoma. J. Pediatr. Surg. 11:247-252, 1976.

Azzopardi, J. G. and Williams, E. D. Pathology of "non-endocrine" tumors associated with Cushing's syndrome. Cancer 22:274-286, 1968.

Becker, D. and Schumacher, P. O. o,p'DDD therapy in invasive adenocortical carcinoma. Ann. Int. Med.

82:677-679, 1975.

Benaily, M., Schweisguth, O., and Job, J. C. Les tumeurs cortico-surrenales de L'enfant. Etude retrospective de 34 cas observes de 1954 a 1973. Arch. Fr. Pediatr. 32:441-453, 1975.

Bennington, J. L. and Beckwith, J. B. Tumors of the Kidney, Renal Pelvis, and Ureter, p. 126. Fascicle 12, Second Series, Atlas of Tumor Pathology. Washington: Armed Forces Institute of Pathology, 1975.

Birke, G., Franksson, C., Gemzell, C-A., Moberger, G., and Plantin, L-O. Adrenal cortical tumours. Acta Chir. Scand. 117:233-246, 1959.

Cassan, P., Baglin, A., Coulbois, J., et al. Corticosurrénalomes malins non-sécrétants révélés par une fièvre prolongée. Nouv. Presse Med. 7:2153-2156, 1978.

DeSchryver-Kecskemeti, K., Kraus, F. T., Engleman, W., and Lacy, P. E. Alveolar soft-part sarcoma — a malignant angioreninoma. Am. J. of Surg. Pathol. 6:5-18, 1982.

DHEW Publication No. (NIH)75-787. Third National Cancer Survey: Incidence Data. Natl. Cancer Inst. Monogr. 41, 1975.

Didolkar, M. S., Bescher, R. A., Elias, E. G., and Moore, R. H. Natural history of adrenal cortical carcinoma. Cancer 47:2153-2161, 1981.

Friedland, R. P. and Whetsell, W. O., Jr. Adrenal cortical carcinoma with Cushing's syndrome, organic psychosis, and aphasia in a seventy-one-year-old woman. Mt. Sinai J. Med. 45:509-523, 1978.

Gabrilove, J. L., Sharma, D. C., Wotiz, H. H., and Dorfman, R. I. Feminizing adreno-cortical tumors in the male. Medicine 44:37-79, 1965.

Gorgas, K., Böck, P., and Wuketich, S. Fine structure of a virilizing adrenocortical adenoma. Beitr. Pathol. 159:371-397, 1976.

Hajjar, R. A., Hickey, R. C., and Samaan, N. A. Adrenal cortical carcinoma. Cancer 35:549-554, 1975.

Halmi, K. A. and Lascari, A. D. Conversion of virilization to feminization in a young girl with adrenal cortical carcinoma. Cancer 27:931-935, 1971.

Harrison, J. H., Mahoney, E. M., and Bennett, A. H. Tumors of the adrenal cortex. Cancer 32:1227-1235, 1973.

Hoffman, D. L. and Mattox, V. R. Treatment of adrenocortical carcinoma with o,p'-DDD. Med. Clin. North Am. 56:999-1012, 1972.

Hough, A. J., Hollifield, J. W., Page, D. L., and Hartmann, W. H. Prognostic factors in adrenal cortical tumors. Am. J. Clin. Pathol. 72:390-399, 1979.

Hutter, A. M., Jr., and Kayhoe, D. E. Adrenal cortical carcinoma. Am. J. Med. 41:572-580, 1966.

Huvos, A. G., Hajdu, S. I., Brasfield, R. D., and Foote, F. W., Jr. Adrenal cortical carcinoma. Cancer 25:354-361, 1970.

Ibanez, M. L. The Pathology of Adrenal Cortical Carcinoma: Study of 22 Cases, pp. 231-239. In: Endocrine and Nonendocrine Hormone-Producing Tumors. Chicago: Year Book Medical Publishers, 1971.

Javadpour, N., Woltering, E. A., and Brennan, M. F. Adrenal neoplasms. Cur. Probl. Surg. 17:3-52, 1980.

Kelly, W. F., O'Hare, M. J., Loizou, S., Davies, D., and Laing, I. Hypermineralocorticism without excessive aldosterone secretion: an adrenal carcinoma producing deoxycorticosterone. Clin. Endocrinol. 17:353-361, 1982.

King, D. R. and Lack, E. E. Adrenal cortical carcinoma. Cancer 44:239-244, 1979.

Lewinsky, B. S., Grigor, K. M., Symington, T., and Neville, A. M. The clinical and pathologic features of "non-hormonal" adrenocortical tumors. Cancer 33:778-790, 1974.

Liddle, G. W. Tests of pituitary-adrenal suppressibility in the diagnosis of Cushing's syndrome. J. Clin. Endocrinol. Metab. 20:1539-1560, 1960.

Lipsett, M. B., Hertz, R., and Ross, G. T. Clinical and pathophysiologic aspects of adrenocortical carcinoma. Am. J. Med. 35:374-383, 1963.

Lynch, H. T., Katz, D. A., Bogard, P. J., and Lynch, J. F. The sarcoma, breast cancer, lung cancer, and adrenocortical carcinoma syndrome revisited. Am. J. Dis. Child. 139:134-136, 1985.

Macfarlane, D. A. Cancer of the adrenal cortex. Ann. R. Coll. Surg. Engl. 23:155-186, 1958.

Mackay, A. Atlas of Human Adrenal Cortex Ultrastructure, pp. 346-489. In: Functional Pathology of the Human Adrenal Gland. Symington, T. (Ed.). Baltimore: The Williams & Wilkins Company, 1969.

McKenna, T. T., Miller, R. B., and Liddle, G. W. Plasma pregnenolone and 17-OH-pregnenolone in patients with adrenal tumors, ACTH excess, or idiopathic hirsutism. J. Clin. Endocrinol. Metab. 44:231-236, 1977.

Meador, C. K., Liddle, G. W., Island, D. P. et al. Cause of Cushing's syndrome in patients with tumors arising from "nonendocrine" tissue. J. Clin. Endocrinol. Metab. 22:693-703, 1962.

Miller, R. W. Peculiarities in the occurrence of adrenal cortical carcinoma. Am. J. Dis. Child. 132:235-236, 1978.

Mitschke, H., Saeger, W., and Breustedt, H-J. Zur ultrastruktur der nebennierenrindentumoren beim Cushingsyndrom. Virchows Arch. [Pathol. Anat.] 360:253-264 1973.

Neville, A. M. and O'Hare, M. J. Aspects of Structure, Function, and Pathology, pp. 1-65. In: The Adrenal Gland. James, V. H. T. (Ed.). New York: Raven Press, 1979.

O'Hare, M. J., Monaghan, P., and Neville, A. M. The pathology of adrenocortical neoplasia: a correlated structural and functional approach to the diagnosis of malignant disease. Hum. Pathol. 10:137-154, 1979.

Orth, D. N. and Liddle, G. W. Results of treatment in 108 patients with Cushing's syndrome. N. Engl. J. Med. 285:243-247, 1971.

Ostuni, J. A. and Roginsky, M. S. Metastatic adrenal cortical carcinoma. Arch. Int. Med. 135:1257-1258, 1975.

Powell-Jackson, J. D., Calin, A., Fraser, R. et al. Excess deoxycorticosterone secretion from adrenocortical carcinoma. Br. Med. J. 2:32-33, 1974.

Rees, L. H. and Ratcliffe, J. G. Ectopic hormone production by non-endocrine tumours. Clin. Endocrinol. (Oxf.) 3:263-299, 1974.

Schteingart, D. E., Seabold, J. E., Gross, M. D., and Swanson, D. P. Iodocholesterol adrenal tissue uptake and imaging in adrenal neoplasms. J. Clin. Endocrinol. Metab. 52:1156-1161, 1981.

Scott, H. W., Jr., Foster, J. H., Liddle, G., and Davidson, E. T. Cushing's syndrome due to adrenocortical tumor. Ann. Surg. 162:505-516, 1965.

Shipkey, F. H., Lieberman, P. H., Foote, F. W., and Stewart, F. S. Ultrastructure of alveolar soft part sarcoma. Cancer 17:821-830, 1964.

Shons, A. R. and Gamble, W. G. Nonfunctioning carcinoma of the adrenal cortex. Surg. Gynecol. Obstet. 138:705-709, 1974.

Strauch, G. O. and Vinnick, L. Persistent Cushing's syndrome apparently cured by ectopic adrenalectomy. J.A.M.A. 221:183-184, 1972.

Strott, C. A., Nugent, C. A., and Tyler, F. H. Cushing's syndrome caused by bronchial adenomas. Am. J. Med. 44:97-104, 1968.

Sullivan, M. Boileau, M., and Hodges, C. V. Adrenal cortical carcinoma. J. Urol. 120:660-665, 1978.

Symington, T. Functional Pathology of the Human Adrenal Gland. Baltimore: The Williams & Wilkins Company, 1969.

Tang, C. K. and Gray, G. F. Adrenocortical neoplasms. Urology 5:691-695, 1975.

———, Harriman, B. B., and Toker, C. Myxoid adrenal cortical carcinoma. Arch. Pathol. Lab. Med. 103:635-638, 1979.

Tannenbaum, M. Ultrastructural pathology of the adrenal cortex. Pathol. Annu. 8:109-156, 1973.

Telner, A. H. Adrenal cortical carcinoma: an unusual cause of hyperaldosteronism. Can. Med. Assoc. J. 129:731-732, 1983.

Valente, M., Pennelli, N., Segato, P., Bevilacqua, L., and Thiene, G. Androgen producing adrenocortical carcinoma. Virchows Arch [Pathol. Anat.] 378:91-103, 1978.

Visser, H. K. A. The adrenal cortex in childhood. Arch. Dis. Child. 41:113-136, 1966.

Weiss, L. M. Comparative histologic study of 43 metastasizing and nonmetastasizing adrenocortical tumors. Am. J. Surg. Pathol. 8:163-169, 1984.

Welsh, R. A., Bray, D. M. III, Shipkey, F. H., and Meyer, A. T. Histogenesis of alveolar soft part sarcoma. Cancer 29:191-204, 1972.

METASTATIC CARCINOMA

Incidence. Metastases to the adrenal glands are frequently seen at autopsy. As many as 27 percent of patients dying with carcinomas have been found to harbor adrenal metastases at autopsy (Abrams et al.). Carcinomas of the lung and breast, as well as malignant melanoma, are the tumors with the highest incidence of adrenal metastases. In one recorded series, 26 of 95 patients with breast cancer undergoing adrenalectomy had adrenal metastases (Brown et al.). Cho and Choi reported a 36 percent incidence of mammary carcinoma metastatic to adrenal at autopsy. Auerbach and associates found lung carcinoma metastatic to adrenal in 34 percent of autopsied patients. Retrospective studies of patients dying with esophageal, gastric, and colorectal cancer have shown 10.3, 16, and 14 percent adrenal involvement, respectively, at autopsy (Cedermark et al.). Metastases are found in the adrenal glands of 7 to 19 percent of autopsied patients who died of renal cell carcinoma (Campbell et al.) Not surprisingly, autopsy studies of adrenal metastases from other countries reflect the common tumors of the particular locale. For example, Burkitt's lymphoma is the most common adrenal metastasis in Nigeria (Ejeckman and Attah).

Clinical Diagnosis. Metastases to the adrenal glands are usually clinically inapparent (Zornoza et al.) even when bilateral, but instances of adrenal insufficiency due to this cause have been reported (Vieweg et al.; Seidenwurm et al.). The rarity of adrenal insufficiency associated with bilateral adrenal metastases is due to the fact that residual cortex is almost always present. Massive bilateral adrenal metastases are often detectable by computerized axial tomography (fig. 127) or selective arteriography (fig. 128). In the relatively unusual cases of adrenal insufficiency due to carcinomatosis, a low plasma cortisol unresponsive to ACTH infusion is present.

Gross. The appearance of adrenals bearing metastatic tumors varies considerably, according to the type of tumor present (pl. X). As a rule, total destruction of the cortex does not take place and residual foci of cortex may be appreciated. Renal cell carcinoma, which may invade the ipsi- or contralateral adrenal, is characteristically coarsely nodular, while squamous cell carcinoma is gray white. Both may attain considerable size without causing adrenal insufficiency (pl. X). Small cell undifferentiated (oat cell) carcinoma from the lung may produce a composite pattern of adrenal enlargement

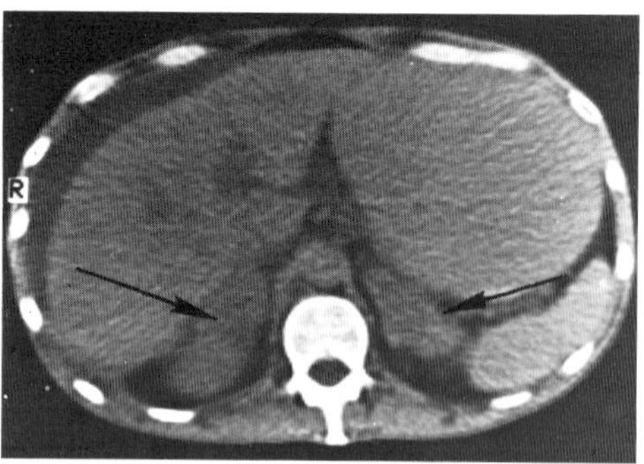

Figure 127
(Figures 127 and 128 from same patient)
METASTATIC CARCINOMA
Computerized axial tomographic (CAT) scan demonstrates bilateral adrenal masses (arrows) adjacent to vertebral column in a 49 year old man with metastatic squamous cell carcinoma of bronchogenic origin (see pl. X-E). The patient had hypocortisolism unresponsive to ACTH stimulation.

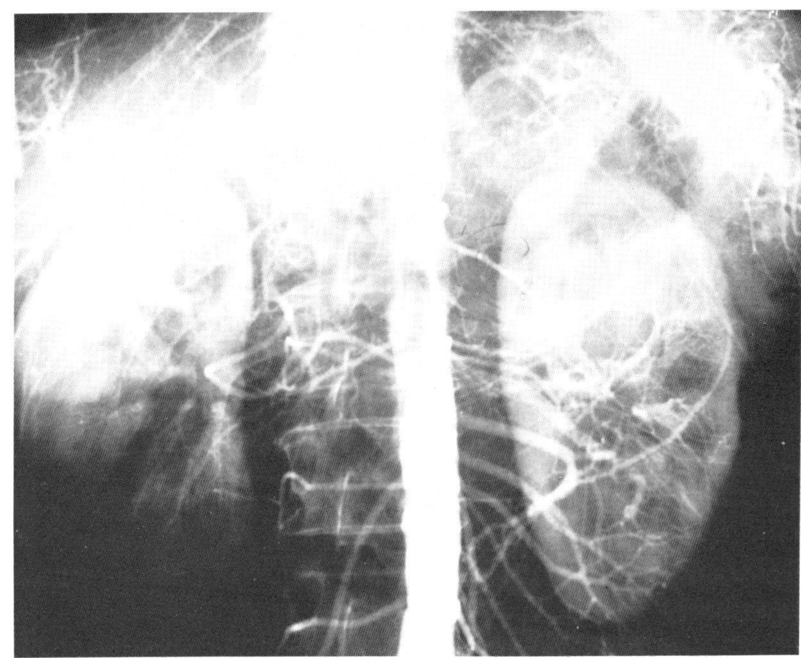

Figure 128
METASTATIC CARCINOMA
Aortic arteriogram demonstrates bilateral hypervascular suprarenal masses.

by a combination of metastasis and hyperplasia due to ectopic ACTH production. Adenocarcinomas may infiltrate the gland, producing diffuse enlargement.

Microscopic. The histologic appearance of carcinoma metastatic to the adrenal gland resembles that of the primary tumor. Bronchogenic carcinomas are among the leading causes of adrenal metastases (fig. 129). In the case of poorly differentiated neoplasms, this may be of little aid in localizing the site of the primary tumor. Squamous cell and adenocarcinomas (fig. 130) of bronchogenic origin characteristically metastasize to the adrenal gland, occasionally attaining large dimensions. Residual adrenal tissue can usually be identified. This is often in the region of the central vein and outer cortex. In some instances, the original outline of the glands is totally obscured by massive tumor involvement (fig. 131). Small cell undifferentiated carcinoma characteristically widely infiltrates the gland. In some cases, ACTH production by the tumor produces bizarre enlargement of adjacent adrenocortical cells (fig. 132). In contrast, such changes are absent surrounding metastatic squamous cell (fig. 129) or large cell undifferentiated carcinomas (fig. 133). Other neuroendocrine pulmonary tumors may metastasize to the adrenal glands. These metastases may obliterate the gland (figs. 134–136), producing a confusing picture often solved only by electron microscopy.

PLATE X
METASTATIC CARCINOMA

(Plate X-A and figure 91 from same case)

A. Metastatic renal cell carcinoma to adrenal produced massive expansion and destruction. Note multinodularity. X.33. (Courtesy of Dr. G. Gray, New York, NY.)

B. Renal cell carcinoma invades adrenal by direct continuity. Note adrenal extending to left and downward from upper, white tumor nodule. X.33.

C. Solitary metastasis from renal carcinoma attenuates cortical tissue at upper and lower portions of picture. X2.5.

D. Squamous carcinoma of lung replaces much of adrenal. Note dull cut surface and small amounts of remaining brown cortical tissue (arrows). X1.5.

E. Poorly differentiated squamous carcinoma of lung expands and replaces each adrenal, producing clinical hypocorticism in this patient. X.33.

F. This markedly hyperplastic adrenal is characteristic of ectopic ACTH production from small cell carcinoma of lung. Metastatic tumor is present in small white translucent foci (arrows). No medulla is present in this cross section. Actual size.

G. Hepatocellular carcinoma is metastatic within the adrenal gland. Dark brown color, although characteristic of primary liver tumors, resembles some adrenal cortical neoplasms, but contrasts with the surrounding adrenal tissue (a). X1.25.

PLATE X

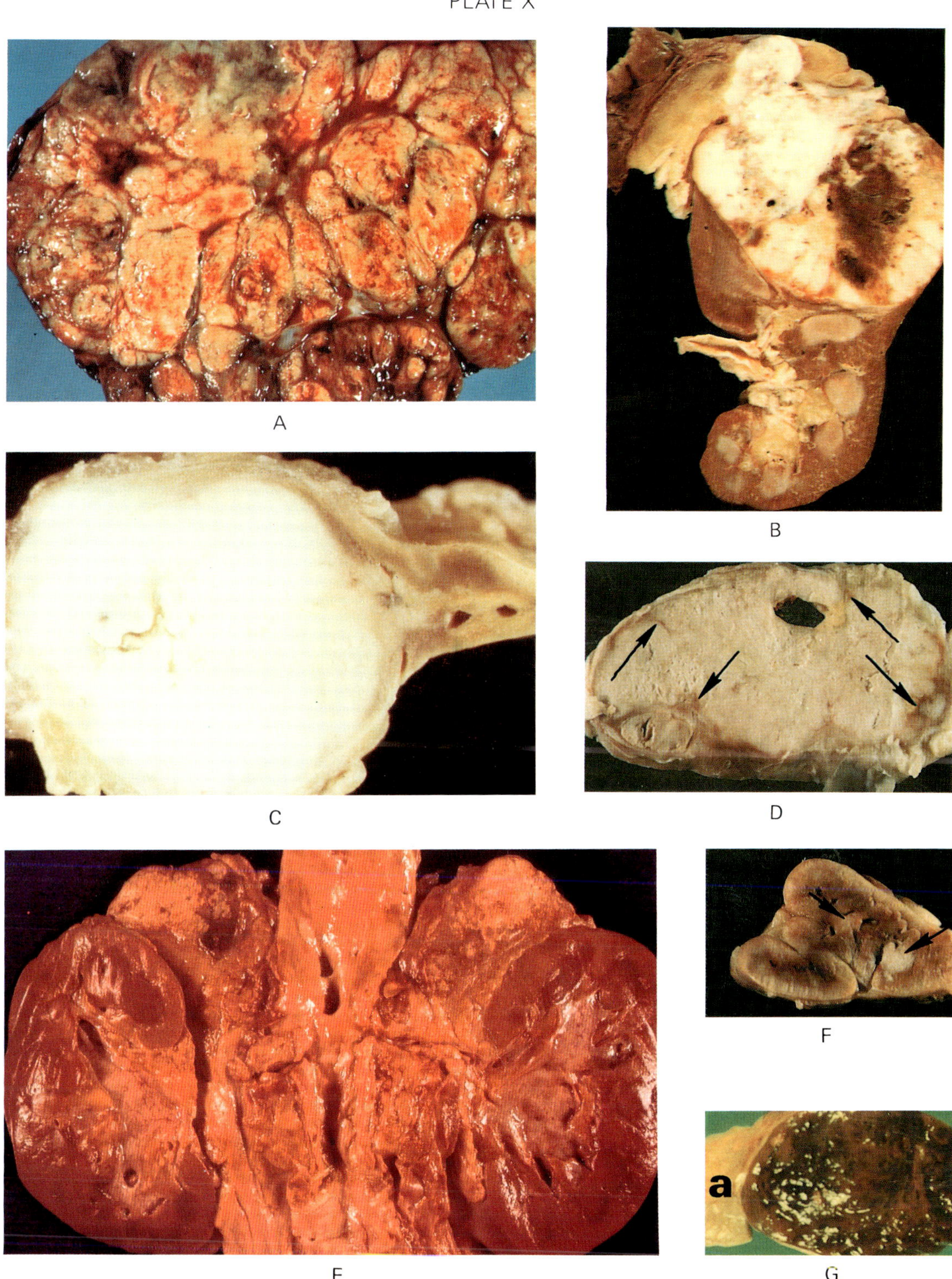

A

B

C

D

E

F

G

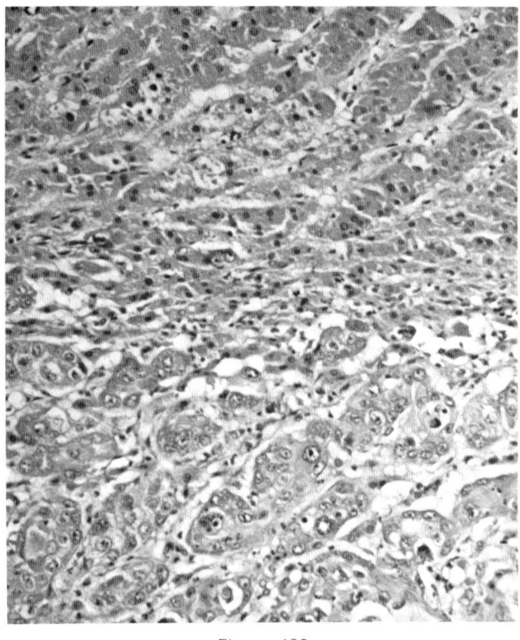

Figure 129
METASTATIC CARCINOMA
Squamous cell carcinoma of bronchogenic origin is
metastatic to adrenal gland. Note sharp demarcation
between tumor (lower) and adrenal (upper), as well as lack
of reactive changes in the adrenal cells. X160.

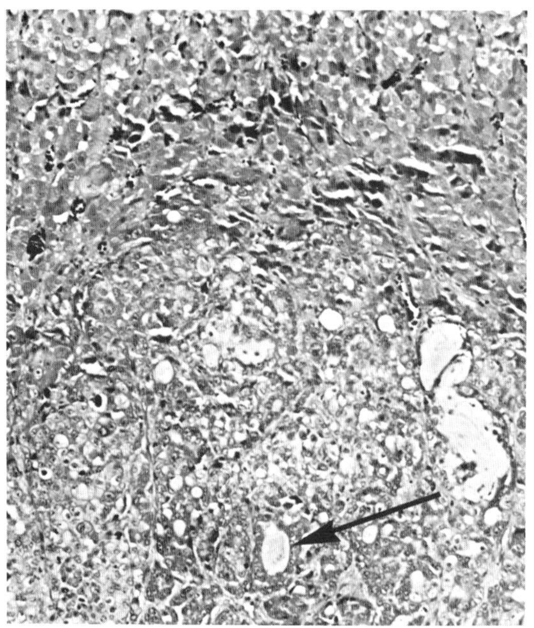

Figure 130
METASTATIC CARCINOMA
Gland formation (arrow) is apparent in this metastasis
from adenocarcinoma of lung. X120.

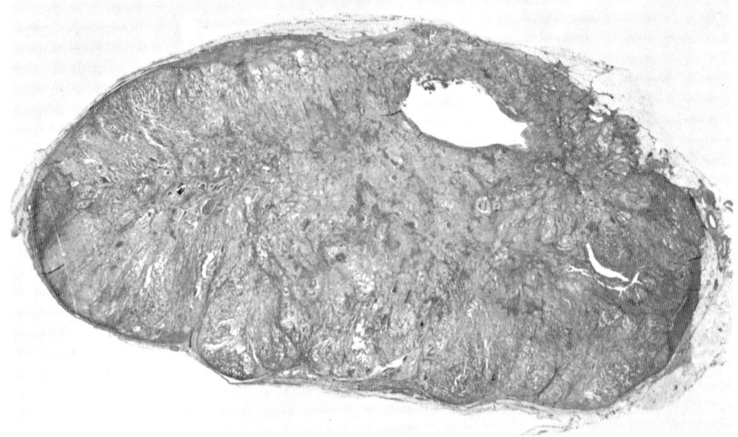

Figure 131
METASTATIC CARCINOMA
Note dilatation of central vein. Residual adrenal tissue survived in this region and
in several subcapsular areas despite extensive involvement by pulmonary squamous
carcinoma. The patient was not Addisonian. X1.5.

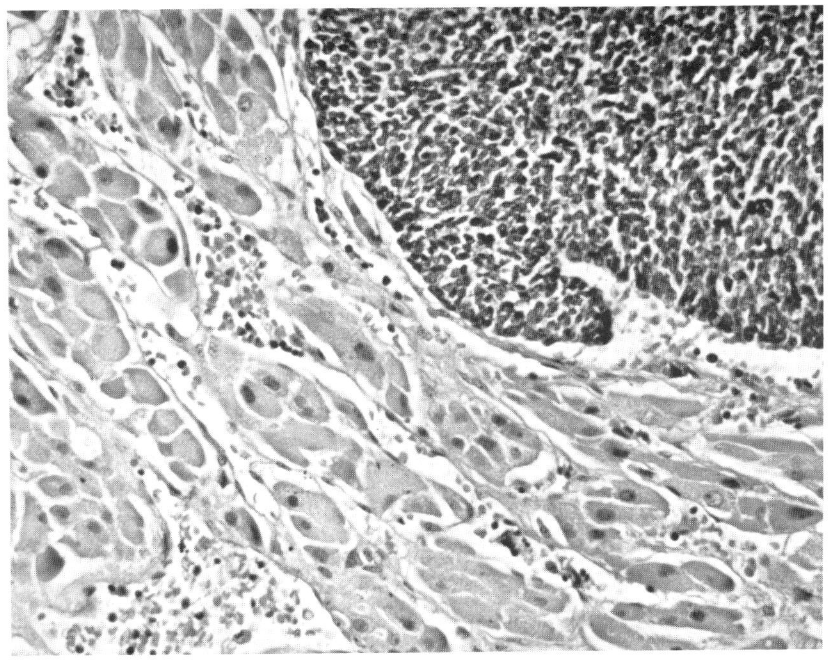

Figure 132
METASTATIC CARCINOMA
Adrenal cells are bizarre and hypertrophic adjacent to metastatic oat cell carcinoma from lung. Tumor produced the ectopic ACTH syndrome. X160.

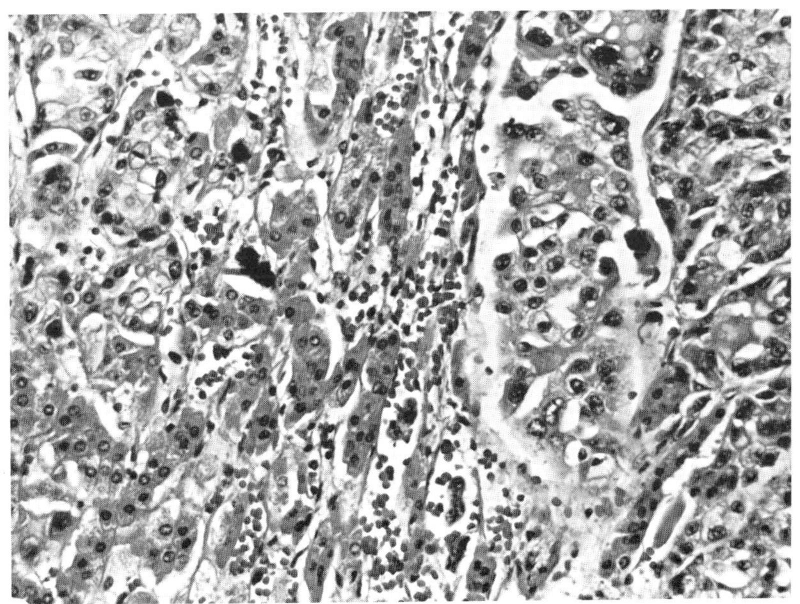

Figure 133
METASTATIC CARCINOMA
Large cell undifferentiated carcinoma of lung metastatic to adrenal gland is seen at right. Note resemblance to adrenal cells on left. X210.

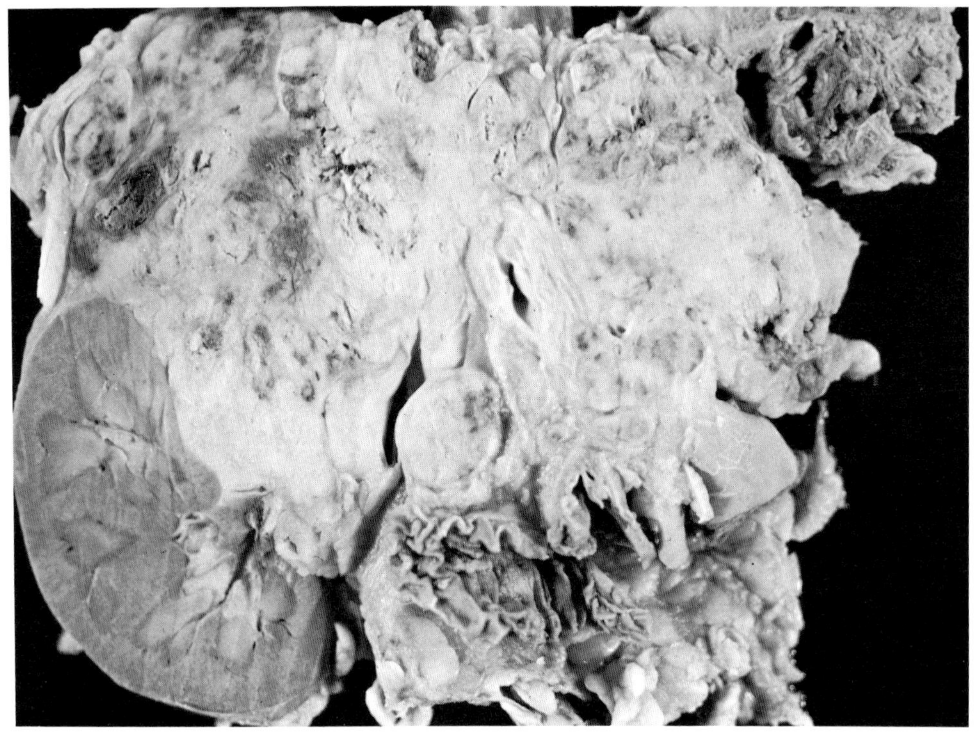

Figure 134
(Figures 134–136 from same patient)
METASTATIC CARCINOMA
Extensive metastasis of mediastinal carcinoid tumor obliterates both adrenal glands. View is from anterior, with right kidney still in place. Patient had neither hypo- nor hypercortisolism clinically.

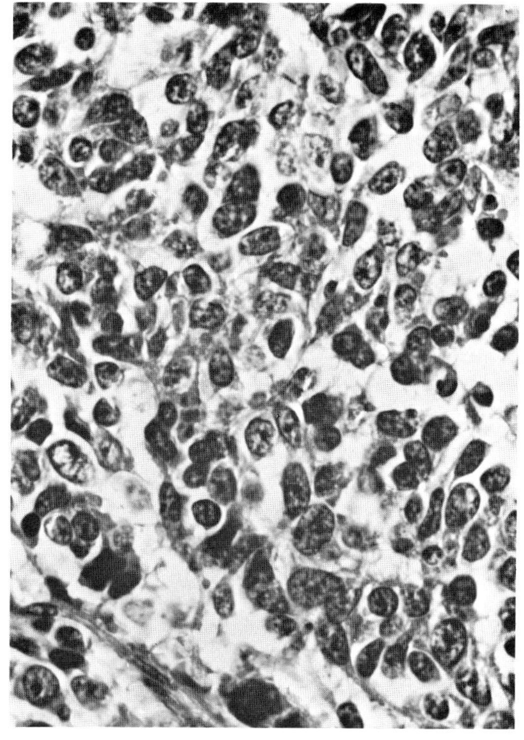

Figure 135
METASTATIC CARCINOMA
Photomicrograph of tumor demonstrates high nuclear-cytoplasmic ratio without evidence of differentiation. X525.

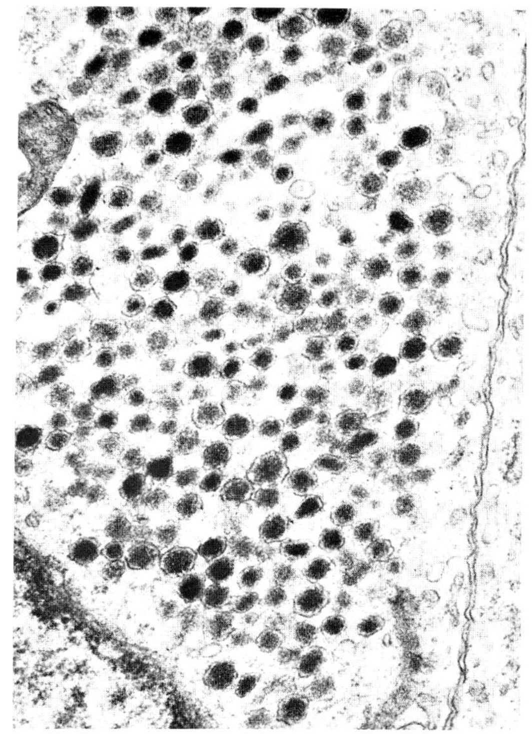

Figure 136
METASTATIC CARCINOMA
Numerous dense core neurosecretory granules are present in this electron micrograph of tumor. Uranyl acetate-lead citrate. X39,000. (Courtesy of Dr. A. Glick, Nashville, TN.)

Metastatic hepatocellular carcinoma to the adrenal gland may cause diagnostic confusion with a primary adrenal cortical carcinoma (fig. 137). However, electron microscopy will usually demonstrate mitochondrial inclusions and bile canaliculi characteristic of the former. Renal cell carcinoma (fig. 138) has a tendency toward solitary adrenal metastasis (Foucar and Dehner) which, on occasion, may resemble a primary adrenal tumor. Renal cell carcinoma may also develop after radiation for primary adrenal carcinoma (Andler et al.).

Diffuse microscopic involvement of the adrenal glands is characteristic of metastatic breast cancer (fig. 139). Although this condition is not often associated with clinical symptomatology, it may be encountered commonly in surgical material if endocrine ablation is attempted (Brown et al.).

Electron microscopic examination may be valuable in establishing the nonadrenal cortical nature of a neoplasm in the gland. Many large cell undifferentiated carcinomas of pulmonary origin metastasize to the adrenal glands. These carcinomas resemble dysplastic adrenal cortical cells (fig. 133), but lack ultrastructural characteristics of adrenal cells such as specialized mitochondria or smooth endoplasmic reticulum.

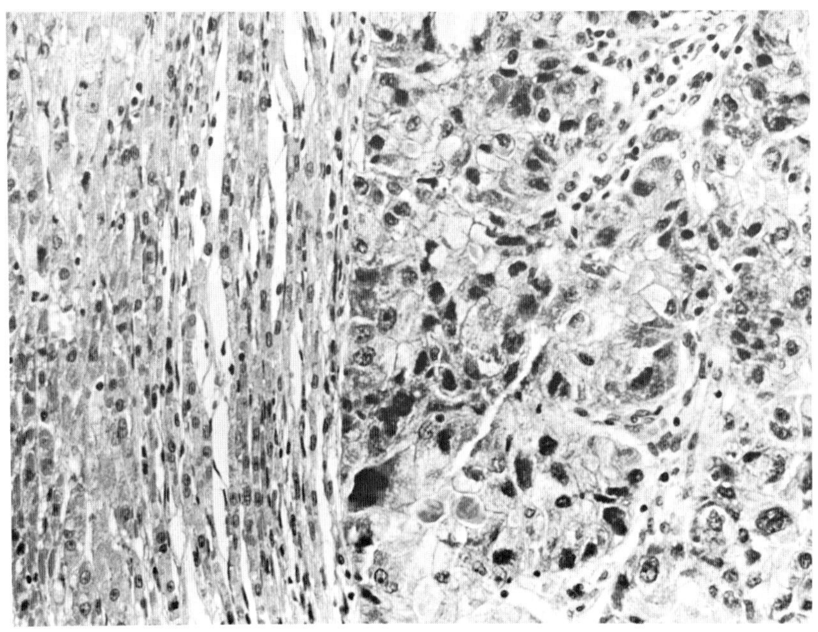

Figure 137
METASTATIC CARCINOMA
Pleomorphic tumor cells (right) of this metastatic hepatocellular carcinoma could be easily confused with primary adrenocortical carcinoma. Note the compression of the adjacent adrenal cortical cells (left). Bile staining was not present. X260.

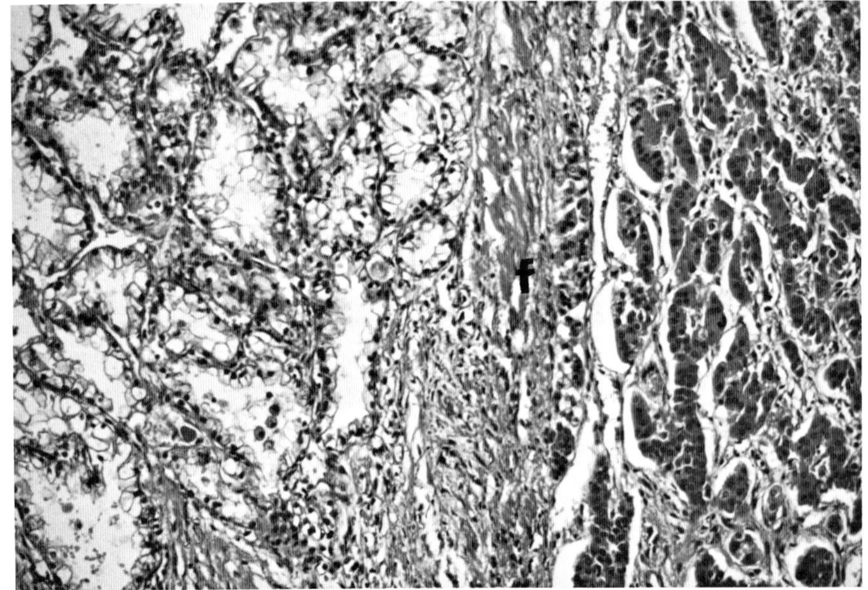

Figure 138
METASTATIC CARCINOMA
Clear glycogen-filled tumor cells (left) from this metastatic renal cell carcinoma encroach upon adrenal tissue at the right. A fibrotic pseudocapsule (f) separates the two. X210.

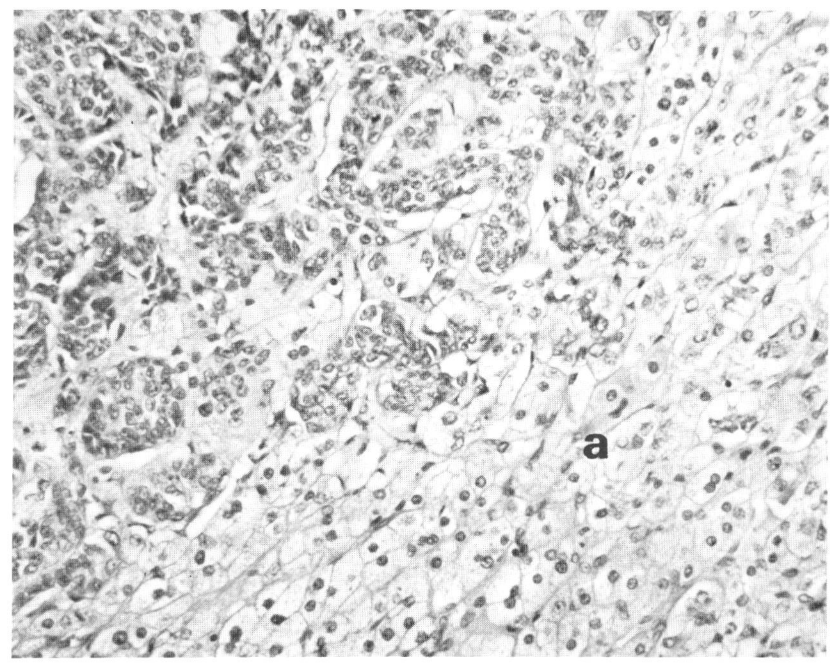

Figure 139
METASTATIC CARCINOMA
Nests and columns of breast carcinoma cells infiltrate the adrenal tissue (a) (right). Such
infiltration is characteristic of most mammary carcinoma metastases in the gland. X160.

Poorly differentiated squamous cell carcinomas of bronchogenic origin may also resemble a primary adrenal carcinoma. However, the ultrastructural appearance of cytoplasmic vacuoles surrounded by tonofilaments is characteristic of these tumors (fig. 140).

Differential Diagnosis. Primary adrenocortical carcinomas may be confused with a metastatic lesion only in special cases when the histologic appearance bears some resemblance to a poorly differentiated adrenocortical primary tumor. Examples of such neoplasms include hepatocellular carcinoma (fig. 127), large cell undifferentiated lung carcinoma (fig. 133), and malignant melanoma (fig. 141). Rarely, endometrial carcinoma may cause confusion in an adrenal metastasis (Nakano et al.). Even more

rarely, paragangliomas or adrenal medullary tumors may metastasize to the contralateral adrenal (figs. 142, 143). This situation can cause considerable diagnostic confusion, especially if the primary adrenal medullary tumor is not large. In this case, it may be impossible to distinguish a metastasis from multifocal primary adrenal medullary tumors. The clinical circumstances, histochemistry, and electron microscopic findings characteristic of these metastatic tumors usually allow prompt distinction from primary adrenal cortical tumors.

References

Abrams, H. L., Spiro, R., and Goldstein, N. Metastases in carcinoma. Cancer 3:74-85. 1950.
Andler, W., Havers, W., Stambolis, C., Medrano, J., and Stollmann, B. Renal cell carcinoma following radiation therapy for an adrenal cortical carcinoma. J. Pediatr. 93:634-636, 1978.

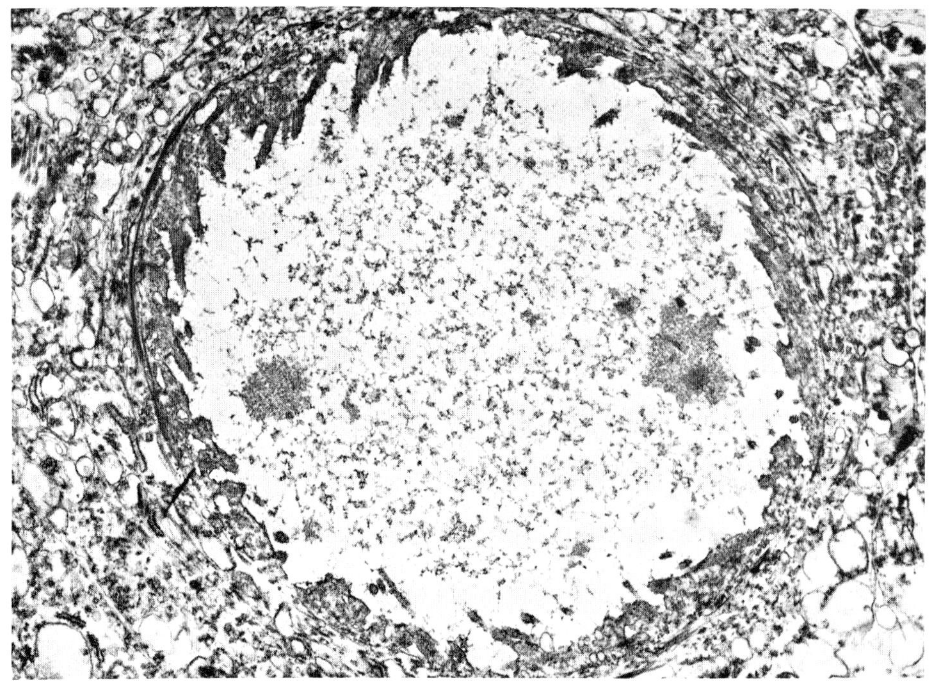

Figure 140
METASTATIC CARCINOMA
Poorly differentiated squamous cell carcinomas of lung frequently contain vesicles surrounded by tonofilaments, as depicted here. Primary adrenal carcinomas never manifest these structures. Uranyl acetate-lead citrate. X70,000. (Courtesy of Dr. A. Glick, Nashville, TN.)

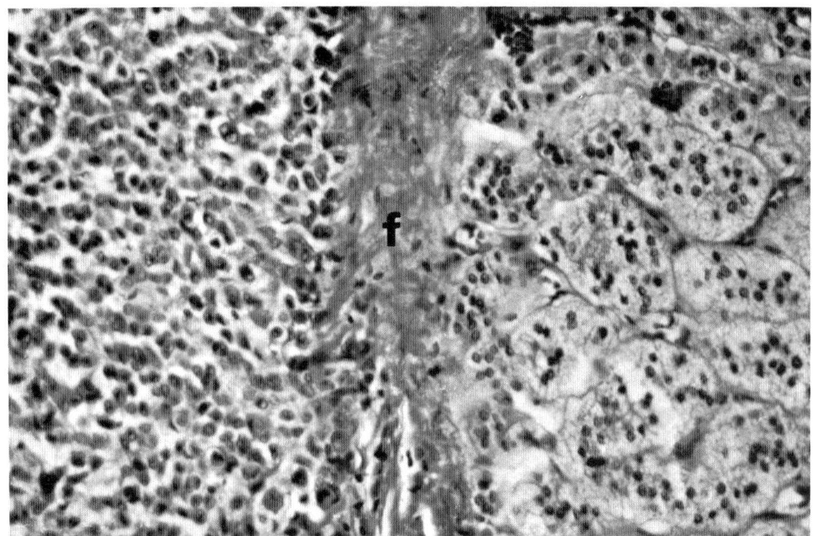

Figure 141
METASTATIC CARCINOMA
Adrenal tissue (right) is separated by a narrow band of connective tissue (f) from metastatic malignant melanoma. Stains of tumor revealed melanin. Primary tumor was removed many years previously. X250.

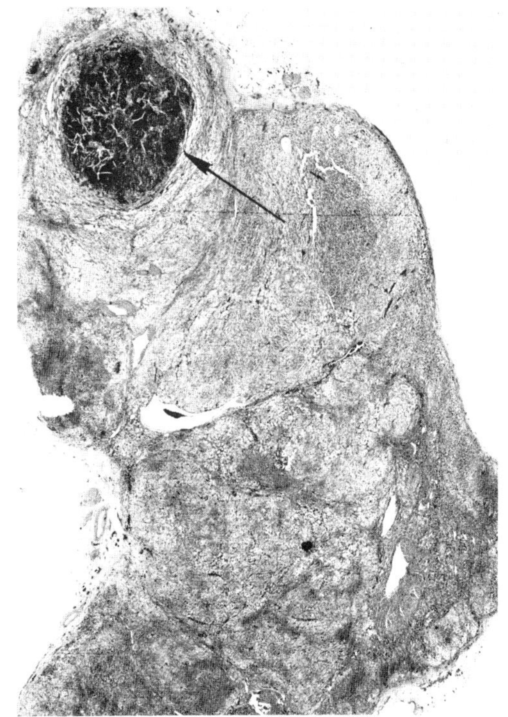

Figure 142
(Figures 142 and 143 from same patient)
METASTATIC CARCINOMA
Low power view of adrenal that contains metastases
(arrow) from a paraganglioma of the opposite adrenal. Note
sharp demarcation of tumor deposit. X3.5.

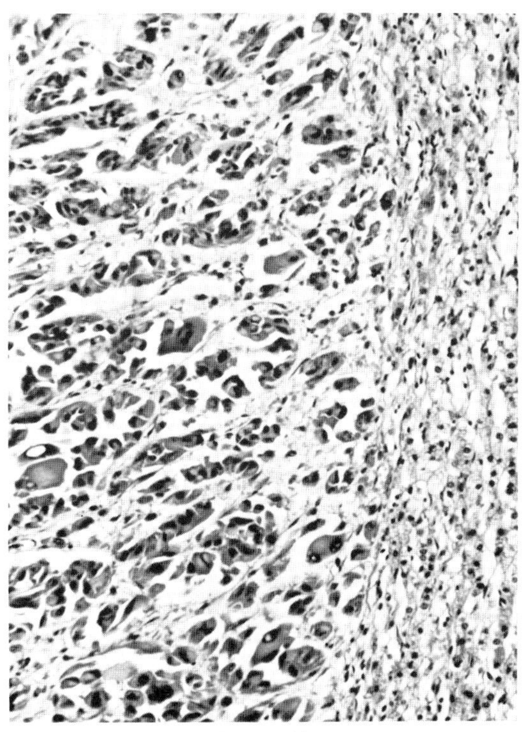

Figure 143
METASTATIC CARCINOMA
Note the pleomorphic pattern of neoplasm (left). Tumor
cells superficially resemble those of an adrenal cortical carcinoma, but fluorescence was demonstrated in cytoplasmic
granules after exposure to formaldehyde vapor. X120.

Auerbach, O., Garfinkel, L., and Parks, V. R. Histologic
type of lung cancer in relation to smoking habits, year
of diagnosis and sites of metastases. Chest 67:382-387,
1975.

Brown, P. W., Terz, J. J., King, R., and Lawrence, W., Jr.
Bilateral adrenalectomy for metastatic breast carcinoma. Arch. Surg. 110:77-81, 1975.

Campbell, C. M., Middleton, R. G., and Rigby, O. F.
Adrenal metastasis in renal cell carcinoma. Urology
21:403-405, 1983.

Cedermark, B. J., Blumenson, L. E., Pickren, J. W., and
Elias, E. G. The significance of metastases to the
adrenal gland from carcinoma of the stomach and
esophagus. Surg. Gynecol. Obstet. 145:41-48, 1977.

———, Blumenson, L. E., Pickren, J. W., Holyoke, D. E.,
and Elias, E. G. The significance of metastases to the
adrenal glands in adrenocarcinoma of the colon and
rectum. Surg. Gynecol. Obstet. 144:537-546, 1977.

Chu, S. Y., and Choi, H. Y. Causes of death and metastatic
patterns in patients with mammary cancer. Am. J.
Clin. Pathol. 73:232-234, 1980.

Ejeckam, G. C. and Attah, Ed'B. Pattern of secondary
adrenal tumors in Ibadan, Nigeria. Int. Surg.
60:368-369, 1975.

Foucar, E. and Dehner, L. P. Renal cell carcinoma occurring with contralateral adrenal metastasis. Arch. Surg.
114:959-963, 1979.

Nakano, K. K. and Schoene, W. C. Endometrial carcinoma
with a predominant clear-cell pattern with metastases
to the adrenal, posterior mediastinum and brain. Am.
J. Obstet. Gynecol. 122:529-530, 1975.

Seidenwurm, D. J., Elmer, E. B., Kaplan, L. M., Williams,
E. K., et al. Metastases to the adrenal glands and the
development of Addison's disease. Cancer 54:552-557,
1974.

Vieweg, W. V. R., Reitz, R. E., and Weinstein, R. L.
Addison's disease secondary to metastatic carcinoma:
an example of adrenocortical and adrenomedullary insufficiency. Cancer 31:1240-1243, 1973.

Zornoza, J., Bracken, R., and Wallace, S. Radiologic features of adrenal metastases. Urology 8:295-299, 1976.

UNUSUAL TUMORS OF THE ADRENAL CORTEX

MYELOLIPOMA AND RELATED LESIONS

SYNONYMS AND RELATED TERMS: Bone marrow heterotopia; myeloid metaplasia.

Definition. Adrenal myelolipomas are benign tumors or tumor-like lesions composed of mature fat and bone marrow.

Incidence. Myelolipomas (Oberling; De-Navasquez) are uncommonly encountered at autopsy, where they are usually incidental findings. They are usually seen in mature adults as incidental findings. Although most tumors are small, less than 4 cm. in diameter (Boudreaux et al.), larger tumors have presented with abdominal discomfort. The incidence at autopsy has been estimated at 0.08 to 0.4 percent (Olsson et al.).

Clinical Diagnosis. Larger myelolipomas likely to cause discomfort are usually readily apparent on CAT scans, intravenous pyelography, or arteriography (fig. 144), where they are seen as vascular masses

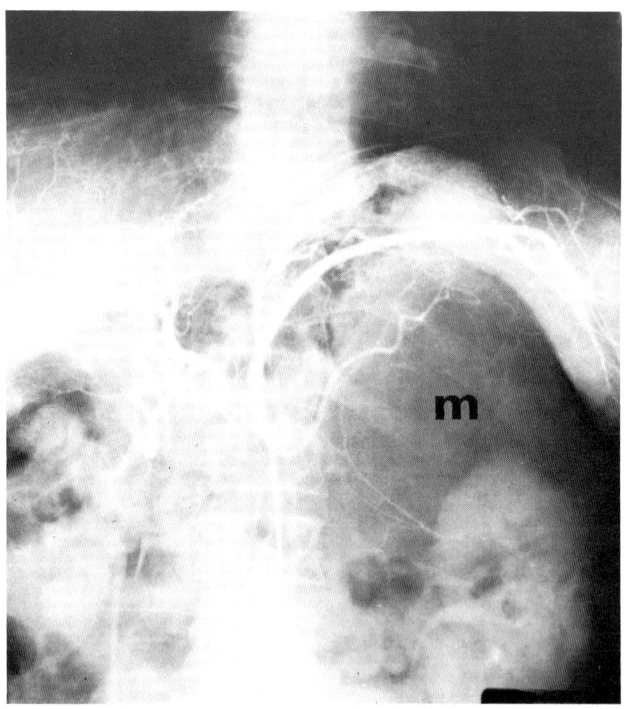

Figure 144
(Figures 144 and 147 from same patient)
MYELOLIPOMA
Celiac arteriogram demonstrates a large avascular mass (m) between spleen and kidney. Surgical exploration revealed a large myelolipoma. (From Bennett, B.D., McKenna, T.J., Hough, A.J., Dean, R., and Page, D.L. Adrenal myelolipoma associated with Cushing's disease. Am. J. Clin. Pathol. 73:443-447, 1980.)

displacing major vessels (Gee et al.). Rarely, rupture of the lesions may occur, causing severe abdominal hemorrhage (Dyckman and Freedman, Parsons and Thompson).

Endocrine dysfunction of various types has been associated with the development of these lesions. In two reported instances, prolonged ACTH stimulation was thought to be causal (Bennett et al.; Boudreaux et al.). It is of interest that microscopic myelolipomatous foci are seen in adrenal cortical hyperplasia associated with Cushing's disease (Collins), in experimental states of increased ACTH secretion (Selye and Stone), and in burn patients (Delarue and Monsaingeon). Myelolipomatous foci have also been described in adenomas (Cussen; McDonnell; Nicod), however, the distinction between adenoma and a nodular adrenal is not always clear.

Gross. Lesions are usually pale yellow with interspersed foci of red or pink representing hematopoietic components (Plate XI-A, C). Larger lesions may have a lobulated appearance (Plate XI-B). The lesions are unencapsulated, but may be multiple and bilateral (figs. 145, 146).

Microscopic. Lesions are composed of mature fat and proliferating hematopoietic tissue (fig. 147). Although lesions usually displace adrenal cortical tissue, at times

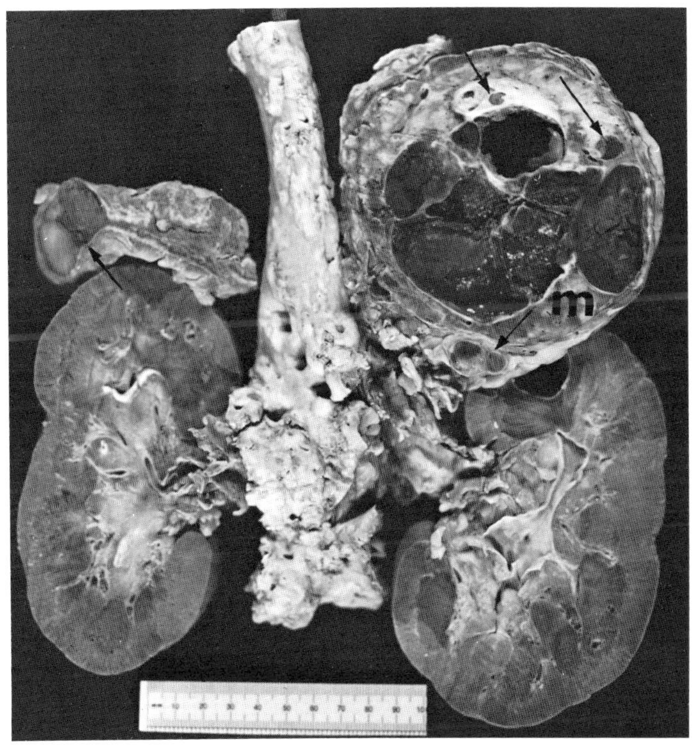

Figure 145
(Figures 145, 146, and 148 from same patient)
MYELOLIPOMA
Multiple myelolipomas (arrows) are seen in this case. Large cystic mass (m) is adrenal medullary tumor producing ectopic ACTH syndrome. Note hyperplastic contralateral adrenal. X.33.

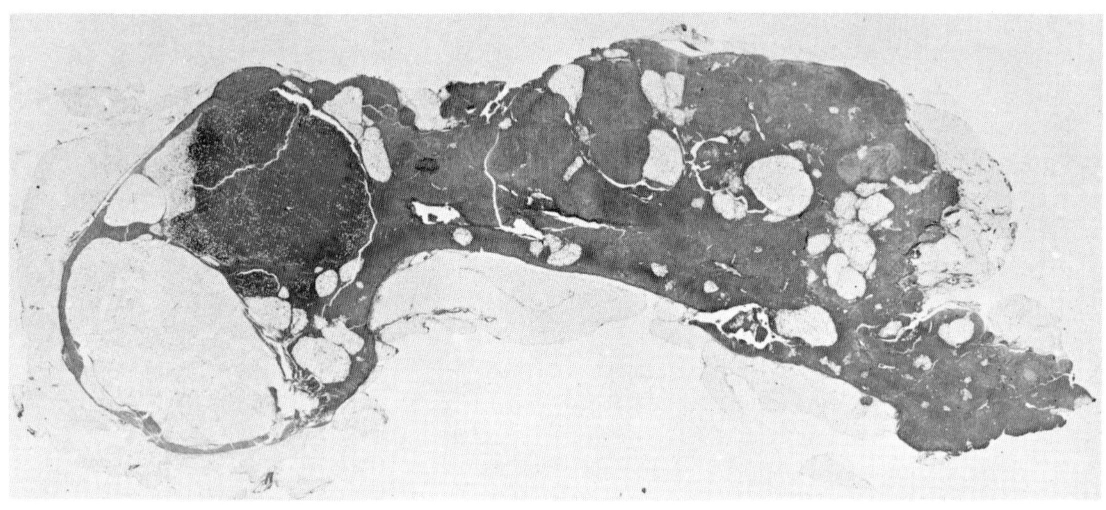

Figure 146
MYELOLIPOMA
Multiple myelolipomas, as denoted by clear areas, are present in hyperplastic adrenal gland. X3.2.

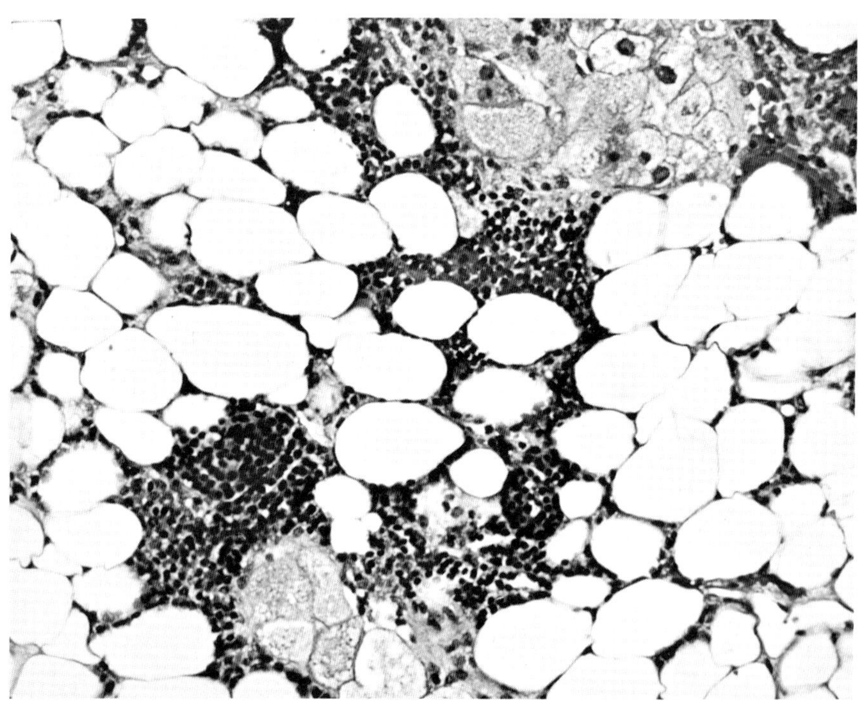

Figure 147
MYELOLIPOMA
Intimate arrangement of adipose tissue and hematopoietic elements is characteristic of myelolipoma. Note foci of adrenal cortical cells at upper right and lower center. X175.

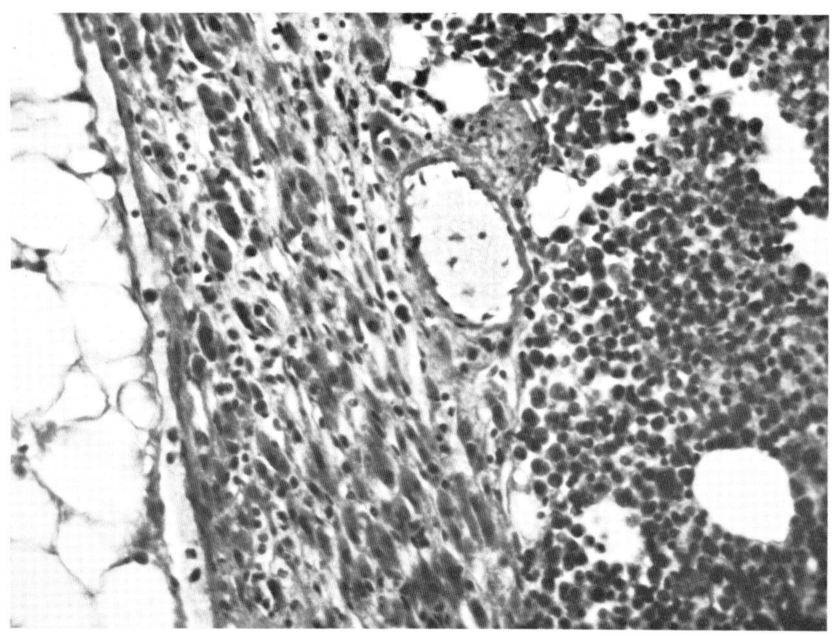

Figure 148
MYELOLIPOMA
More usual pattern of adrenal tissue surrounding the myelolipoma is shown in this photomicrograph. Adrenal tissue is displaced, but not invaded by the hematopoietic tissue. X160.

adrenal cortical cells may be intimately involved with the substance of the myelolipoma (figs. 147–149), as described by Boudreaux and colleagues and Bennett and associates. Adrenal cortical cells may be bizarre in appearance (fig. 149), especially in those cases associated with excess ACTH secretion. The hematopoietic tissue resembles active bone marrow and contains the various cell lines in different stages of maturation (fig. 150).

Natural History. Although there is debate as to the neoplastic or hyperplastic nature of myelolipomas, most current evidence favors a reactive or hyperplastic origin. This evidence includes the production of similar lesions in rats by ACTH and/or androgens (Selye and Stone) and the association of large myelolipomas with increased ACTH secretion in such states as Cushing's disease (Bennett et al.), congenital adrenal hyperplasia (Boudreaux et al.), and ectopic ACTH syndrome (fig. 145). At any rate, the tumors do not invade or behave in an aggressive manner. With the exception of displacement of viscera or the rare examples of rupture, complications are not seen.

Differential Diagnosis

Lipoma. Rarely, lipomas of the adrenal gland may be confused with myelolipomas. Lipomas contain no hematopoietic tissue. However, the same factors may be active in the causation of both, since lipomatous foci are often found in adrenals from patients with chronic disease.

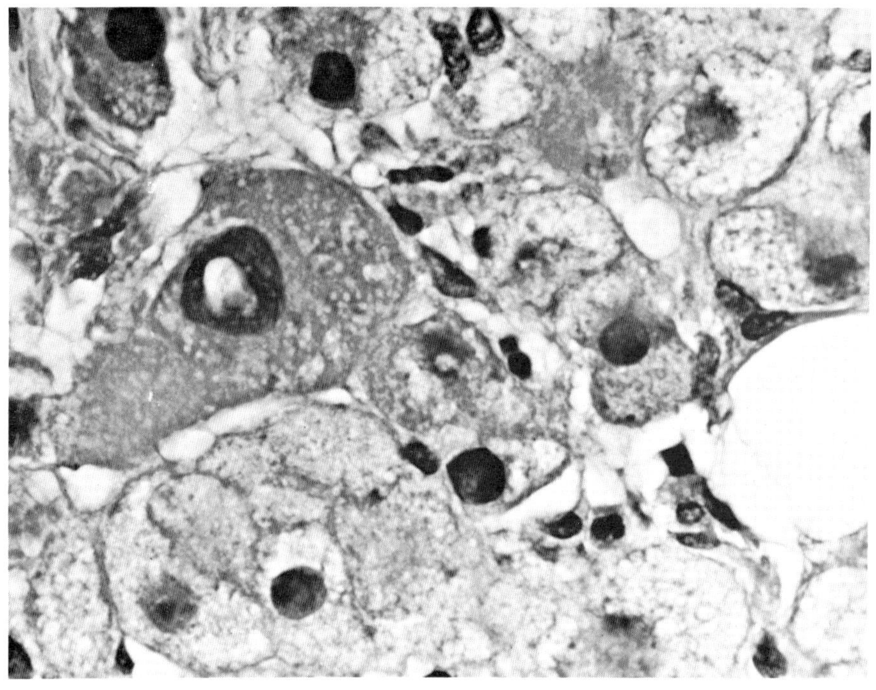

Figure 149
MYELOLIPOMA
Bizarre reactive changes in adrenal cortical cells may be seen in cases of myelolipoma associated with increased ACTH secretion. X800.

Extramedullary Hematopoiesis. In this condition, production of blood cells takes place in sites other than bone marrow. In extreme instances the adrenals may be involved, recapitulating early embryonic life. No fat is present in the gland. There is some evidence that the hematopoietic component in myelolipoma may contribute materially.

Adrenal Cortical Hyperplasia. Myelolipomatous and lipomatous foci are commonly seen in the adrenals in Cushing's disease (figs. 151, 152). These foci may be conspicuous, but should not distract from the basic pathology of Cushing's disease, with increase in thickness of both fasciculate and reticulate zones.

MISCELLANEOUS CONNECTIVE TISSUE TUMORS

ANGIOMAS

Rarely, true connective tissue neoplasms may originate in the adrenal cortex. These may include hemangiomas of both the capillary (fig. 153) and cavernous types (Rothberg et al.; Lang) and lymphangiomas (fig. 154). Clinical diagnosis may be aided by phleboliths and by hypervascularity on radiographic studies (Rothberg et al.). These tumors are usually asymptomatic, but may be mistaken for primary or secondary adrenal malignancy clinically.

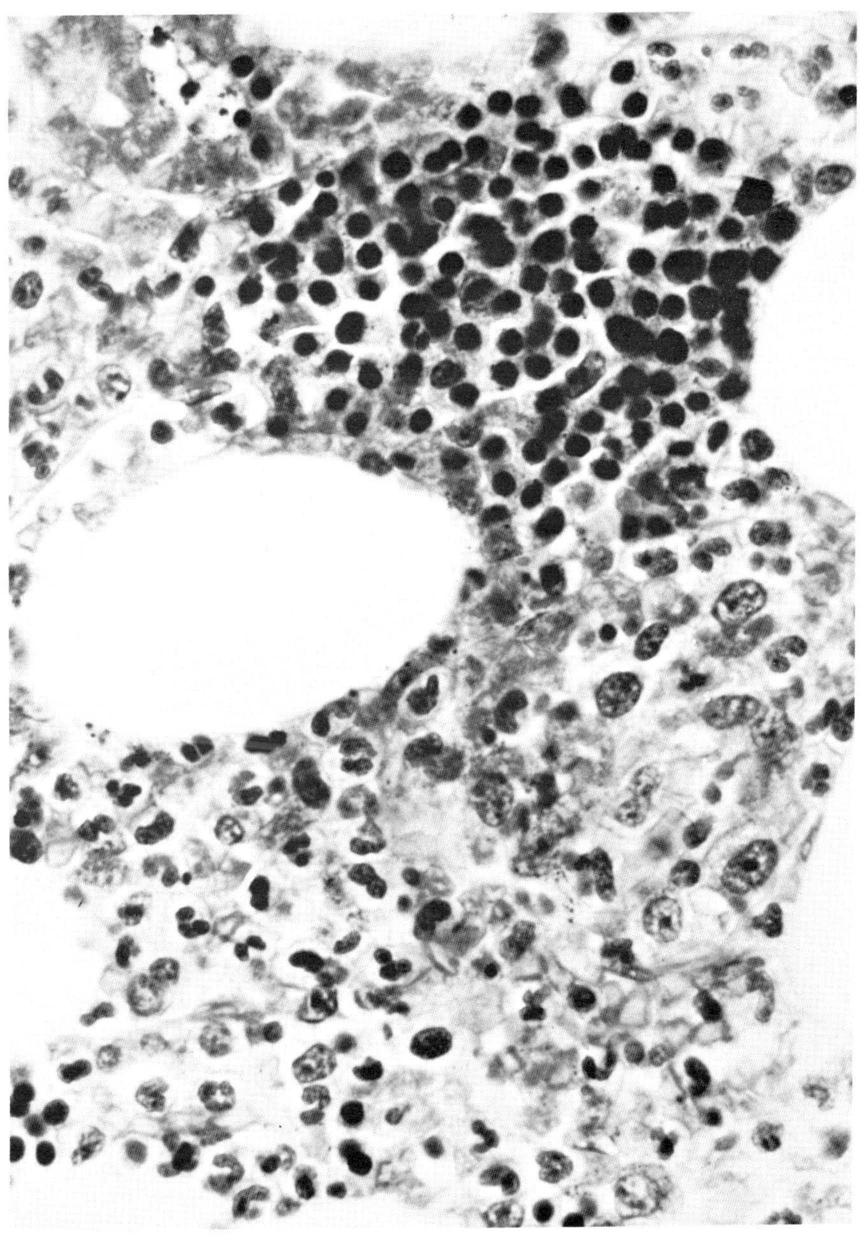

Figure 150
MYELOLIPOMA
A broad range of hematopoietic cell types may be present in myelolipomas. Note island of erythroblasts (upper right) and background of granulocytic precursors. X600.

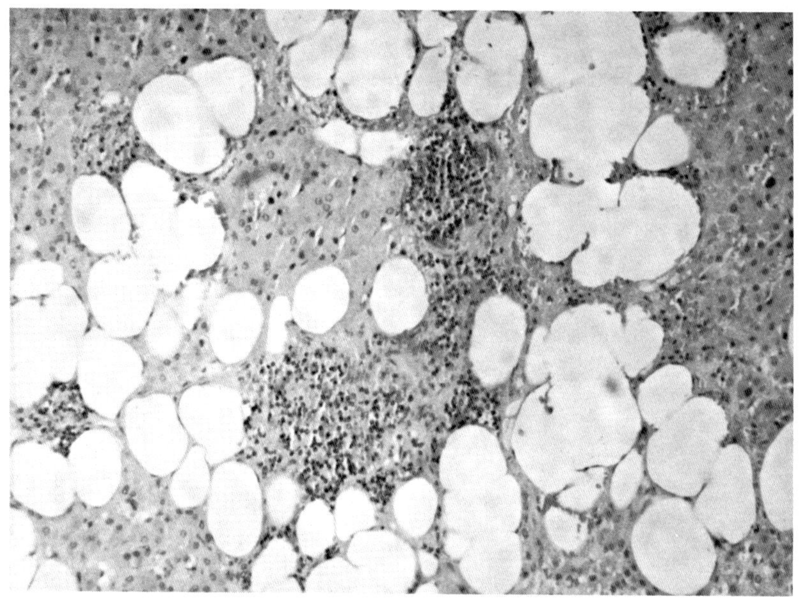

Figure 151
MYELOLIPOMA
Focal myelolipomatous change is seen in this adrenal from 48 year old man with
adrenal hyperplasia due to Cushing's disease. X100.

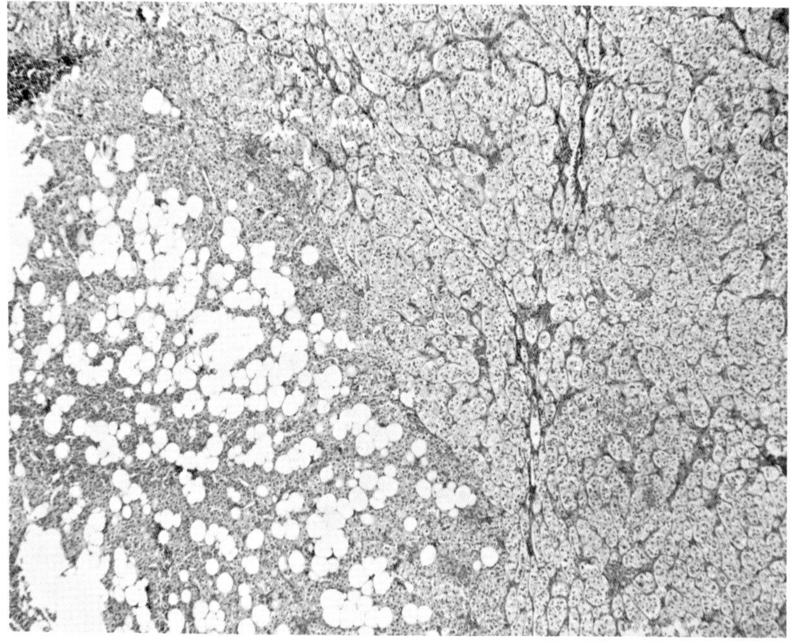

Figure 152
MYELOLIPOMA
Discrete myelolipoma has formed in this adrenal from a 38 year old woman with
Cushing's disease. X45.

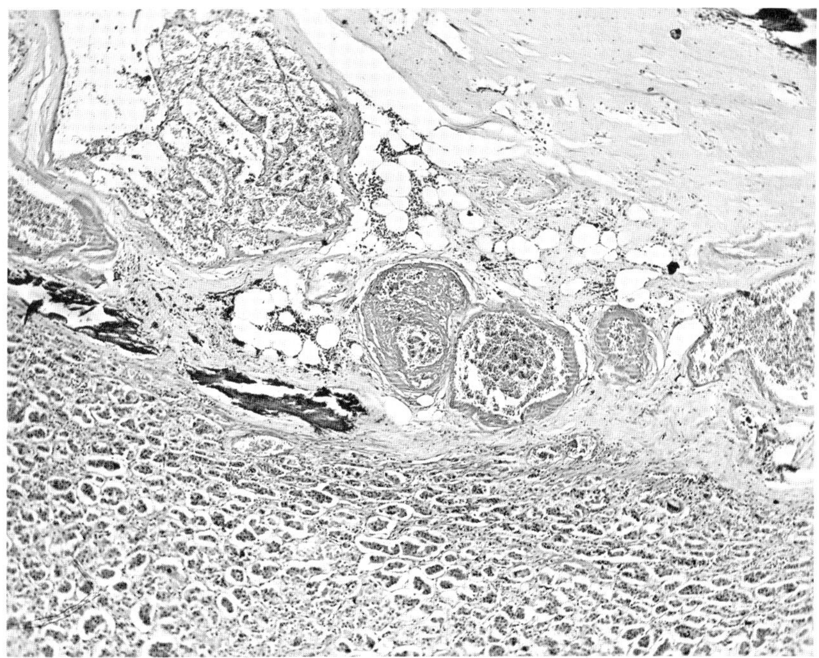

Figure 153
ANGIOMA
Angiomatous proliferation of vessels is noted in the capsule of this adrenal gland. X45.

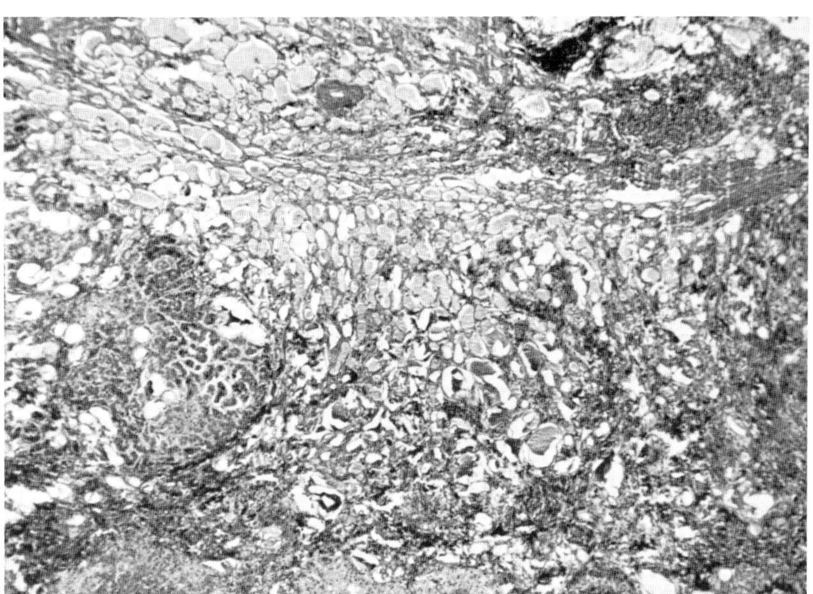

Figure 154
LYMPHANGIOMA
Lymphangioma occupies a considerable portion of this adrenal gland. This was an incidental finding. X63. (Courtesy of Department of Pathology, Johns Hopkins Hospital, Baltimore, MD.)

LEIOMYOMA AND OTHER MESENCHYMAL TUMORS

These tumors presumably originate from the musculature of the adrenal vasculature. At times, a continuity with the adrenal vein can be demonstrated. The tumors are usually small and discovered incidentally at autopsy (figs. 155, 156). Rarely, malignant connective tissue neoplasms, such as leiomyosarcomas (Choi and Liu), may arise in the adrenal cortex (fig. 157). Since these tumors metastasize widely and since adrenal carcinomas may be sarcomatoid, the adrenal origin of sarcomas is often debatable and most are likely metastatic to the adrenal from distant sites instead (Rao et al.).

MALIGNANT LYMPHOMA

With a few exceptions, primary or secondary involvement of the adrenal glands by malignant lymphoma is rare. Burkitt's lymphoma commonly involves the glands (Ejeckham and Attah). However, this is not seen among other types of lymphomas.

Plasmacytomas may be primary in the gland (fig. 158) and produce mass effects on radiographic studies. The histology of these lesions is similar to other extramedullary plasmacytomas (fig. 159). Secondary involvement of the gland by myeloma or by follicular lymphomas (fig. 160) is much more common than localized origin in the gland.

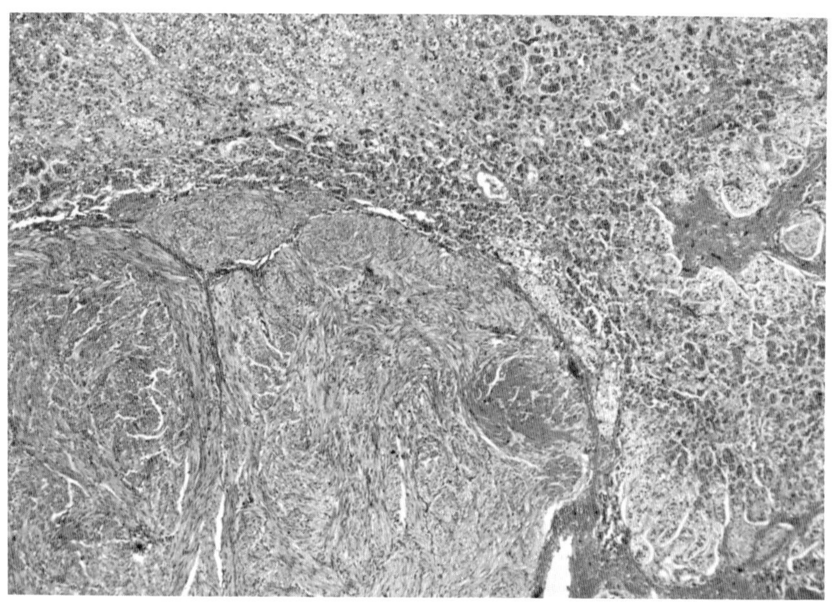

Figure 155
(Figures 155 and 156 from same patient)
LEIOMYOMA
This leiomyoma arose about the central vein (lower center). Note compression of the surrounding gland. X33. (Courtesy of Department of Pathology, Johns Hopkins Hospital, Baltimore, MD.)

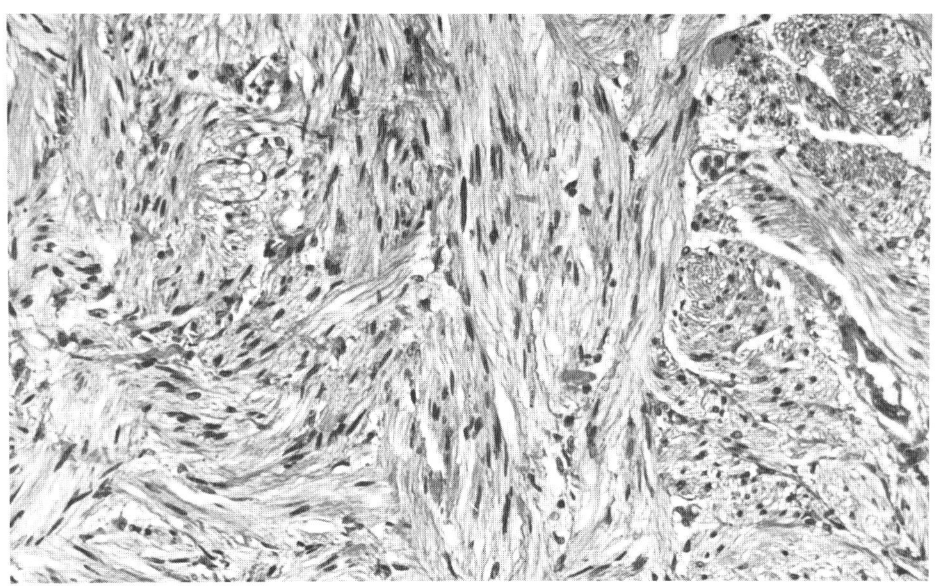

Figure 156
LEIOMYOMA
Higher power view shows characteristic interlacing bundles of leiomyoma. X250.

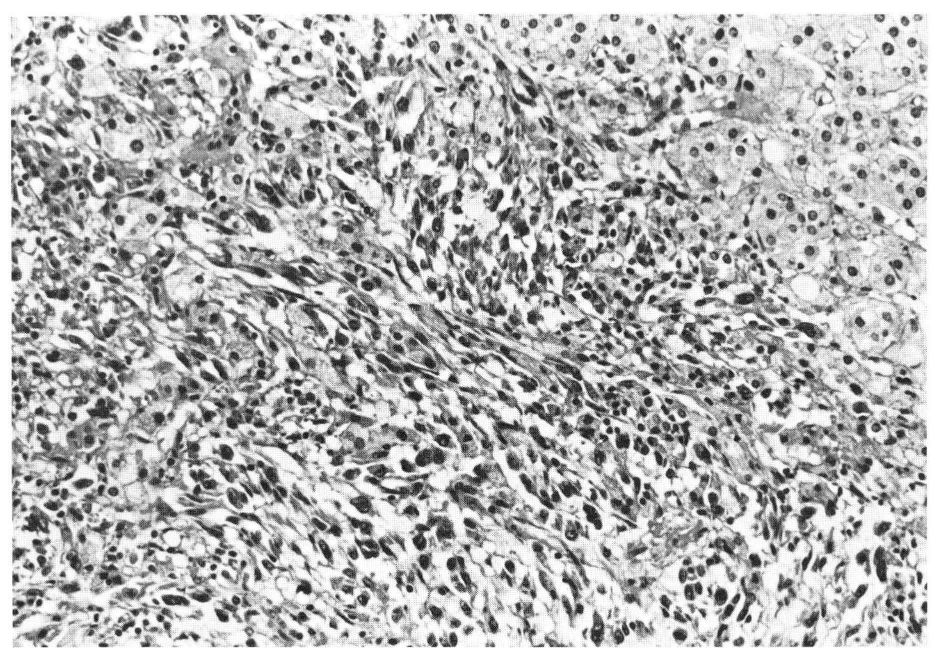

Figure 157
SARCOMA
Primary sarcoma of adrenal gland discovered at autopsy. Note junction with adrenal tissue (upper right). The only other tumor noted was a squamous cell carcinoma of the scalp. X100. (Courtesy of Dr. J. Connolly, Boston, MA.)

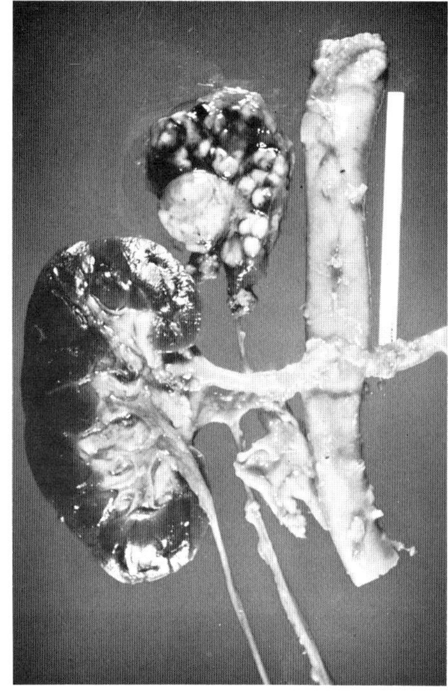

Figure 158
(Figures 158 and 159 from same patient)
PLASMACYTOMA
Extramedullary plasmacytoma of the adrenal distorts the
outline of the gland. Multiple nodules are present. X.33.
(Courtesy of Royal Marsden Hospital, London, England.)

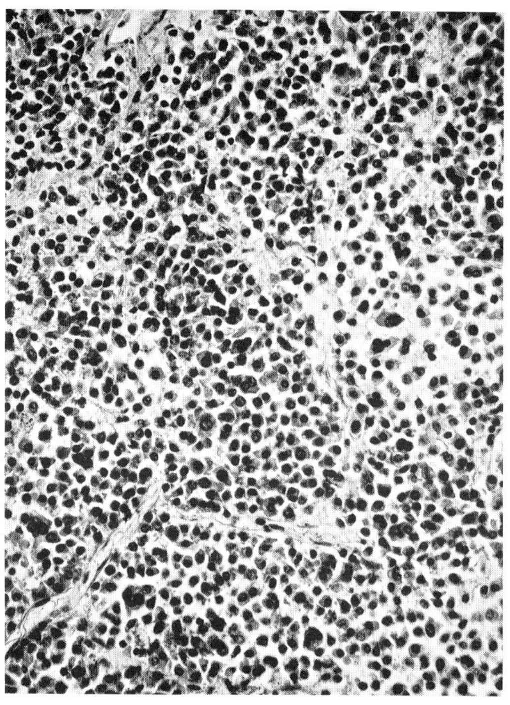

Figure 159
PLASMACYTOMA
Plasmacytoma of adrenal gland demonstrates bizarre
plasma cells separated by thin connective tissue septae of
residual adrenal gland. X160.

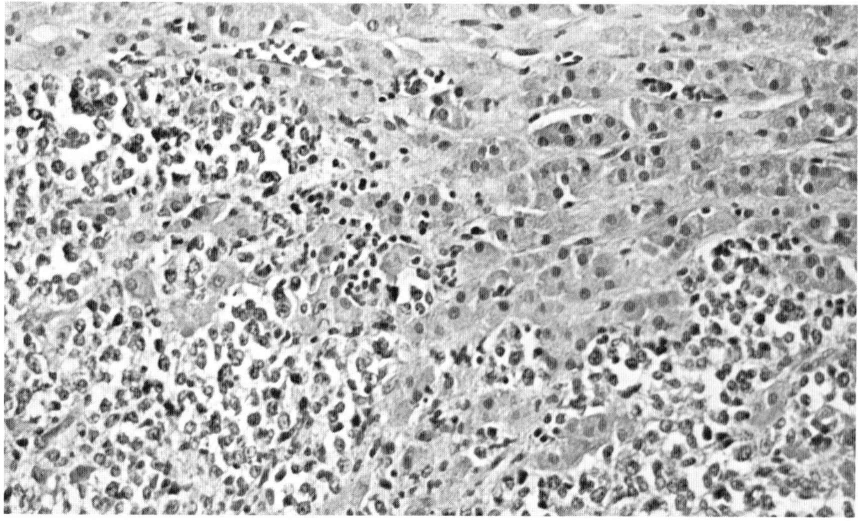

Figure 160
LYMPHOMA
Malignant lymphoma involves adrenal gland. This is uncommon even in advanced cases.
Lymphocytes infiltrate among adrenal cells. X200.

References

Bennett, B.D., McKenna, T.J., Hough, A.J., Dean, R., and Page, D.L. Adrenal myelolipoma associated with Cushing's disease. Am. J. Clin. Pathol. 73:443-447, 1980.

Boudreaux, D., Waisman, J., Skinner, D. G., and Low, R. Giant adrenal myelolipoma and testicular interstitial cell tumor in a man with congenital 21-hydroxylase deficiency. Am. J. Surg. Pathol. 3:109-123, 1979.

Choi, S. H. and Liu, K. Leiomyosarcoma of the adrenal gland and its angiographic features: A case report. J. Surg. Oncol. 16:145-148, 1981.

Collins, D. C. Formation of bone marrow in the suprarenal gland. Am. J. Pathol. 8:97-105, 1932.

Cussen, L. J. Adrenal myelolipoma. Med. J. Aust. 1:641-642, 1964.

Delarue, J. and Monsaingeon, A. Métaplasies myéloides dans la cortico-surrénale des brûlés. C. R. Soc. Biol. (Paris) 114:777-778, 1950.

DeNavasquez, S. A case of myelo-lipoma (bone-marrow heterotopia) of the suprarenal gland. Guy's Hosp. Rep. 88:237-240, 1935.

Dyckman, J. and Freedman, D. Myelolipoma of the adrenal with clinical features and surgical excision. Mt. Sinai Hosp. J. 24:793-796, 1957.

Ejeckam, G. C., and Attah, Ed'B. Pattern of secondary adrenal tumors in Ibadan, Nigeria. Int. Surg. 60:368-369, 1975.

Gee, W. F., Chikos, P. M., Greaves, J. P. Ikemoto, N., and Tremann, J. A. Adrenal myelolipoma. Urology 5:562-566, 1975.

Lang, E. K. The roentgenographic diagnosis of suprarenal masses. Radiology 87:35-45, 1966.

McDonnell, W.V. Myelolipoma of adrenal. Arch. Pathol. 61:416-419, 1956.

Nicod, J-L. Adénome, lipome et myélolipome de la cortico-surranale. Bull Cancer (Paris) 50:109-122, 1963.

Oberling, C. Les formations myélo-lipomateuses. Bull. Cancer (Paris) 18:234-246, 1929.

Olsson, C. A., Krane, R. J., Klugo, R. C., and Selikowitz, S. M. Adrenal myelolipoma. Surgery 73:665-670, 1973.

Parsons, L., Jr. and Thompson, J.E. Symptomatic myelolipoma of the adrenal gland. N. Engl. J. Med. 260:12-15, 1959.

Plaut, A. Myelolipoma in the adrenal cortex (myelo-adipose structures). Am. J. Pathol. 34:487-515, 1958.

Rao, N. G., Krishnaswami, S., Cherian, G. and Krishnaswami, H. Sarcoma of the pulmonary artery with metastases to pancreas and adrenal glands. Chest 66:459-462, 1974.

Rothberg, M., Bastidas, J., Mattey, W. E., and Bernas, E. Adrenal remangiomas: angiographic appearance of a rare tumor. Radiology 126:341-344, 1978.

Selye, H. and Stone, H. Hormonally induced transformation of adrenal into myeloid tissue. Am. J. Pathol. 26:211-233, 1950.

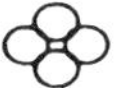

PLATE XI

(Plate XI-A and C from same patient)

A. MYELOLIPOMA

Myelolipomas are often incidentally removed at operation or discovered at autopsy, as in this case. Pale red areas are hematopoietic. X1.5.

B. MYELOLIPOMA

Myelolipomas may attain massive proportions. This specimen, removed from an adult male with Cushing's disease, measured 17 cm in largest dimension. The dark red areas represent hematopoietic tissue. X0.5.

C. MYELOLIPOMA

Histologic appearance of myelolipoma reveals interspersed hematopoietic and adipose tissue. As in this case, adrenal cortical cells are sometimes scattered throughout the lesion (left). X125.

D. CYST

Cysts may be complicated by hemorrhage, as in this case. This is a rare cause of acute abdominal pain. X.085. (Courtesy of Dr. G. Gray, New York, NY.)

E. CYST

This simple cyst of the adrenal gland contains a smooth wall without excresences. These are usually incidental findings and are of no endocrine significance. X1.33. (Courtesy of Dr. W.A. Gardner, Jr., Nashville, TN.)

PLATE XI

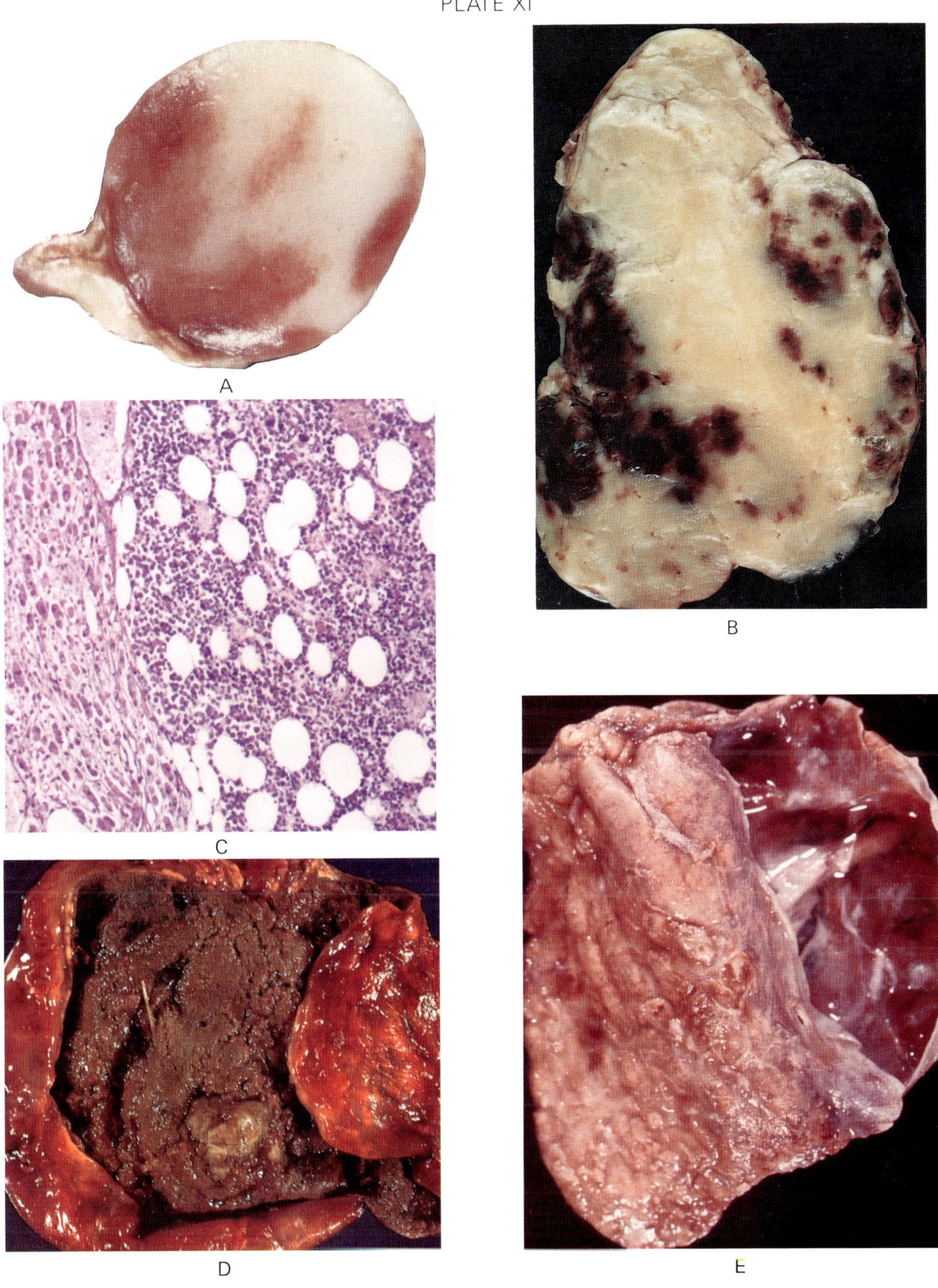

A

B

C

D

E

NONNEOPLASTIC ADRENAL ENLARGEMENT

CYSTS

Definition. Cysts are enclosed, fluid filled masses of the adrenal.

Incidence. Cysts of over several centimeters in diameter are uncommon, with approximately 300 cases recorded in the medical literature. Occasional cysts reach very large size, containing several liters of fluid. Most of these are technically pseudocysts, as no epithelial or endothelial lining is apparent. Occasional cysts caused by parasitic disease, particularly ecchinococal disease, are associated with cysts at the more usual locations as well.

Most adrenal cysts are small and constitute incidental findings at time of necropsy. Larger ones present as mass lesions associated with lumbar pain and are resected (Kearney et al.; Gisserot et al.). At times, hypertension has been ameliorated by removal of large adrenal cysts (Geelhoed and Spiegel). Many cysts have diffuse calcification within the wall, which is a helpful radiographic finding (Costandi et al.). Clinical presentation of adrenal cysts in neonates is rare (Levin et al.).

Gross. These lesions vary from being microscopic in size to weighing several kilograms and containing several liters of fluid. The larger cysts are usually filled with a brown or bloody fluid (pl. XI-D). The cyst wall is usually less than a centimeter in thickness, consisting of firm, fibrous tissue with foci of brown hemosiderin deposition and calcification (fig. 161). Islands of adrenal cortical tissue may be apparent as small yellow islands in the cyst wall.

The so-called lymphangiectatic cyst less frequently presents as a mass lesion during life and is most frequently found as an incidental finding at autopsy (fig. 162; Incze et al.). These are regularly multiloculated, with the various cystic spaces measuring from 1 to 15 mm in diameter and containing clear or slightly milky fluid. Occasionally, and certainly more often in larger examples of this condition, areas of scar and old organizing hemorrhage may be present.

Microscopic Appearance. The walls of the larger cysts consist of well organized fibrous tissue with foci of hemosiderin deposition and collection of macrophages (fig. 163). The inner surface has no endothelial or epithelial lining, but, rather, fibroblasts adjacent to areas of organizing hemorrhage and fibrin deposits.

The lymphangiectatic cysts have a flattened endothelial lining with delicate fibrous tissue and smooth muscle bundles in the walls (Incze et al.). Areas of organizing hemorrhage and scar may be apparent, as noted in the pseudocysts of hemorrhagic type described above.

An extremely rare occurrence is a true epithelial cyst lined by a cuboidal and occasionally ciliated epithelium (Foster).

Pathogenesis. The most common cyst presenting as a clinical problem appears by anatomic evaluation to be the end result of organization of a hemorrhagic event occurring within the adrenal (Foster). The common occurrence of hemorrhage within the adrenal is discussed below. The so-called lymphangiectatic cysts probably represent neoplasms or malformations of the lymphatic

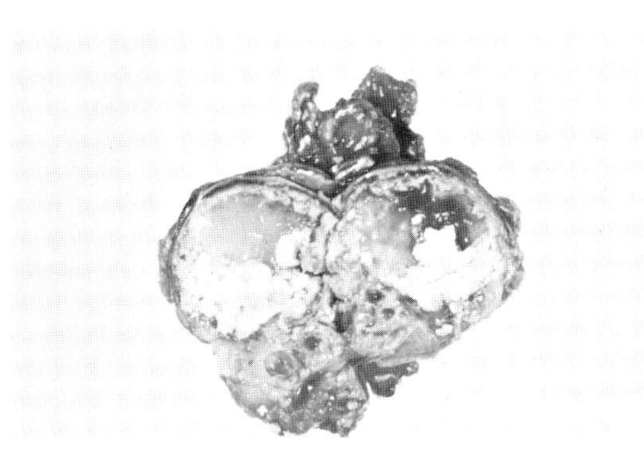

Figure 161
(Figures 161 and 163 from same patient)
ADRENAL CYST
Adrenal cyst contains gelatinous material, evidently resulting from old local hemorrhage. White areas are calcification. Smaller cysts with clear fluid present below larger cyst.

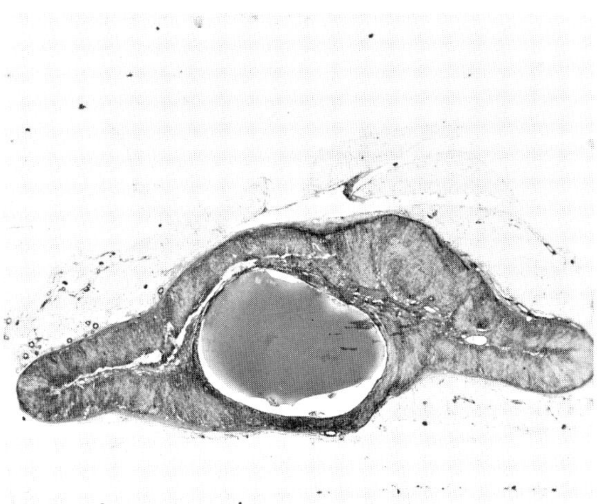

Figure 162
ADRENAL CYST
This smooth walled cyst presented as an incidental finding at autopsy. A delicate lining of flattened cells adjacent to a narrow band of fibroblasts lines the wall. X3.

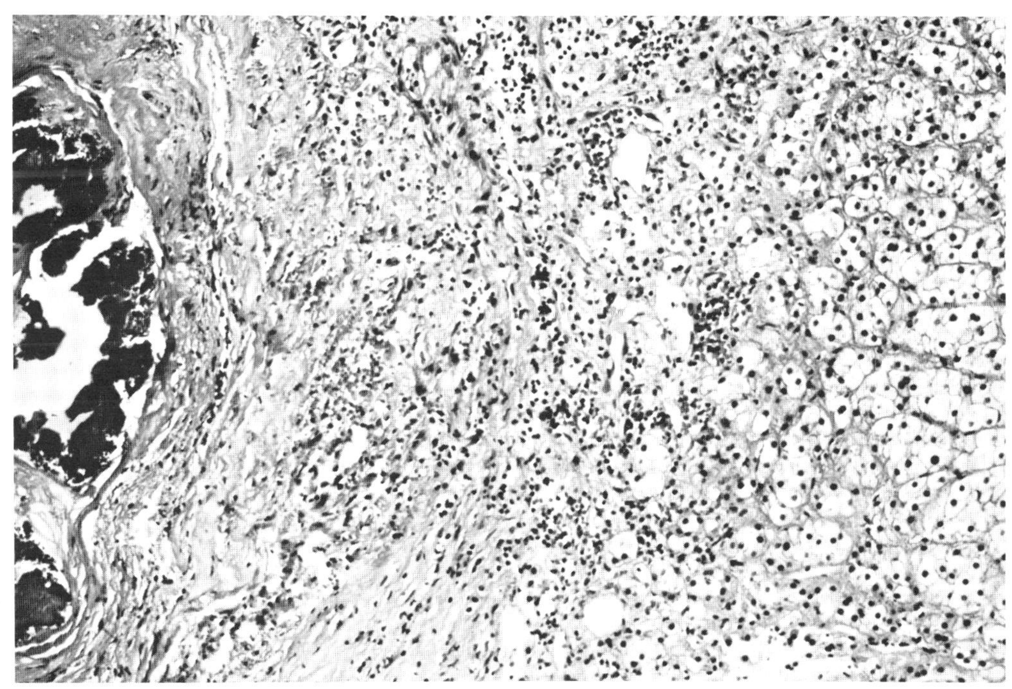

Figure 163
ADRENAL CYST
Calcification in cyst wall is seen at left. Normal cortical cells are present at right. X225.

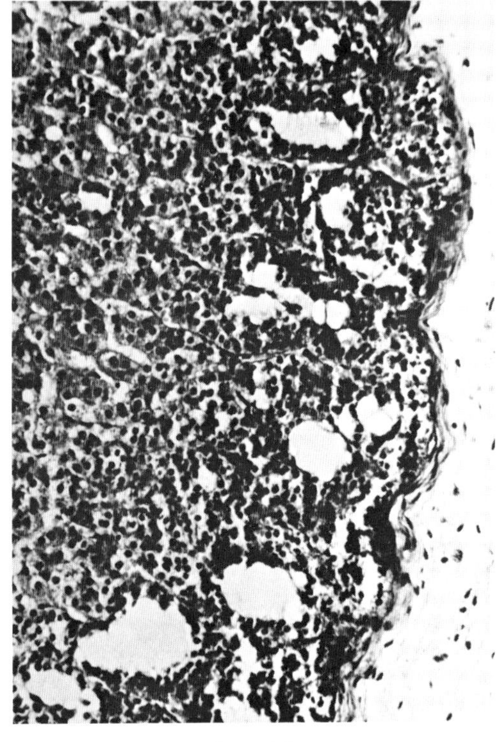

Figure 164
MICROCYSTS
Microcystic alteration of outer cortical zone is seen from a stillborn infant of 32 weeks' gestation. X175. (Courtesy of the late Dr. E.H. Oppenheimer, Baltimore, MD.)

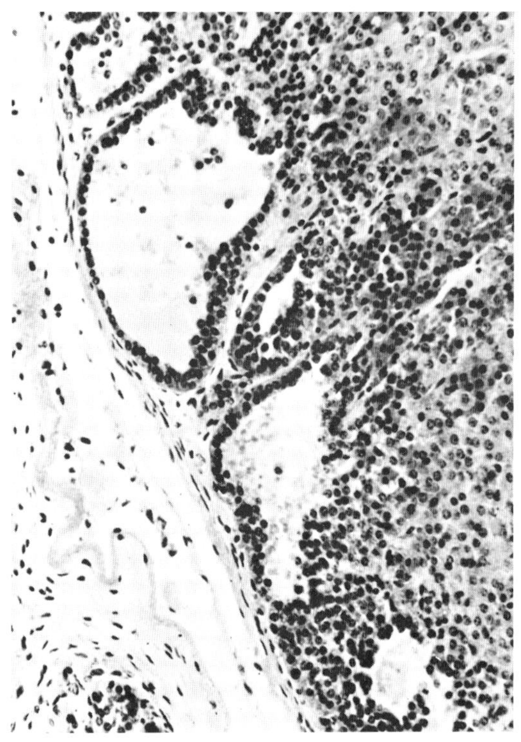

Figure 165
MICROCYSTS
Microcysts of outer cortex are seen from stillborn infant of 25 weeks' gestation with severe amnionitis. Cysts are lined by regular small cells of the outer zone, with some erythrocytes, protein, and rare necrotic cells in the center of the cysts. X175. (Courtesy of the late Dr. E.H. Oppenheimer, Baltimore, MD.)

system (Incze et al.) and are analagous to those occurring elsewhere. The rare epithelial cysts with well developed cuboidal or ciliated epithelium are probably developmental abnormalities and may well represent displaced tissue from the urogenital anlage with cystic transformation.

The relatively common presence of microscopic cysts (pl. XI-E) in the permanent cortices of infants (figs. 164, 165) is a finding of no known clinical significance (Oppenheimer), although many believe they are related to stress (Rodin et al.).

HEMORRHAGE AND NECROSIS

Small foci of necrosis, sometimes associated with hemorrhage, are relatively frequently found in the adrenal at time of necropsy. They most commonly occur with other signs of hypoperfusion and hypotension, such as centrilobular necrosis in the liver and renal tubular necrosis (Kuhajda and Hutchins). Extensive hemorrhage is best known and seen most dramatically in association with septicemia, associated with the so-called Waterhouse-Friderich-

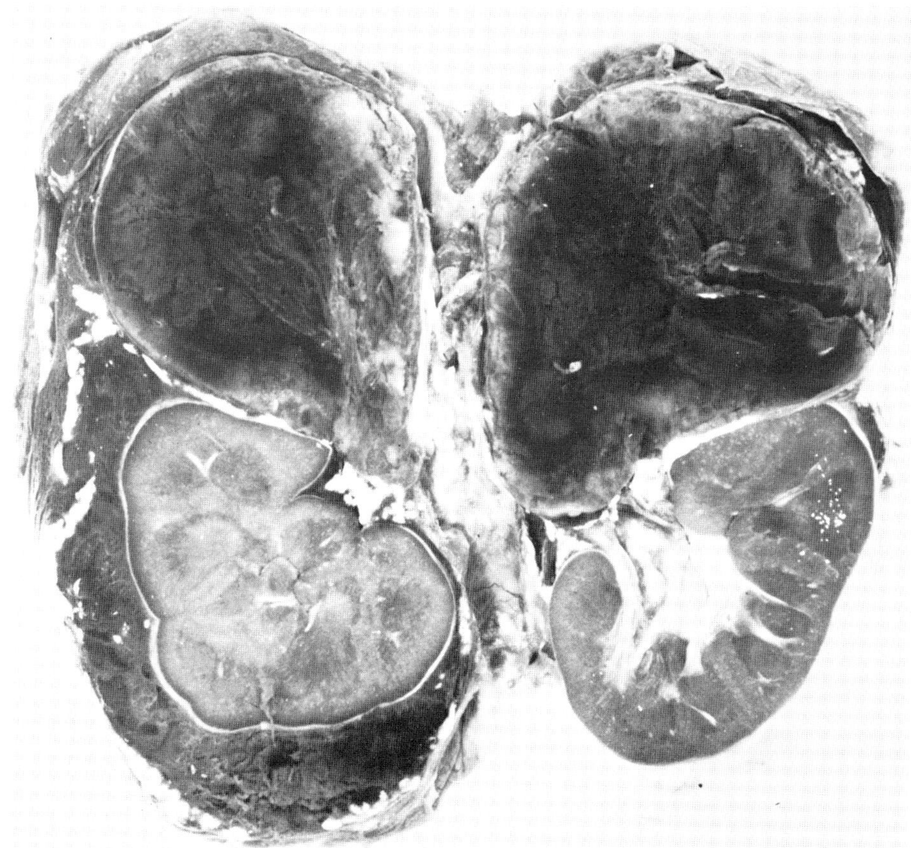

Figure 166
EXTENSIVE ADRENAL HEMORRHAGE
Infarction and local hemorrhage produce bilateral enlargement of adrenal area, with extension of hemorrhage around the kidney at lower left. The patient was a two year old girl who died with Waterhouse-Friderichsen syndrome 12 hours after onset of malaise and 2 hours after onset of petechial rash. Approximately actual size. (Courtesy of Department of Pathology, Radcliffe Infirmary, Oxford, England.)

sen syndrome (fig. 166). Areas of necrosis and hemorrhage are usually associated with perinatal stress, generalized bleeding tendency, disseminated intravascular coagulation, septicemia, or trauma (Xarli et al.; Clark). Massive retroperitoneal hemorrhage of life threatening proportions may present in the clinical background noted or appear without apparent predisposing cause (Page and Scully; Clark et al.). Survival of such a hemorrhagic event will eventuate in the

formation of an adrenal cyst of posthemorrhagic type (see Cysts).

Smaller areas of necrosis appear as ghost adrenal cells, usually in the cortex, with local hemorrhage. Usually, few acute inflammatory cells are apparent, except when the areas of necrosis are relatively large extending through the full thickness of the cortex in a segmental fashion. The medulla is usually spared, except when virtually the entire gland is involved (fig. 167).

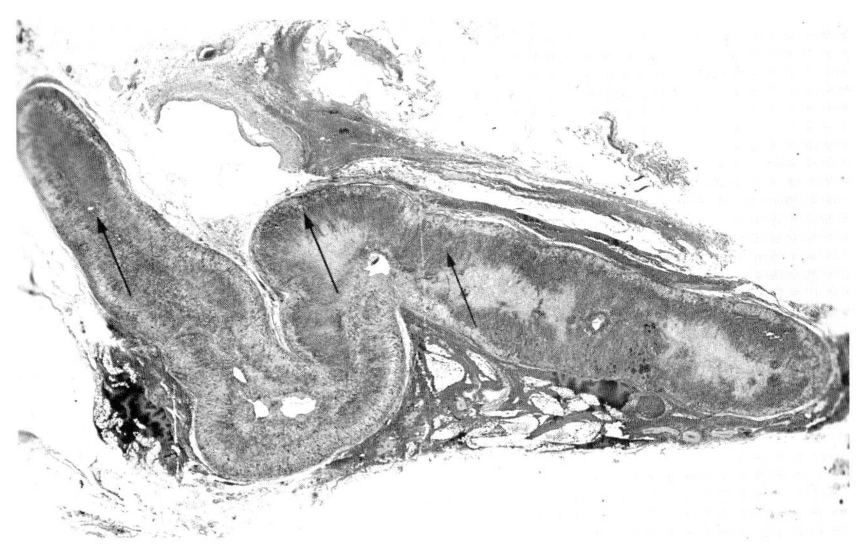

Figure 167
MICROSCOPIC INFARCTION AND HEMORRHAGE
Subcapsular zone is spared. Hemorrhagic infarcted zones are dark and are present through-
out the gland (arrow). A small amount of spared medullary tissue is at lower left. X4.

GRANULOMATOUS INFECTION

Definition. Adrenal involvement by infections producing a granulomatous reaction
usually results in an enlargement of the
adrenals. The most common infections in
the United States producing this condition
are tuberculosis and histoplasmosis. Adrenal destruction leading to Addison's disease is often a result of this process. Prior
to a reduction in the overall incidence of
tuberculosis in this century, this was the
most common cause of Addison's disease.

Anatomic Appearance. The adrenal
involved by granulomatous infection appears to be inflated like a balloon, producing rounded contours, usually with
caseous material making up most of the
mass (fig. 168). The borders are grossly
smooth, but the adrenal is characteristically
adherent to surrounding structures. The
picture is quite characteristic, contrasting
with that produced by malignant neoplasms
in its complete involvement of the adrenal

and lack of invasion into adjacent structures, although adherence to kidney and
other structures is characteristic. Histologically, there are few, if any, recognizable
adrenal cells to be found, and most of these
will be at the subcapsular area.

We mention amyloid deposition briefly
here because it produces adrenal enlargement most often when present in association with chronic granulomatous infection,
so-called secondary amyloidosis. The interstitial infiltration by amyloid may triple the
size of the glands (O'Donnell), producing
an almost homogeneous, waxy gross appearance. Addison's disease is produced
when the preferential deposition of amyloid
in the inner cortical zones is extensive
(Kaufman), and this can occur without
enlarging the glands (Heller and Camarata).
The more common type of amyloidosis
which is associated with plasma cell disorders (Glenner) usually produces only
focal, vascular amyloid deposits in the
adrenal.

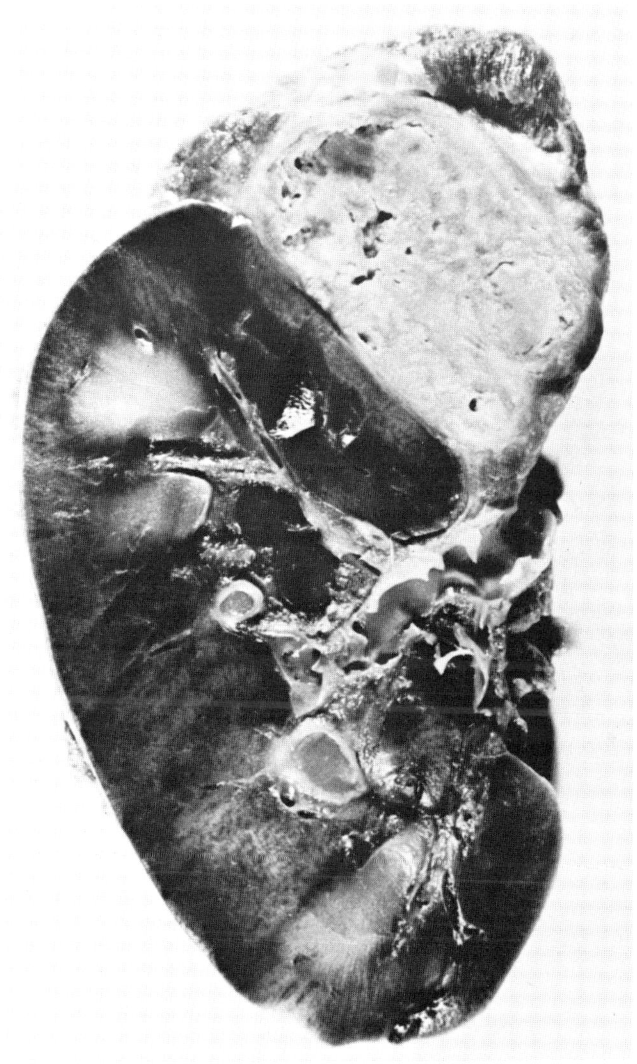

Figure 168
GRANULOMATOUS INFECTION
Enlarged adrenal adherent to kidney surface is largely replaced by caseous material. The infection caused by tuberculosis has also produced adherence to the diaphragm seen as fragments of muscle at uppermost portion of picture. Approximately actual size. (Courtesy of Department of Pathology, University of Leeds, Leeds, England.)

References

Clark, O. H. Postoperative adrenal hemorrhage. Ann. Surg. 182:124-129, 1975.

———, Hall, A. D. and Schambelan, M. Clinical manifestations of adrenal hemorrhage. Am. J. Surg. 128:219-224, 1974.

Costandi, Y. T., Inaba, Y., Kerr, A., Wendel, R. G., Henning, D. C., and Evans, A. T. Calcified adrenal cysts. Urology 5:777-779, 1975.

Foster, D. G. Adrenal cysts. Arch. Surg. 92:131-143, 1966.

Geelhoed, G. W. and Spiegel, C. T. "Incidental" adrenal cyst. South. Med. J. 74:626-630, 1981.

Gisserot, D., Poupée, J. C., Doury, J. C., Gourrion, M., Jan, P., and Huguet, J. F. Un pseudo-kyste de la surrenale. J. Radiol. Electrol. Med. Nucl. 60:63-69, 1979.

Glenner, G. G. Amyloid deposits and amyloidosis: the beta-fibrilloses. N. Engl. J. Med. 302:1283-1292, 1330-1343, 1980.

Heller, E. L. and Camarata, S. J. Addison's disease from amyloidosis of adrenal glands. Arch. Pathol. 49:601-604, 1950.

Incze, J. S., Lui, P. S., Merriam, J. C., Austen, G., Widrich, W. C., and Gerzof, S. G. Morphology and pathogenesis of adrenal cysts. Am. J. Pathol. 95:423-432, 1979.

Kaufmann, E. Pathology for Students and Practitioners, pp. 1286-1287. Philadelphia: P. Blakiston's Son and Co., 1929.

Kearney, G. P., Mahoney, E. M., Maher, E., and Harrison, J. H. Functioning and nonfunctioning cysts of the adrenal cortex and medulla. Am. J. Surg. 134:363-368, 1977.

Kuhajda, F. P. and Hutchins, G. M. Adrenal corticomedullary junction necrosis: a morphologic marker for hypotension. Am. Heart J. 98:294-297, 1979.

Levin, S. E., Collins, D. L., Kaplan, G. W., and Weller, M. H. Neonatal adrenal pseudocyst mimicking metastatic disease. Ann. Surg. 179:186-189, 1974.

O'Donnell, W. M. Changing patterns of Addison's disease. Arch. Intern. Med. 86:266-279, 1950.

Oppenheimer, E. H. Cyst formation in the outer adrenal cortex. Arch. Pathol. 87:653-659, 1969.

Page, L. B. and Scully, R. E. Case records of the Massachusetts General Hospital, Case 14-1969. N. Engl. J. Med. 280:772-776, 1969.

Rodin, A. E., Hsu, F. L., and Whorton, E. B. Microcysts of the permanent adrenal cortex in perinates and infants. Arch. Pathol. Lab. Med. 100:499-502, 1976.

Xarli, V. P., Steele, A. A., Davis, P. J., Buescher, E. S., et al. Adrenal hemorrhage in the adult. Medicine 57:211-221, 1978.

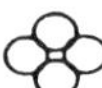

ADRENAL MEDULLARY TUMORS

PHEOCHROMOCYTOMA

SYNONYMS AND RELATED TERMS: Intra-adrenal paraganglioma; chromaffin cell tumor; chromaffinoma; chromophile tumor; cystic medullary struma of adrenal; medullary adenoma of the adrenal; adrenergic tumor; pheochromoblastoma.

Terminology and Definitions. The term pheochromocytoma was first introduced by Pick in 1912 to describe an adrenal medullary tumor which darkened on exposure to dichromate containing fixatives. The subsequent use of this term, both in relationship to tumors of the adrenal medulla and extra-medullary paraganglia, however, has led to considerable confusion and variation in nomenclature. Tumors of the extra-adrenal paraganglia have been divided into chromaffin positive and negative types on the basis of their reactions to solutions of potassium dichromate (Lattes). Despite the lack of a positive chromaffin reaction, however, some of these tumors have been shown to contain catecholamines by sensitive histochemical and biochemical extraction methods. Moreover, some of these chromaffin negative tumors have been associated with typical clinical manifestations of catecholamine hypersecretion. Classifications based on the chromaffin reaction, therefore, may not reflect the catecholamine content or the clinical manifestations associated with the tumor.

In Fascicle 9, Second Series, Tumors of the Extra-adrenal Paraganglion System, Glenner and Grimley have divided the tumors into four major groups on the basis of anatomic distribution, patterns of innervation, microscopic structure, and function. These include the branchiomeric, intravagal, aortico-sympathetic, and visceral-autonomic paragangliomas. Moreover, these authors suggest that the term pheochromocytoma should be restricted to paragangliomas arising solely in the adrenal gland. It should be noted, however, that the concept of extra-adrenal pheochromocytomas is still firmly rooted in the literature and that some authors favor the use of the term pheochromocytoma for any functional chromaffin positive or negative intra- or extra-adrenal paraganglioma. In this Fascicle, the term pheochromocytoma will be reserved for those paragangliomas which arise in the adrenal medulla and which may be demonstrated by a combination of biochemical, histochemical, and/or ultrastructural methods to contain catecholamines.

Incidence. Pheochromocytoma is a rare tumor which has been reported to occur in 0.005 to 0.1 percent of unselected autopsies. In patients with severe sustained hypertension studied by catecholamine assays and pharmacologic testing or subjected to bilateral lumbar sympathectomy, the frequency of pheochromocytoma ranges from 0.4 to 0.6 percent (Manger and Gifford). These tumors may occur at any age, and rare congenital examples have been reported. Pheochromocytomas most commonly become manifest between the third and fifth decades. In patients with familial pheochromocytoma syndromes, most cases are diagnosed within the first two decades.

In adults, the sex incidence is approximately equal, although some studies have suggested a slightly increased incidence in females. In a review of 100 cases of pheochromocytoma in children less than 15 years of age, the male to female ratio was 2:1 (Stackpole et al.). While the tumors in boys were randomly distributed, 62 percent of those in girls occurred between the ages of 11 and 15 years.

Clinical. The clinical manifestations in patients with pheochromocytoma are highly variable. Approximately equal numbers of patients have sustained or paroxysmal hypertension (Remine et al.). Episodes of paroxysmal hypertension are noted frequently in those patients with sustained blood pressure elevations. Occasional patients with profound paroxysmal hypotension and tachycardia have also been described, and have been shown to have predominantly epinephrine secreting pheochromocytomas. Some patients with small tumors may have no characteristic signs or symptoms, while other patients may have some of the clinical and metabolic manifestations without documented hypertension. The development of orthostatic hypotension in a patient with sustained hypertension is suggestive of pheochromocytoma. Pheochromocytoma during pregnancy may masquerade as toxemia.

The most common clinical symptomatology in patients with pheochromocytoma results from excess production of catecholamines by the tumor (Manger and Gifford). Headache is present in over 90 percent of patients with paroxysmal hypertension. It is often severe and throbbing and may be accompanied by nausea and vomiting. The frequency of headache is approximately 70 percent in patients with sustained hypertension associated with pheochromocytoma. Diaphoresis is a common symptom in patients with both paroxysmal and sustained hypertension and occasional patients may present with a history of drenching night sweats. Palpitations with or without tachycardia, anxiety, and tremulousness are more commonly encountered in those patients with paroxysmal hypertension. Less common complaints include chest and abdominal pain, dyspnea, visual disturbances, paresthesias and extremity pains, constipation, and weight loss. Weakness, fatigue, and prostration may be severe at the conclusion of an attack. Pallor and flushing of the face and upper part of the body are common findings. The tremulousness, tachycardia, and hyperventilation may suggest hyperthyroidism. Evidence of hypermetabolism may be manifested by increased fasting blood glucose levels. An enlarged adrenal may be palpated in approximately 15 percent of patients. Pressure on the abdomen may lead to an increase in blood pressure or the onset of diaphoresis in approximately half the patients with pheochromocytoma. The major complications of pheochromocytoma include cardiac arrhythmias, myocardial infarction, cerebrovascular accidents, neuroretinopathy, and benign and malignant nephrosclerosis.

Myocardial damage is seen commonly in patients with pheochromocytoma and undoubtedly plays an important role in causing the death of untreated patients (VanWay et al.). The earliest lesion has been referred to as myofibrillar degeneration of cardiac muscle. These areas of degeneration are subsequently replaced by histiocytes and later by fibrous tissue. The lesions are characteristically multifocal, but tend to occur predominantly in the subendocardial region of the left ventricle. These lesions most closely resemble the so-called catecholamine cardiomyopathy which may be induced in experimental animals by the administration of high doses of vasoactive amines (Alpert et al.). Rarely, pheochromocytoma may masquerade as a cardiomyopathy (Garcia and Jennings).

Cushing's syndrome may be associated with pheochromocytoma (Meloni et al.). In some of these cases, ectopic production of ACTH by the tumors has been documented (Berenyi et al.). In a recently studied patient with an ACTH producing pheochromocytoma, Spark and associates found that levels of plasma ACTH varied directly with urinary catecholamine excretion, suggesting that a common factor regulated peptide and catecholamine secretion. After removal of the pheochromocytoma, urinary catecholamines became normal while plasma ACTH and cortisol levels fell to zero. This finding suggested that ACTH secretion from the pheochromocytoma had suppressed the normal hypothalamic-pituitary-adrenal axis. Sisson and colleagues have shown recently that ACTH-like immunoreactivity is present in some pheochromocytomas unassociated with the ectopic ACTH syndrome. Pheochromocytomas have also been shown to contain a variety of other regulatory peptide products which may be demonstrated by immunohistochemical technics in tissue sections or by radioimmunoassays of tissue extracts (Hassoun et al.). Leu-enkephalin-like immunoreactivity, for example, has been demonstrated in 50 percent of cases of pheochromocytoma (DeLellis et al., 1983). In addition to leu- and met-enkephalin, a variety of other peptide products, including vasoactive intestinal peptide, somatostatin, substance P, and calcitonin have also been found in pheochromocytomas (Linnoila et al.; Lundberg et al.; Weinstein and Ide). In general, isolated tumor cells or small groups of cells are positive for these hormonal products. The release of these peptides may be responsible for some of the unusual symptoms encountered in occasional patients with pheochromocytoma. Hypercalcemia also has been documented in occasional patients with these tumors (Heath and Edis). In at least some instances, hypercalcemia may result from a direct effect of catecholamines on the parathyroid glands.

Occasional patients with pheochromocytoma may be normotensive. At least four mechanisms have been suggested to explain the absence of hypertension in these cases: nonsecretion of catecholamines, minimal secretion of catecholamines, high rates of amine inactivation within the tumor, and increased tolerance of tissue receptors for catecholamines. Recently, a normotensive patient with bilateral pheochromocytomas was found to have a deficiency of dopamine beta hydroxylase within the tumor (Feldman et al.). In this case, although the tumor contained high concentrations of dopamine, the levels of norepinephrine were markedly reduced.

Biochemistry of Pheochromocytomas. Although epinephrine accounts for 80-85 percent of the total normal adrenal medullary catecholamines, most pheochromocytomas secrete more norepinephrine than epinephrine. According to Neville, 29 percent of pheochromocytomas secrete only norepinephrine, while 15 percent of tumors secrete more than 50 percent epinephrine. The remaining tumors secrete both norepinephrine and epinephrine, with a predominance of norepinephrine. The epinephrine content of many extra-adrenal paragangliomas, with the exception of those arising in the organ of Zuckerkandl and renal hilus, is negligible (Neville). The low rates of epinephrine synthesis in extra adrenal paragangliomas have been attributed to decreased activity of phenylethanolamine-N-methyl transferase in tissues distant from the adrenal cortex.

The pheochromocytomas present in patients with type II multiple endocrine neoplasia syndrome have been reported to secrete more epinephrine than norepinephrine (DeLellis; Hamilton et al.). In some kindreds at high risk for the development of this syndrome, increased urinary epinephrine to norepinephrine ratios have been reported to represent one of the earliest manifestations of adrenal medullary hyperfunction. In addition to epinephrine and norepinephrine, pheochromocytomas rarely may secrete dopamine, dopa, and serotonin. Increased levels of dopa and dopamine have been suggested as markers for malignant pheochromocytoma; however, recent studies have indicated that these amines may also be present in benign tumors (Robinson et al.).

Laboratory Tests. Measurements of urinary VMA (Table 2) and metanephrines have been used most extensively in screening patients for pheochromocytoma (Manger and Gifford). With these tests, 80 to 90 percent of cases will be detected. If these tests are negative, assay of urine for catecholamines is indicated. A negative test for urinary catecholamines may be followed by a repeat assay after histamine stimulation with or without use of an alpha adrenergic blocking agent. Recent comparative studies have revealed that measurements of plasma catecholamines had the highest sensitivity for the diagnosis of pheochromocytoma, while urinary VMA levels proved to have the lowest sensitivity (Bravo and Gifford).

Preoperative Localization Procedures. Plain films of the abdomen may be expected

to demonstrate pheochromocytomas in only a small percentage of cases (fig. 169). Intravenous pyelography with or without nephrotomography has been used successfully in the preoperative localization of pheochromocytomas in up to 50 percent of cases. In a recent report from the Mayo Clinic, nephrotomography accurately localized pheochromocytomas in 67 percent of patients (Remine et al.). In no patient, however, did the tumor measure less than 2.5 cm in diameter. Aortography and selective arteriography may be expected to clear-

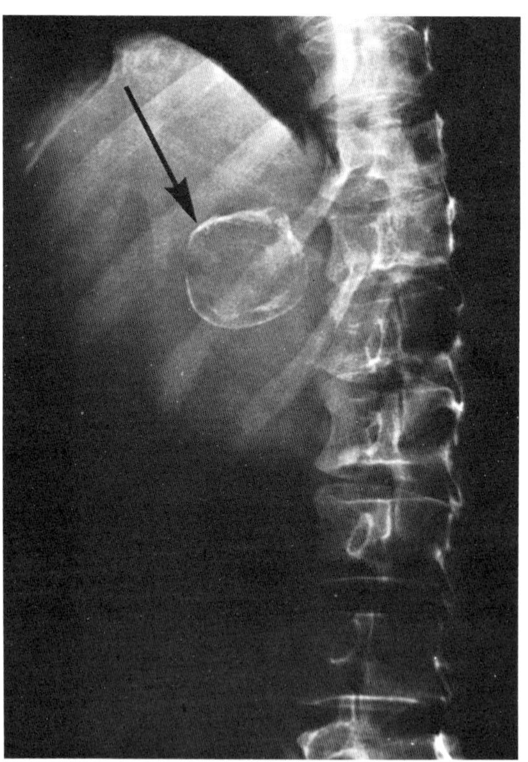

Figure 169
PHEOCHROMOCYTOMA
Plain film of the abdomen was obtained from a patient with a longstanding history of persistent hypertension. A large right suprarenal calcified mass was noted (arrow). Gross and microscopic examination revealed a degenerated cystic pheochromocytoma. The wall was composed of dense fibrous connective tissue that was heavily calcified.

ly delineate tumors in more than 85 percent of cases. The pheochromocytomas characteristically show a fine vascular pattern or tumor blush (fig. 170). Adrenal venography has been most successful for the demonstration of small tumors and for the localization of relatively hypovascular pheochromocytomas. Recent studies indicate that computerized axial tomography (fig. 171) represents a sensitive noninvasive technic for tumor localization (Manger and Gifford). A recent report from the Cleveland Clinic indicates that the relative accuracies of selective angiography and computerized axial tomography (CT) are the same for the

detection of pheochromocytomas. CT scanning has the added advantage of being a noninvasive technic (Bravo and Gifford).

Gross. Data from several large series have indicated that the right adrenal is more commonly involved than the left in patients with nonfamilial pheochromocytoma (Remine et al.; Manger and Gifford; Melicow). Tumor weight has been reported to range from 1.2 to 3600 g. Rare examples of microscopic pheochromocytomas measuring several millimeters in diameter have been reported as incidental autopsy findings (Melicow). In a report from the Mayo Clinic, average tumor weight in patients with sustained or episodic hypertension was 100 g (Remine et al.). The vast majority of tumors measure 3 to 5 cm in diameter. Although it is not possible to define anatomically the site of origin of large tumors within the gland, virtually all smaller tumors arise within the head or body regions of the adrenals.

On external examination, most nonfamilial tumors appear as a single, spherical to ovoid, encapsulated mass (pl. XII-A, C, D; figs. 172–175). Small flecks of bright yellow cortical tissue may be seen just beneath the surfaces. The tumors are gray pink to tan and are usually soft in consistency. Exposure to air may result in spontaneous oxidation of the endogenous catecholamines to adrenochrome and noradrenochrome pigments. Larger tumors are often surrounded by a capsule composed of compressed adrenal cortical tissue together with a fibrovascular connective tissue. Smaller tumors are not encapsulated. Areas of recent hemorrhage, necrosis, and cyst formation are more common in larger tumors (pl. XII-D). Occasional tumors may show considerable calcification, which, in some instances, may be apparent in plain

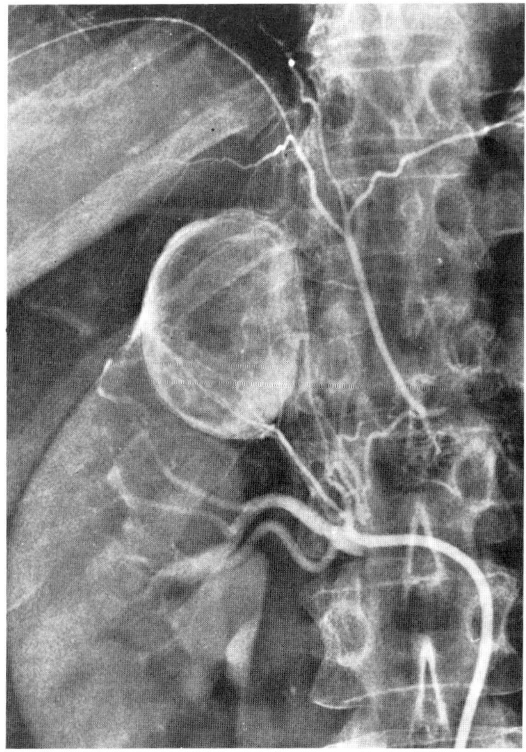

Figure 170
PHEOCHROMOCYTOMA
Selective renal arteriogram shows the characteristic vascular blush typical of a pheochromocytoma.

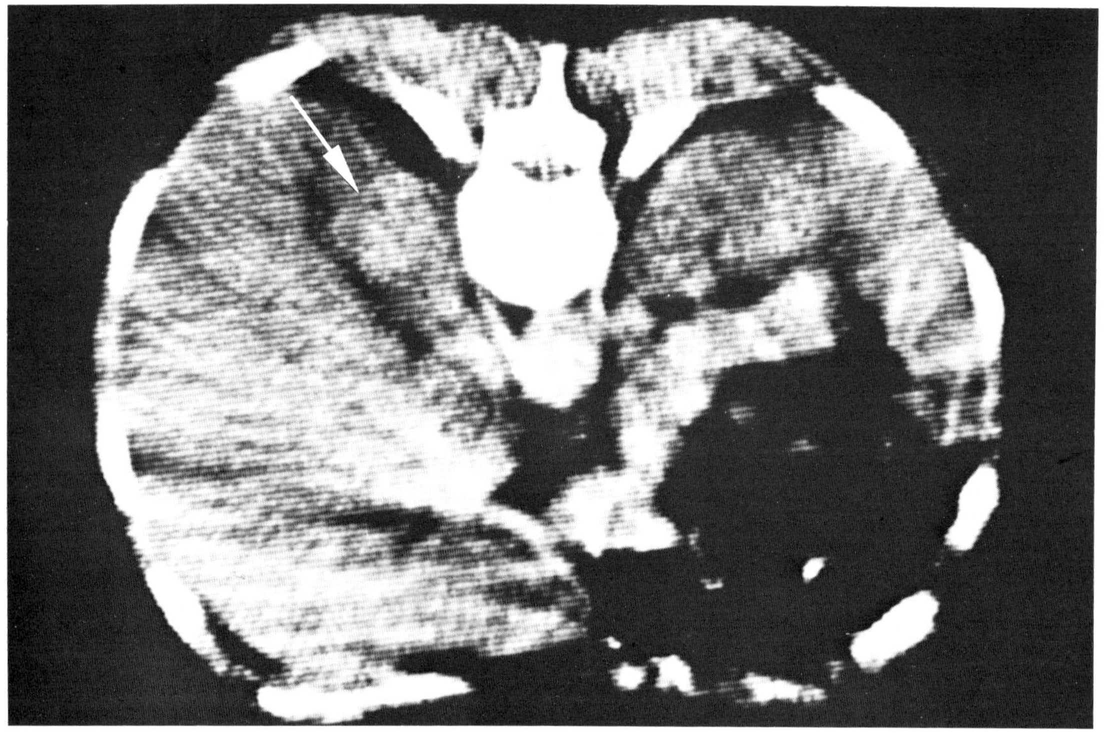

Figure 171
PHEOCHROMOCYTOMA
Computerized axial tomography scan shows a mass lesion above the right kidney (arrow). Excision revealed a pheochromocytoma.

films of the abdomen (fig. 169). Pheochromocytomas may undergo necrosis, with subsequent cyst formation, following arteriography (fig. 175).

Microscopic. Most pheochromocytomas resemble the normal adrenal medulla and are composed of pheochromocytes which are arranged in cords or small or large alveolar patterns ('Zellballen') (figs. 176, 177). Trabecular and diffuse patterns of growth also occur commonly (Medeiros et al.). Adjacent groups of tumor cells are separated by a reticulin rich fibrovascular stroma. Occasional tumors may be composed of cords of small cells intervening between abundant capillary vascular structures that are lined by a single layer of endothelial cells (fig. 178). This pattern may impart an angiomatous appearance to the tumors (Shin et al.). While most pheochromocytomas exhibit a solid alveolar pattern of growth, occasional pseudoacini (fig. 179) containing blood or proteinaceous fluid may be present (VanWay et al.). Most pheochromocytomas are separated from the cortex by a thin band of fibrovascular connective issue. In some patients, however, extension of tumor into the cortex may be apparent (figs. 180, 181). Vascular invasion may also be present in benign tumors. Cyst formation with areas of hemorrhage, necrosis, or myxomatous change are likely to occur in large tumors. In some patients, the cyst wall may become extensively calcified. Rarely, interstitial and/or vascular amyloid deposition may occur (Medeiros et al.).

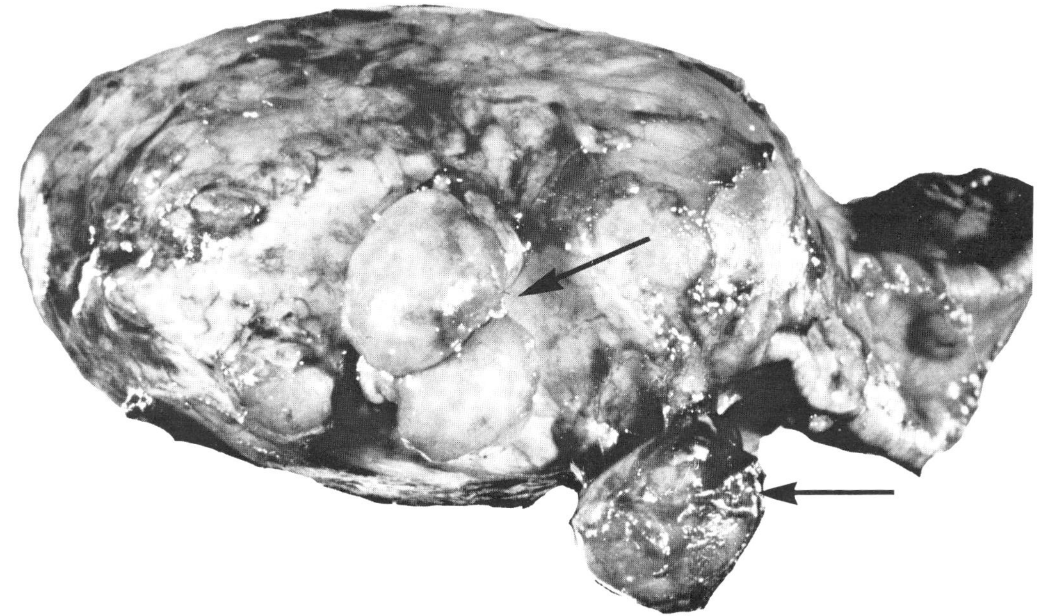

Figure 172
(Figures 172 and 173 from same patient)
PHEOCHROMOCYTOMA

This left adrenal was removed from a 35 year old male with hypertension and high urinary VMA levels. The head and body regions of the gland (left) are replaced with a large mass which showed the typical microscopic features of pheochromocytoma. Several small tumor nodules (arrows) protrude through the capsular surface. The patient also had several periaortic paragangliomas. Despite the presence of overt capsular invasion, there has been no evidence of metastatic disease in five years of follow-up. X2.1.

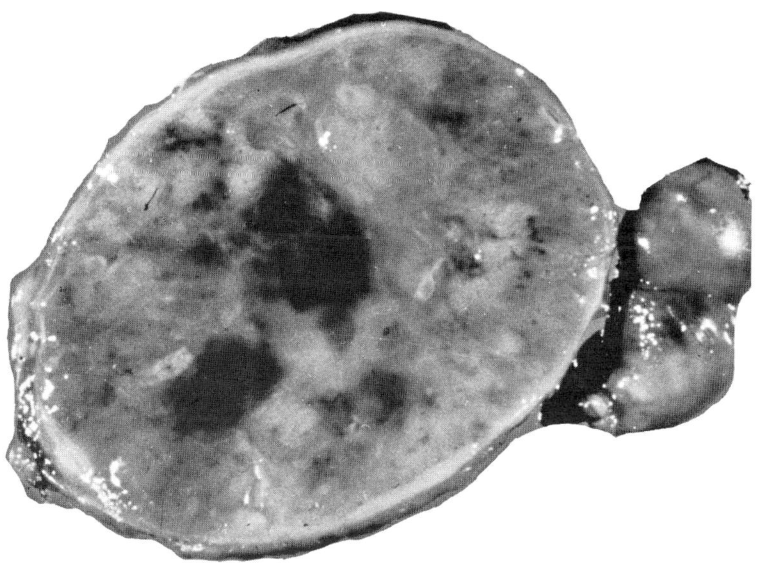

Figure 173
PHEOCHROMOCYTOMA

The figure represents a cross section of the tumor illustrated in figure 172. The tumor shows small foci of hemorrhage. In most areas, a well defined fibrous capsule surrounds the tumor. X2.1.

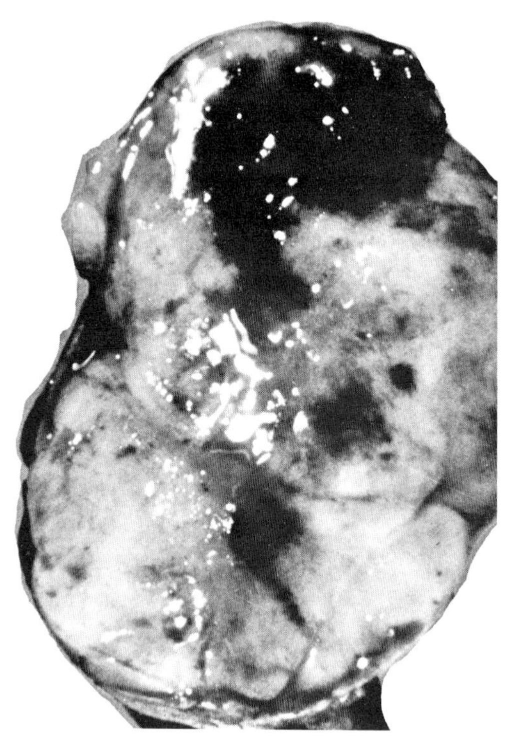

Figure 174
PHEOCHROMOCYTOMA
This pheochromocytoma has a somewhat lobular appearance and a fleshy surface with multiple areas of recent hemorrhage. X2.1.

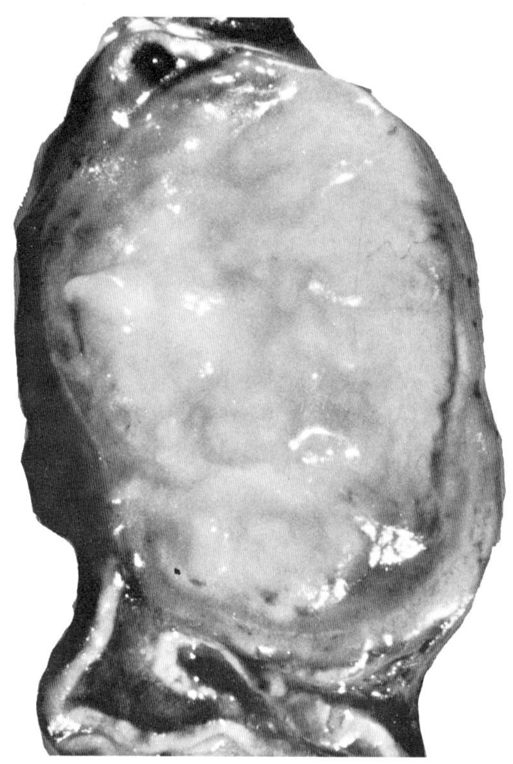

Figure 175
PHEOCHROMOCYTOMA
This pheochromocytoma is from a 28 year old woman and was removed one week after selective arteriographic study. The tumor has become almost completely necrotic. X2.1.

Individual tumor cells generally have a polyhedral shape and are often larger than normal adrenal medullary cells. Depending upon the initial fixation, the cytoplasm varies from eosinophilic to basophilic and is often finely granular (Sherwin, 1968; figs. 177, 181). Occasional tumor cells may have extensively vacuolated cytoplasm. Large numbers of periodic acid-Schiff (PAS) positive droplets may be present within the tumor cell cytoplasm (Dekker and Oehrle; pl. XII-E). The PAS positive inclusions most probably represent giant lysosomal type bodies. Ultrastructural studies have revealed the presence of membrane fragments within these inclusions. The membranous fragments may be derived from catecholamine granules (figs. 182, 183). Considerable nuclear pleomorphism may be present in some tumors, but does not correlate with the biologic behavior (figs. 184, 185). The nuclei are generally round to oval and appear vesicular, with coarsely clumped chromatin and usually a distinct nucleolus. Nuclear "pseudoinclusions" composed of cytoplasmic invaginations into the nucleus may also be found (DeLellis et al., 1980; fig. 186).

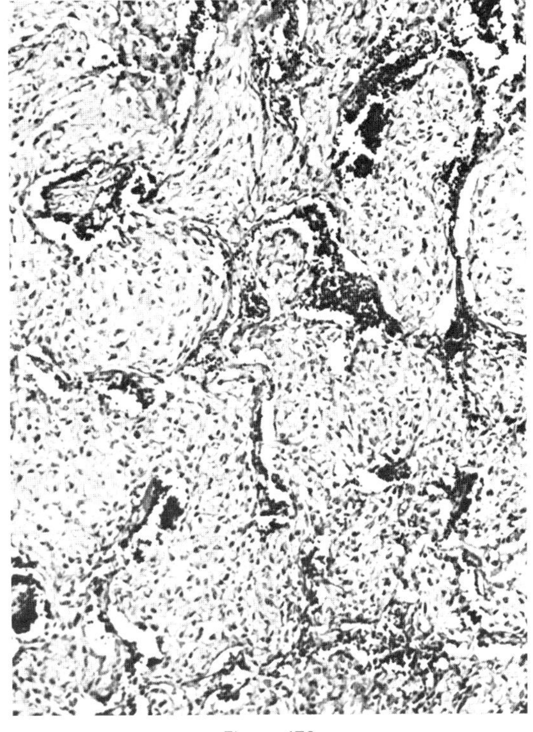

Figure 176
PHEOCHROMOCYTOMA
This pheochromocytoma shows a ''large'' or macronesting (alveolar) pattern of growth. Blood-filled vascular channels are present between the large nests of tumor cells. X125.

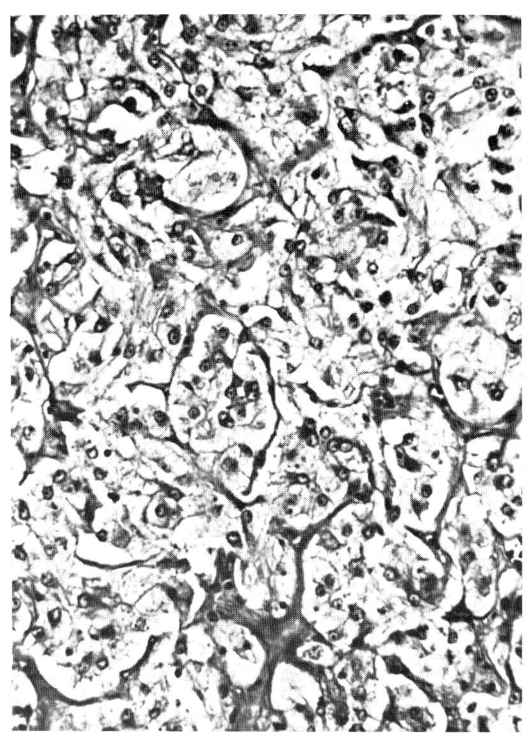

Figure 177
PHEOCHROMOCYTOMA
This pheochromocytoma shows a small nesting (alveolar) pattern of growth with a typical 'Zellballen' appearance. Individual tumor cells have a finely granular cytoplasm. X320.

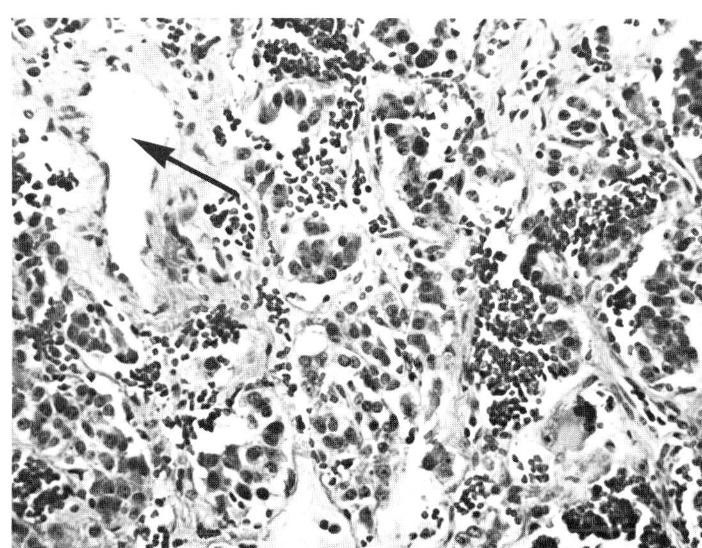

Figure 178
PHEOCHROMOCYTOMA
This pheochromocytoma shows a pronounced vascular or angiomatous appearance. Endothelium lined blood spaces (arrow) separate groups of tumor cells from one another. X320.

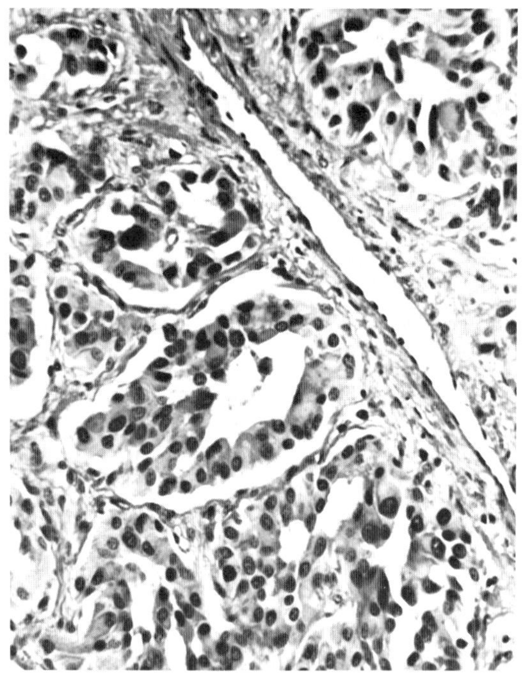

Figure 179
PHEOCHROMOCYTOMA
This tumor shows a pseudoglandular pattern of growth.
Tumor cells are aligned along spaces. X320.

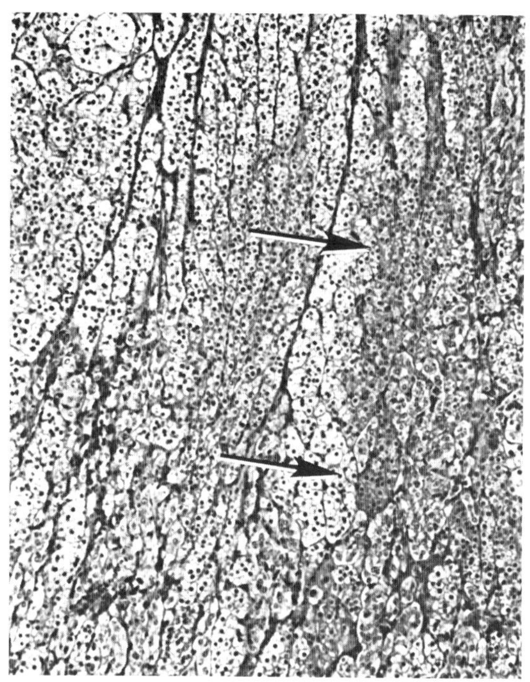

Figure 180
(Figures 180 and 181 from same patient)
PHEOCHROMOCYTOMA
In this pheochromocytoma, groups of tumor cells (arrow)
extend into the surrounding cortex. X125.

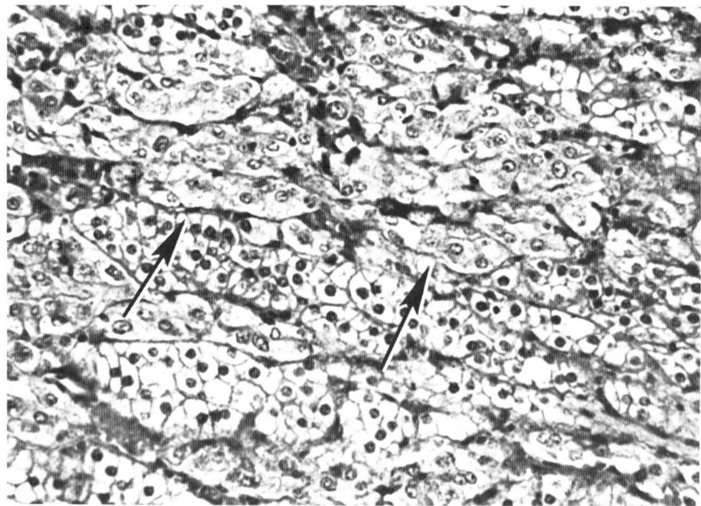

Figure 181
PHEOCHROMOCYTOMA
The figure represents a higher power view of the pheochromocytoma cells illustrated in the previous
figure. The vesicular nuclei and the granular cytoplasm of the tumor cells (arrows) can be readily appreciated. Occasional lesions in which the pheochromocytoma has extended into the cortex have been misinterpreted as mixed cortical-medullary tumors. X320.

Some pheochromocytomas may be composed of relatively small pheochromocytes with round to ovoid hyperchromatic nuclei and small amounts of faintly eosinophilic cytoplasm (fig. 187). These cells resemble the so-called pheochromoblasts. Spindle cell variants of pheochromocytes may be found in less than 5 percent of tumors (fig. 188). Although occasional mitotic figures may be found in benign lesions, the presence of numerous mitoses should alert the pathologist to the possibility of a malignant tumor. Ganglion type cells, which are normal constituents of the adrenal medulla, may also be present within pheochromocytomas. Occasional pheochromocytomas with ganglioneuromatous foci of differentiation have been reported (Dawson and Tapp; figs. 189, 190). In vitro studies of both animal and human pheochromocytomas have established that neoplastic cells derived from these tumors can acquire morphologic and functional characteristics of neurons after culture with nerve growth factor (Tischler and Greene). (See section on Embryology and Postnatal Development/Medulla.) Tumors containing both pheochromocytoma and ganglioneuromatous foci may represent the in vivo counterpart of this phenomenon.

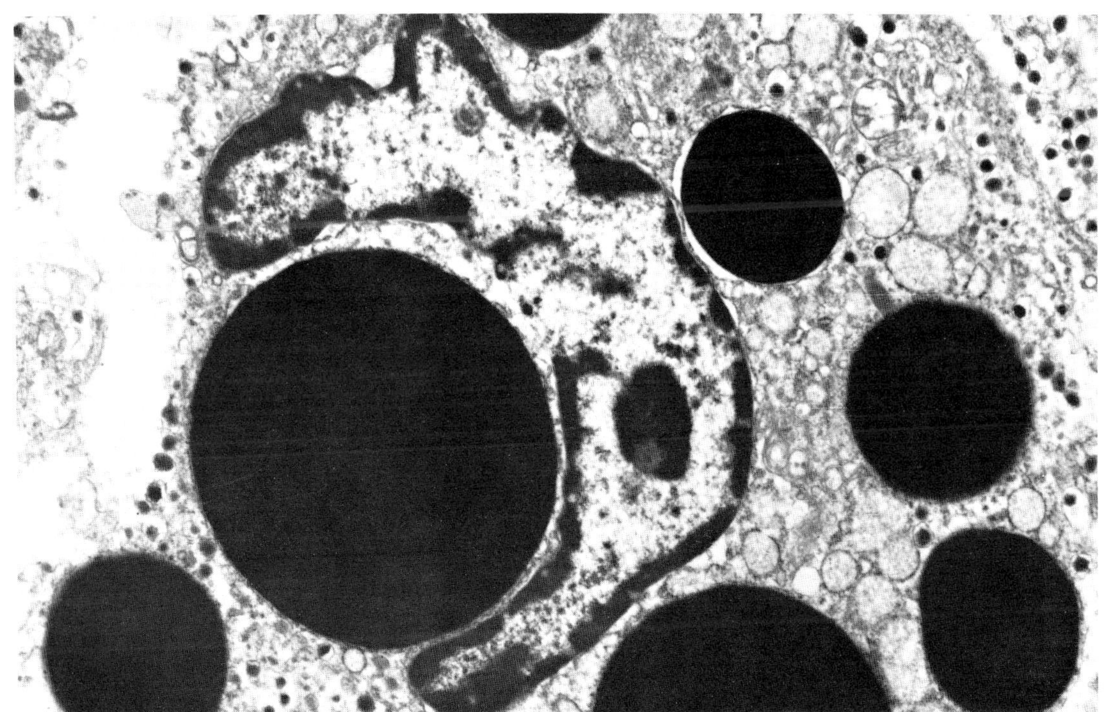

Figure 182
PHEOCHROMOCYTOMA
Electron micrograph illustrates the osmiophilic globules which are often seen in pheochromocytoma cells. One of the globules has indented the nucleus. X9700.

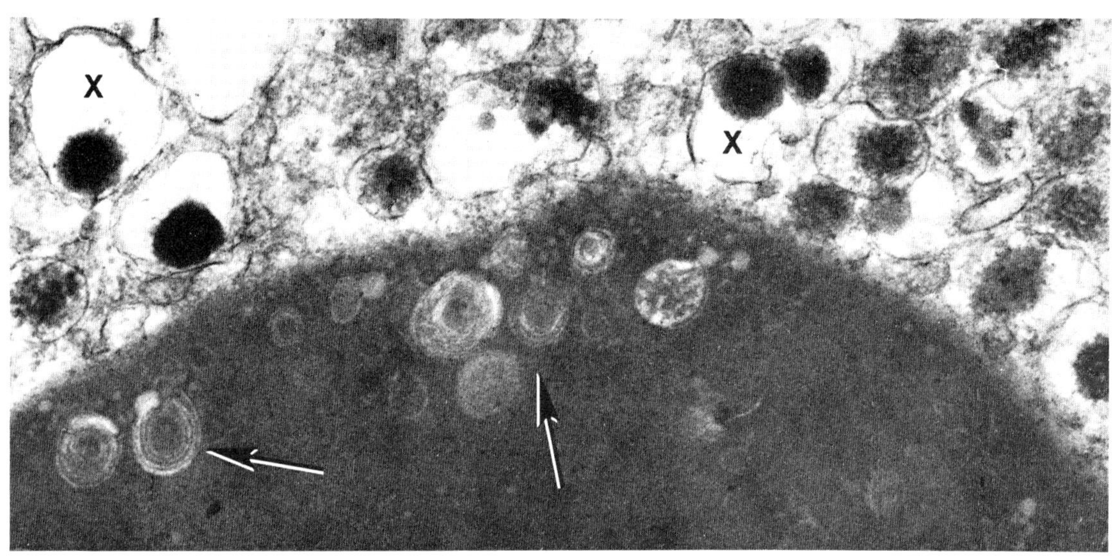

Figure 183
PHEOCHROMOCYTOMA
This pheochromocytoma cell contains a predominance of norepinephrine type granules which are characterized by electron dense cores surrounded by irregular electron lucent spaces (X). A large osmiophilic globule in the lower portion of the field contains membrane-like whorls (arrows), which may represent the membranes of the chromaffin granules. X41,000.

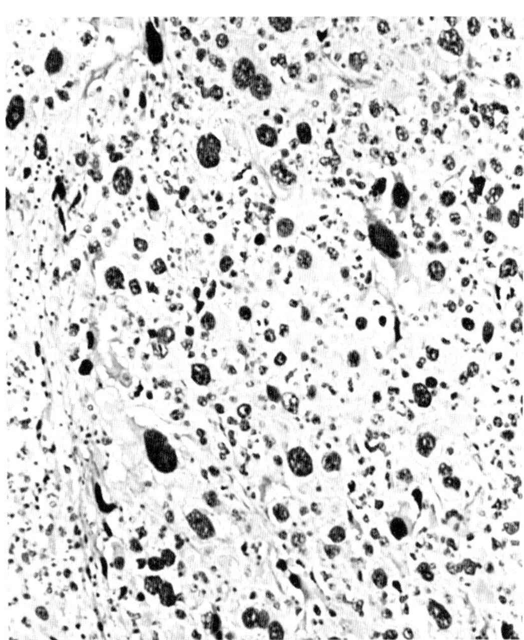

Figure 184
(Figures 184 and 185 from same patient)
PHEOCHROMOCYTOMA
Benign pheochromocytoma shows a striking degree of nuclear pleomorphism with numerous hyperchromatic and irregularly shaped nuclei. X125.

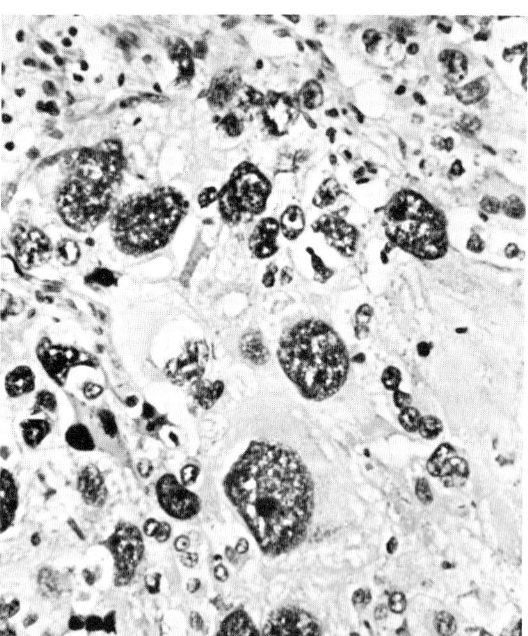

Figure 185
PHEOCHROMOCYTOMA
This figure represents a higher magnification of the previous illustration. The tumor cell nuclei contain coarsely clumped chromatin and large nucleoli. The cytoplasm is abundant. X320.

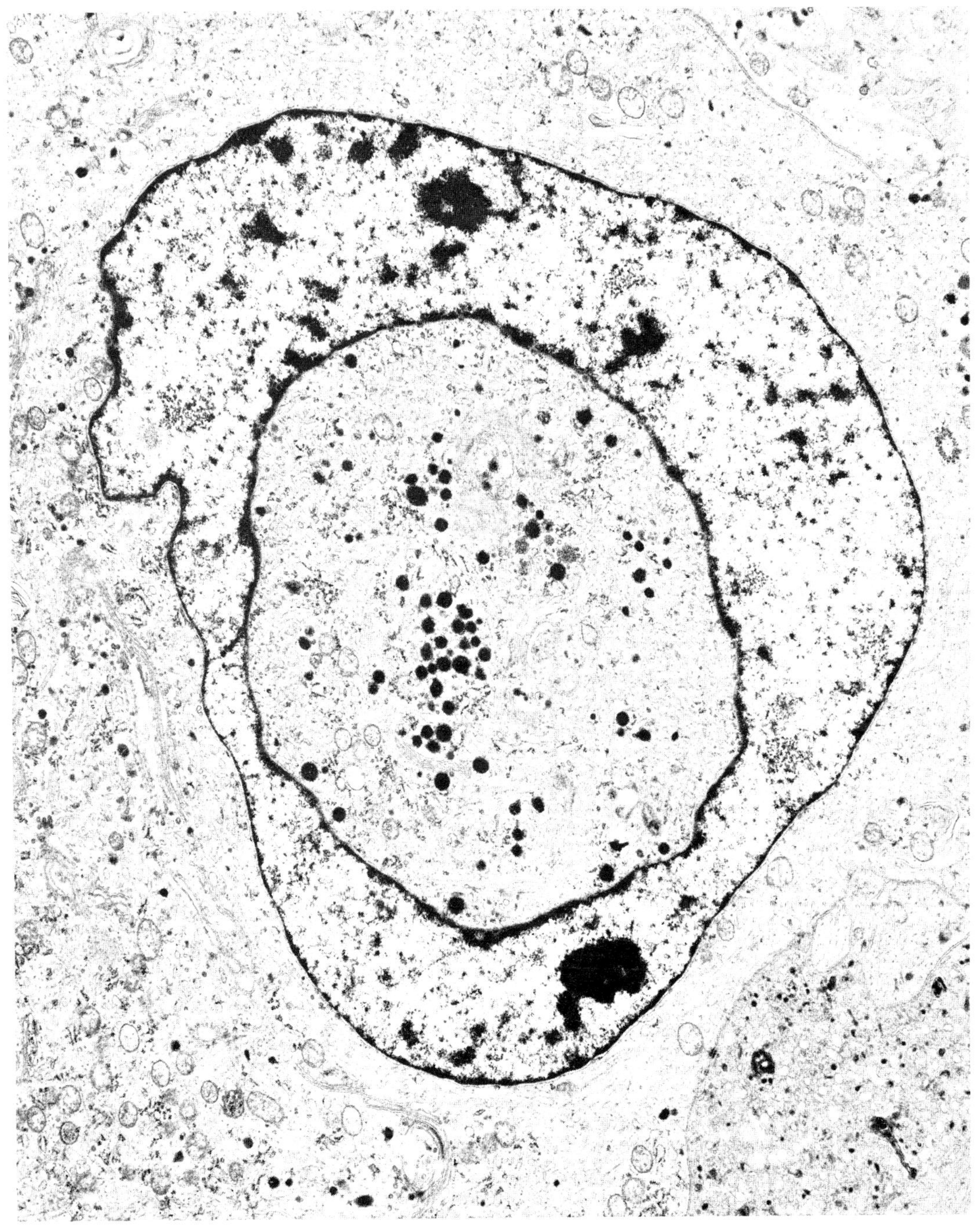

Figure 186
PHEOCHROMOCYTOMA

Many of the tumor cells in this pheochromocytoma contain numerous nuclear inclusions. At the ultrastructural level, the inclusions represent deep cytoplasmic invaginations into the nucleus. In this section, numerous dense core secretory granules are present within the "inclusion." X8100. (From DeLellis, R.A., Suchow, E., and Wolfe, H.J. Ultrastructure of nuclear "inclusions" in pheochromocytoma and paraganglioma. Hum. Pathol. 11:205-207, 1980.)

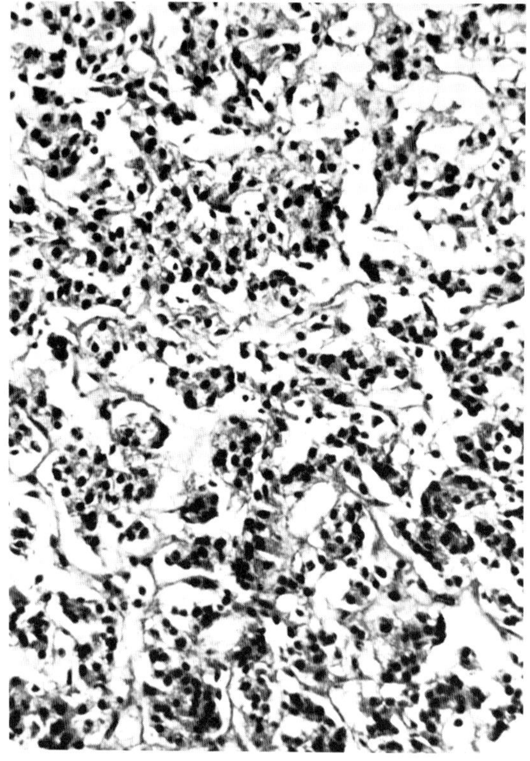

Figure 187
PHEOCHROMOCYTOMA
This pheochromocytoma shows a small nesting (alveolar)
pattern of growth. Individual tumor cells are quite small,
with hyperchromatic nuclei and scanty cytoplasm. X320.

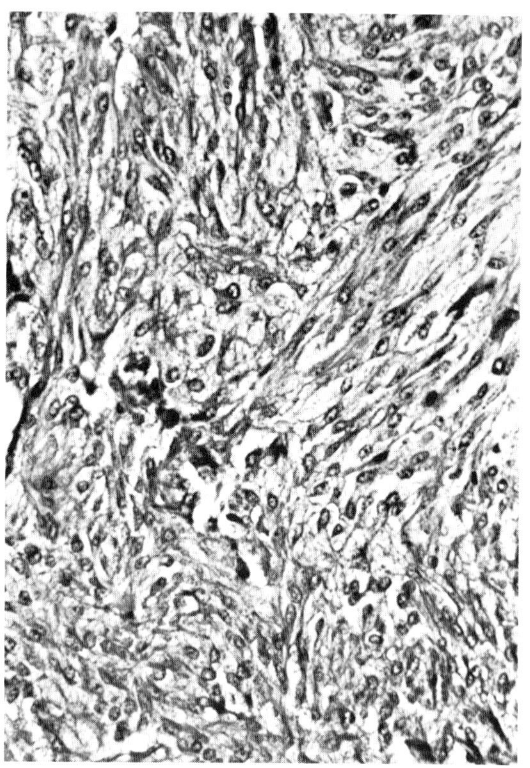

Figure 188
PHEOCHROMOCYTOMA
This pheochromocytoma shows a predominant spindle
pattern of growth. There has been no evidence of recurrent
or metastatic disease in five years of follow-up. X320.

Clusters of mature lymphocytes may also be found within pheochromocytomas (fig. 191). The significance of these inflammatory cells, both within normal and neoplastic medulla, however, remains uncertain. Brown fat has been reported in the retroperitoneal adipose tissue surrounding pheochromocytomas, but the significance of this finding remains obscure (Sherwin, 1968). Periadrenal accumulations of brown fat have also been described in the absence of pheochromocytoma (Medeiros et al.).

The differential diagnosis of pheochromocytomas is discussed in the section on cortical tumors.

Tissue Analysis for Catecholamines. Tumor tissue may be easily stored for later extraction and analysis of catecholamines. Quantitative biochemical methods may confirm a diagnosis of pheochromocytoma or document epinephrine:norepinephrine ratios in the tumor. Five to 10 g of tumor should be weighed, minced, and placed in 3 ml of 0.01N HCl for later analysis

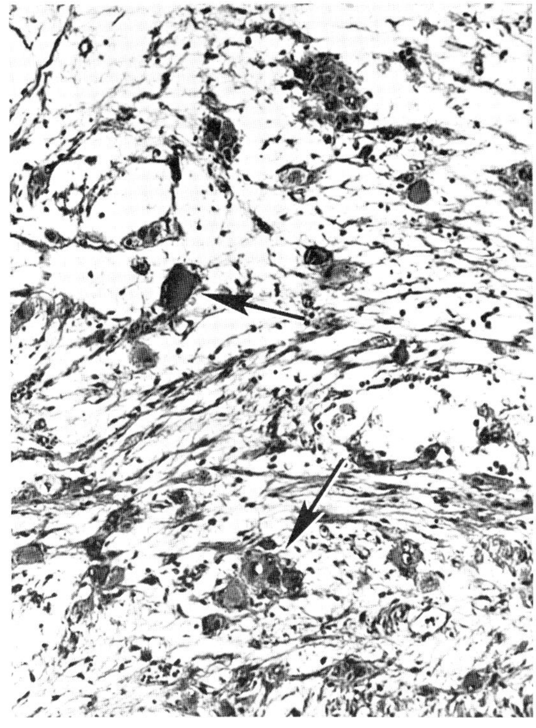

Figure 189
(Figures 189 and 190 from same patient)
PHEOCHROMOCYTOMA
This pheochromocytoma shows a large focus of ganglio-neuromatous differentiation. In this area, the stroma appears edematous and is composed of Schwann cells, occasional ganglion cells (arrows), and scattered lymphocytes. X125.

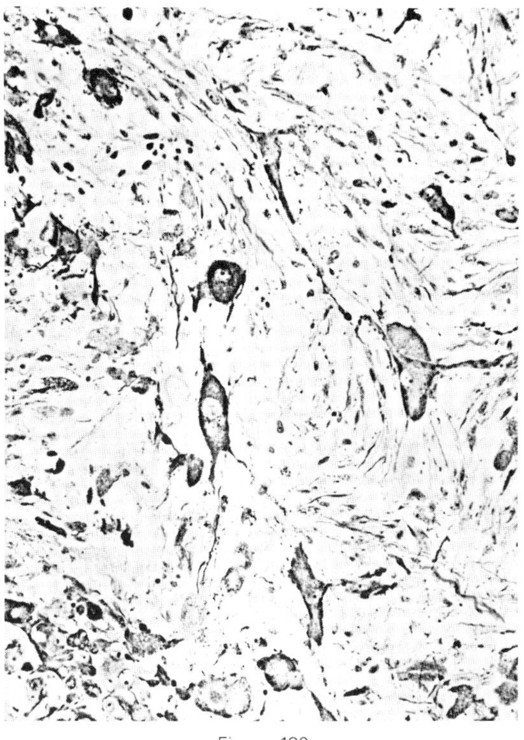

Figure 190
PHEOCHROMOCYTOMA
In this Bodian stain of the ganglioneuromatous focus illustrated in the previous figure, individual ganglion cells with elongated processes are apparent. X320.

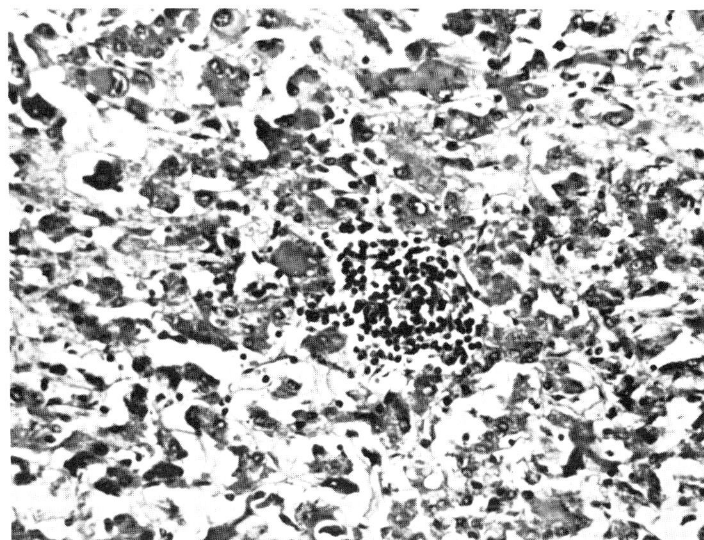

Figure 191
PHEOCHROMOCYTOMA
In this pheochromocytoma, a small collection of lymphocytes is apparent. X320.

(Kennedy et al.). Subsequent analysis will be valid even after storage for several months.

Histochemistry. The ability to accurately diagnose an adrenal tumor as a pheochromocytoma depends in part on methods to demonstrate the catecholamine content of the lesions. Some of the more commonly employed histochemical methods for this purpose are summarized below:

Chromaffin Reaction and its Modifications. The classic chromaffin reaction must be performed on fresh tissue specimens with 5 to 10 percent aqueous solutions of potassium dichromate or with one of the chromate containing fixatives such as Zenker's (without acetic acid) or Orth's fluid (Sherwin, 1968). Under these conditions, potassium dichromate serves as an oxidant, with the formation of adrenochrome and noradrenochrome pigments from epinephrine and norepinephrine, respectively (pl. XII-A, B). A positive chromaffin reaction is obtained from phenolic compounds containing two hydroxyl or amino groups which are ortho or para to one another. The adrenochrome pigment produced by the oxidation of epinephrine has a dark brown color, while the oxidation product of norepinephrine has a pale yellow color that may be difficult to differentiate from the background. When tissues containing high concentrations of catecholamines are placed in dichromate solutions, clouds of red brown pigment may diffuse from the cut surfaces. Subsequent washing, dehydration, and paraffin embedding may lead to considerable extraction of chromogenic pigments. This loss of pigment may lead to a negative microscopic chromaffin reaction, while the gross chromaffin reaction is strongly positive. The

high solubility of the adrenochrome and noradrenochrome pigments limits the sensitivity of the classic chromaffin reaction. Embedding tissues in Carbowax following the chromaffin reaction may lead to less pigment loss. Selective oxidation of norepinephrine-containing cells has been reported in studies employing dichromate solutions at pH 4.1 (Sherwin). This method has been used to differentiate epinephrine and norepinephrine containing granules at the ultrastructural level. Potassium iodate may also be used to demonstrate norepinephrine containing cells selectively. Catecholamines may also be demonstrated with immunohistochemical procedures (Verhofstad et al.).

Substitute Chromaffin Reactions. A variety of technics have been developed for the demonstration of epinephrine and norepinephrine in formalin fixed tissue sections. In general, these methods lack specificity and demonstrate a wide variety of reducing substances, including melanin, lipofuscin, and tissue components containing a high proportion of sulfhydryl groups (Sherwin, 1968). Substitute chromaffin reactions include the standard argentaffin and argyrophil methods, Sevki's modification of the Giemsa technic, and the ferric cyanide method. Fixation of tissues in glutaraldehyde, followed by staining with ammoniacal silver leads to a selective demonstration of norepinephrine-containing cells (Tramezzani et al.). The glutaraldehyde reacts with the primary amine groups of the norepinephrine with the formation of a yellow colored compound which represents the Schiff base or azomethine. The monocondensation product of glutaraldehyde and norepinephrine has an aldehyde group which is responsible for the silver reduction.

Fluorescence Methods. The most significant advance in the histochemical demonstration of catecholamines was the development and refinement of the formaldehyde induced fluorescence technic by Falck and Owman. The basic chemical reaction involves the formation of highly fluorescent derivatives after the condensation of formaldehyde gas with catecholamines and indolylethlamines (pl. XII-F). The successful application of this method depends upon rapid immobilization of the amines within the tissues by freeze drying or rapid air drying and subsequent condensation of the amines with gaseous formaldehyde. Catecholamines form isoquinoline derivatives with an emission maximum of 470 μm which is visible as a green fluorescence. This technic possesses both high specificity and high sensitivity and produces a positive reaction in tissues which are known to contain catecholamines, but which have given negative or equivocally positive chromaffin reactions. Touch preparations are particularly useful for the demonstration of amines in a variety of tumors (DeLellis). The glyoxylic acid method is based on the same principles as the formaldehyde induced fluorescence technic and possesses similar high sensitivity and specificity. A glyoxylic acid method employing cryostat cut frozen sections has been developed recently and has proved to be most useful in the rapid diagnosis of pheochromocytoma and related tumors (de la Torre and Surgeon).

Protein Methods. The chromogranin components of the adrenal medullary cells have been shown to have a predominant random coil conformation and a high proportion of glutamic acid residues (Solcia et al.). Other proteins with these properties include a wide variety of polypeptide hormones such as calcitonin, ACTH, and gastrin. Both toluidine blue and coriophosphine O have been used extensively to demonstrate these hormonal products in the dispersed endocrine cell system (Solcia et al.). Acid hydrolysis prior to staining with these dyes not only removes basic substances such as DNA and RNA, but also converts side chain carboxamido groups to carboxyls which are then free to react with the basic dyes. Lead hematoxylin is thought to react in a similar fashion. Both normal and neoplastic adrenal medullary cells show intense staining with toluidine blue and coriophosphine O. This property has been referred to as masked metachromasia.

The chromogranin component of both normal and neoplastic adrenal medullary cells as well as other cells of the neuroendocrine system may be demonstrated with the use of polyclonal antisera or monoclonal antibodies (Lloyd and Wilson; O'Connor et al.). Immunohistochemical technics employing these reagents have been particularly useful in the distinction of cortical and medullary tumors. In contrast to the distribution of chromogranin in chromaffin type cells, S-100 protein is present in the sustentacular cell components of these tumors (Blaivas et al.). Pheochromocytomas are rich in neurofilament type proteins, in contrast to cortical tumors which are variably positive for cytokeratins and vimentin (Miettinen et al.).

Neuron specific enolase (protein 14-3-2) was first localized in the chromaffin cells of the normal adrenal medulla by Schmechel and associates and was also reported in pheochromocytomas by Tapia and coworkers. Using immunoperoxidase technics, neuron specific enolase typically exhibits a granular cytoplasmic immunoreactivity within

PLATE XII
PHEOCHROMOCYTOMA

A. This figure demonstrates the gross appearance of a positive chromaffin reaction (gross Henle reaction). After immersion in aqueous potassium dichromate, the tumor developed a black brown coloration, due to the oxidation of catecholamines to adrenachrome and noradrenochrome pigments (lower half of figure). The cortex remained unreactive. X1.6. (Courtesy of Dr. G. Gray, New York, NY.)

B. After dehydration and routine embedding, much of the pigment is extracted from tissues. The tumor cells in this illustration contain small amounts of yellow brown pigment, indicative of a positive chromaffin reaction. X320.

C. This pheochromocytoma is sharply demarcated from the adjacent adrenal tissue and has a dusky discoloration. The adjacent medullary tissue appears normal. X1.4.

D. This pheochromocytoma has undergone extensive cystic degeneration. The parenchyma is composed of fibrous connective tissue, which appears trabeculated. X1.

E. This pheochromocytoma contains abundant intracytoplasmic periodic acid-Schiff positive globules (arrows). X250.

F. Touch preparations of this pheochromocytoma were exposed to formaldehyde vapor for one hour. The individual tumor cells show intense yellow green cytoplasmic fluorescence, indicative of high concentrations of catecholamines. X400.

PLATE XII

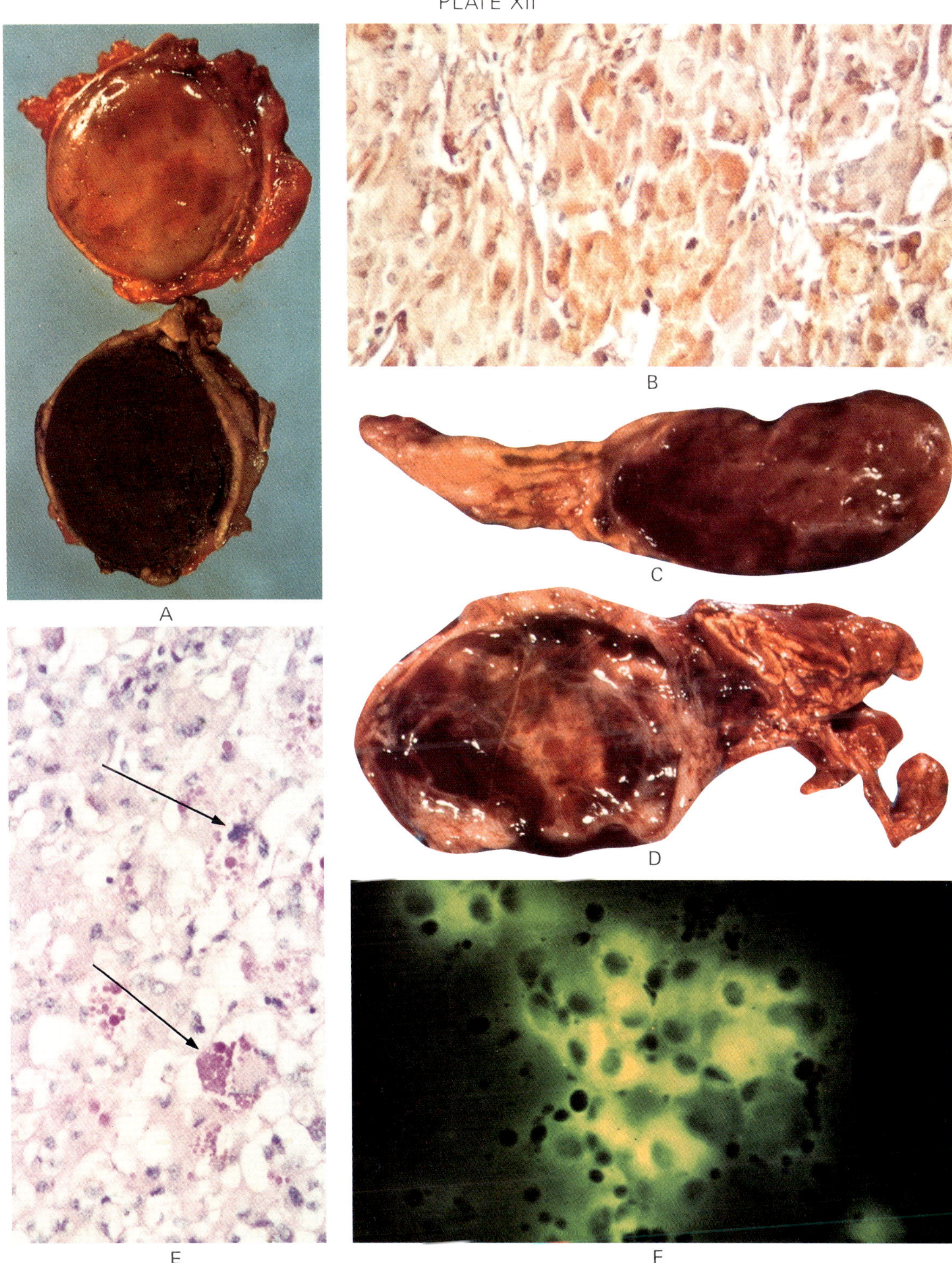

201

the cytoplasm of normal and neoplastic chromaffin cells (Lloyd and Warner). Although this isoenzyme is present characteristically in tumors of neuroendocrine cell origin, it is absent from normal and neoplastic adrenal cortical tissue. The demonstration of neuron specific enolase in a poorly differentiated primary adrenal neoplasm, therefore, should provide evidence of its medullary origin.

Ultrastructure. Similar to cells of the normal adrenal medulla, pheochromocytoma cells contain varying numbers of membrane bound dense core secretory granules. Studies of Yokoyama and Takayasu have indicated that pheochromocytoma cells may be divided into two major groups on the basis of the presence (type I) or absence (type II) of secretory granules. The type I cells were further subdivided into three groups on the basis of the numbers and sizes of secretory granules and vesicles. Type IA cells contained large numbers of vesicles, but relatively few secretory granules that measured 180 $\pm$ 75 mm in diameter. Type IB cells had more numerous granules that measured 130 $\pm$ 70 nm. Finally, the type IC cells had the largest number of granules, which measured 220 $\pm$ 100 nm in diameter and which filled the cytoplasm of individual tumor cells. Although the secretory granules tended to be larger than those found in normal medullary cells, there were no apparent differences in granule morphology between those tumors secreting norepinephrine or epinephrine. It should be remembered, however, that these tumors were fixed initially in osmium tetroxide rather than glutaraldehyde, which forms an insoluble complex with norepinephrine.

Using tumors initially fixed in glutaraldehyde, Tannenbaum was able to find charac-

teristic differences between norepinephrine and epinephrine containing tumors. Pure norepinephrine tumors had highly electron dense secretory granules which were separated from their limiting membranes by a wide electron lucent space (fig. 183). Epinephrine containing tumors contained secretory granules with less dense finely granular contents closely applied to their limiting membranes (fig. 192). These ultrastructural characteristics are similar to those noted in normal adrenal medullary cells. The pheochromocytoma secretory granules, however, tended to be somewhat larger than their normal counterparts. The studies of Lauper and associates showed that pheochromocytomas were composed of dark and light cells, both of which were capable of storing catecholamines. In this study, the numbers and types of norepinephrine and epinephrine granules showed a positive correlation with the type of catecholamines extracted from the tumors. In many cases, however, granules of indeterminant or atypical morphology may be seen (Medeiros et al.).

Recent studies of Watanabe and associates have demonstrated a wide variety of mitochondrial abnormalities in pheochromocytomas. Although large mitochondria have been reported to occur in extra-adrenal paragangliomas, these authors found large elongated mitochondria measuring up to 3 μ in length in a series of pheochromocytomas. In addition to mitochondria with small numbers of cristae, intramitochondrial spheroidal bodies, possibly representing atypical cristae, were also noted. Rare mitochondrial rodlets as well as septate desmosome-like structures between adjacent mitochondria were also found. Watanabe and colleagues suggested that the decreased levels of the mitochondrial en-

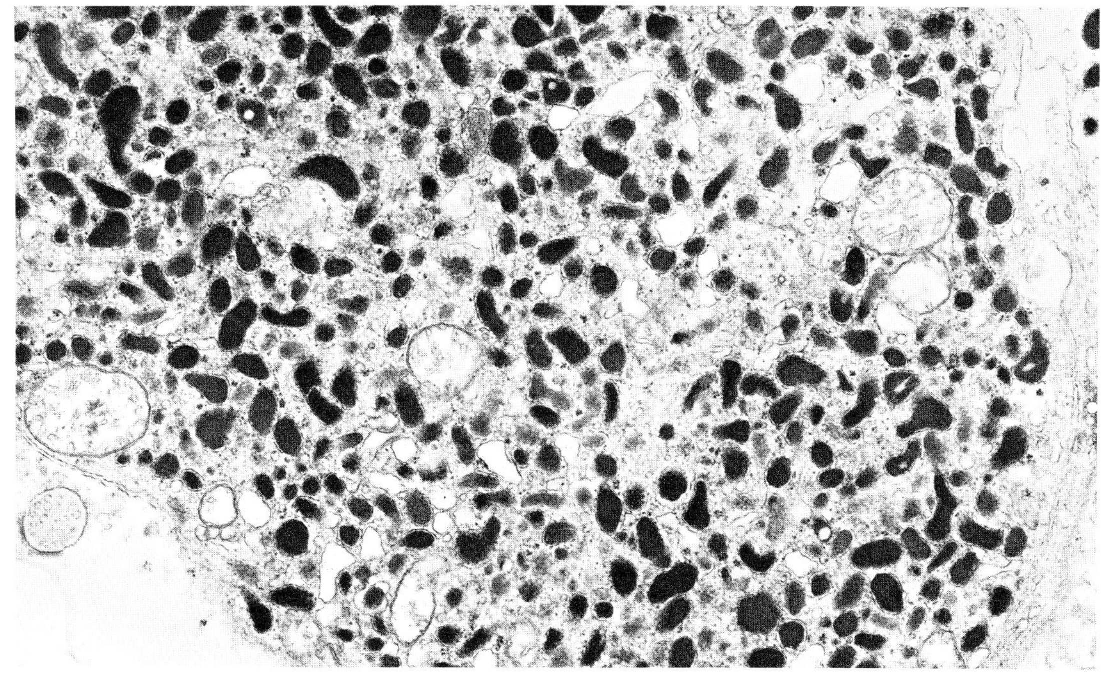

Figure 192
PHEOCHROMOCYTOMA
This pheochromocytoma, which produced epinephrine almost exclusively, contains a population of moderately pleomorphic electron dense epinephrine granules. These granules lack the highly electron dense cores and irregular electron lucent space of norepinephrine granules. X18,000.

zymes, monoamine oxidase and succinic dehydrogenase, were related to these mitochondrial abnormalities.

RECURRENT AND MALIGNANT PHEOCHROMOCYTOMA

The vast majority of patients treated surgically for pheochromocytoma will be cured. Particularly in children and in patients with a family history of pheochromocytoma, however, the recurrence of catecholamine abnormalities following the original operation should prompt a careful search for a second tumor either in the opposite adrenal or in an extra-adrenal site (Harrison et al.). In other patients, increased levels of catecholamines following the primary operation may indicate either local recurrence of tumor or the development of distant metastases. In a report of 138 patients with pheochromocytoma, the tumor recurrence rate was 9.8 percent (Remine et al.). Most of these patients had evidence of recurrence within five to six years from the date of original operation. In general, however, it was not possible to predict on the basis of gross and microscopic characteristics which tumors would recur or metastasize. In the Mayo Clinic series (Remine et al.), the malignant pheochromocytomas tended to be larger than the benign ones. This tendency is supported by Medeiros and associates, who reported a mean weight of 759 g for malignant tumors as compared to 156 g for the benign tumors.

The frequency of malignant pheochromocytomas has been reported to range from 2 to 15 percent. Although a number of gross and microscopic features have been suggested as criteria for differentiating benign and malignant pheochromocytomas, most authors agree that the presence of secondary tumor deposits in sites where chromaffin tissue is not normally present is the only absolute criterion of malignancy (Sherwin, 1968). Using the presence of metastases as a criterion for malignancy, less than 5 percent of pheochromocytomas may be considered to be malignant, as determined by metastatic spread to lymph nodes, liver, or bone.

Cytologically, benign pheochromocytomas may exhibit considerable variation in nuclear size and shape, with numerous giant hyperchromatic nuclei (figs. 184, 185). Malignant pheochromocytomas, on the other hand, may show less nuclear pleomorphism (figs. 193–195). In a cytomorphometric study of benign and malignant pheochromocytomas, Lewis found that benign tumors had a mode corresponding to a diploid (2 n) DNA content and a wide range of values, with nuclei measuring up to 40 n. Malignant pheochromocytomas, on the other hand, had a hyperdiploid or triploid mode with a smaller range of values. This study indicates, therefore, that the finding of striking nuclear pleomorphism favors an interpretation of benign pheochromocytoma. Although mitoses may be seen in adrenal medullary hyperplasia and benign pheochromocytoma, they are rarely numerous. The presence of large numbers of mitoses should alert the pathologist and clinician to the possibility of either future local recurrence or metastatic disease (fig. 195). Vascular and capsular invasion, criteria for malig-

nancy in many other organ systems, occur in both benign and malignant pheochromocytomas and cannot, therefore, be used to assess malignant potential (figs. 172, 173). Finally, the cytologic pattern of tumor cell growth has been suggested as a determinant in predicting malignant potential. Sherwin (1968), for example, suggested that a predominant spindle cell pattern of growth was suggestive of malignancy. Subsequent studies have failed to confirm this hypothesis (Medeiros et al.). The studies of Medeiros and colleagues have indicated that large tumor size, the presence of confluent areas of necrosis, and small tumor cell size are indicative of malignant potential.

Malignant pheochromocytomas are generally slowly growing tumors. When they do metastasize, however, the most common sites of secondary spread include liver (figs. 196, 197), lymph nodes, and bones (fig. 193), particularly the vertebrae, ribs, and skull (Neville). Histologic examination of the metastases should be accompanied by appropriate histochemical, ultrastructural, or biochemical tests for catecholamines. Secondary tumor deposits may resemble completely benign pheochromocytomas or may exhibit considerable pleomorphism (fig. 197). In considering lymph node metastases, all efforts should be directed toward distinguishing concurrent extra-adrenal paragangliomas, which may compress adjacent lymph nodes, from true metastatic deposits.

In patients with multiple endocrine neoplasia type II, metastasis from the medullary thyroid carcinoma may resemble metastatic deposits of pheochromocytoma. In these cases, immunohistochemical staining for calcitonin should permit specific identification of medullary carcinoma.

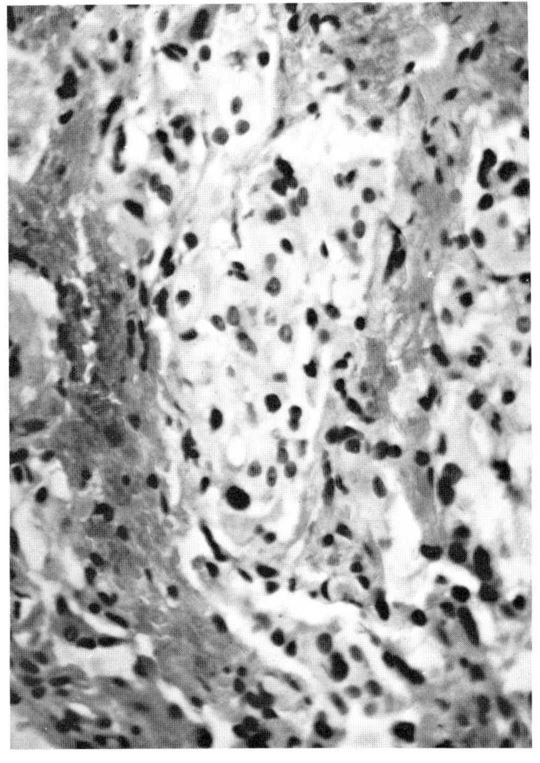

Figure 193
PHEOCHROMOCYTOMA
This metastatic pheochromocytoma in the skull shows a typical nesting pattern of growth. There is relatively little variation in nuclear size or shape. X400.

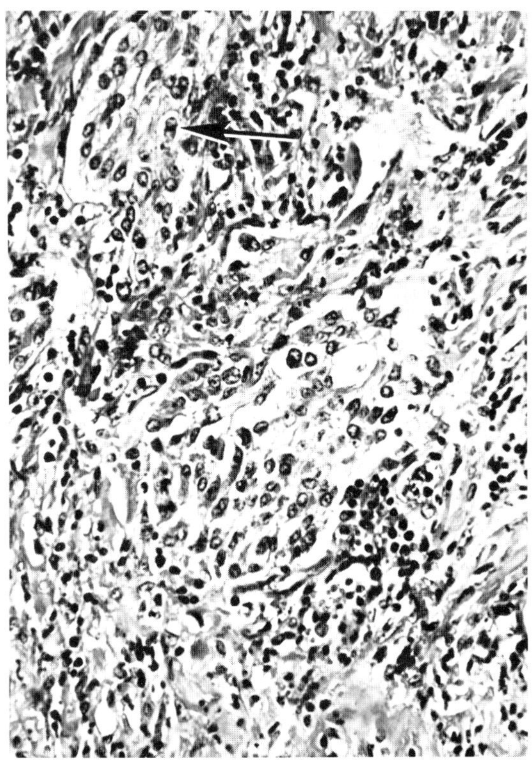

Figure 194
PHEOCHROMOCYTOMA
Locally invasive pheochromocytoma extended beyond the adrenal capsule into the retroperitoneal fat. There is a striking fibroblastic and lymphocytic reaction. The pheochromocytoma cells (arrow) exhibit relatively little pleomorphism. X320.

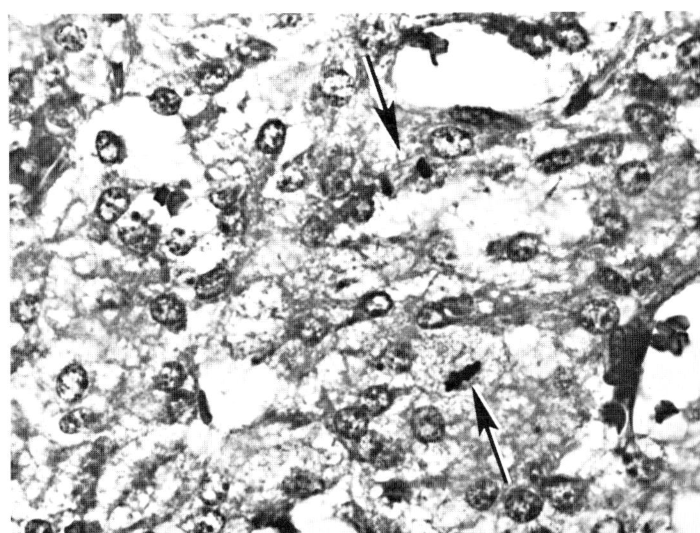

Figure 195
PHEOCHROMOCYTOMA
This malignant pheochromocytoma was associated with retroperitoneal lymph node metastases. The tumor showed a predominant spindle pattern of growth. Two mitotic figures (arrows) are evident in this field. X1000.

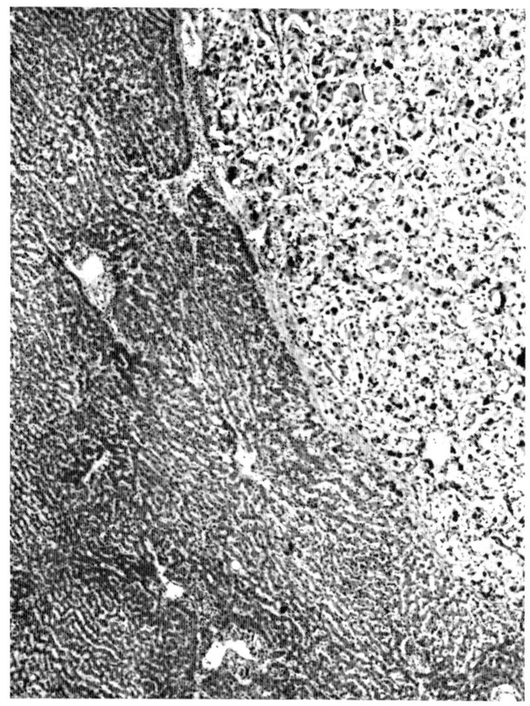

Figure 196
(Figures 196 and 197 from same patient)
PHEOCHROMOCYTOMA
Liver specimen from a patient with malignant pheochromocytoma contained multiple metastatic deposits. In many areas, the tumor nodules were separated from the hepatic parenchyma by a thin fibrous capsule. X50.

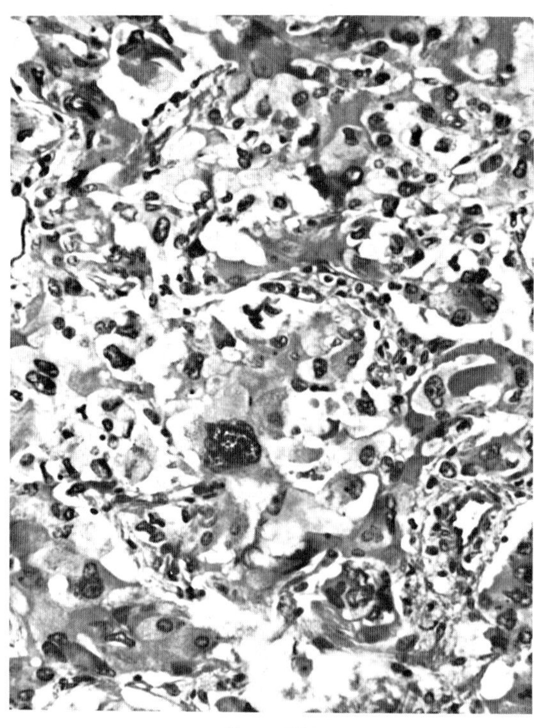

Figure 197
PHEOCHROMOCYTOMA
The individual tumor cells in this metastatic pheochromocytoma show a marked degree of nuclear pleomorphism and hyperchromasia. X400.

Pheochromocytomas may exhibit considerable local invasive growth without the development of distant metastases (fig. 194). Sellwood and associates have described the case of a 45 year old man with recurrent catecholamine abnormalities 11 years after resection of a left sided pheochromocytoma. On re-exploration, the perirenal fibroadipose tissue contained multiple red brown tumor nodules which measured up to 8 mm in diameter. Detailed histologic examination revealed 15 separate tumor nodules. Of considerable interest was a focal foreign body giant cell reaction in the region of the tumor recurrence. Examination of this area with polarized light revealed the presence of multiple birefringent talc crystals. The finding of the talc crystals in the periadrenal adipose tissue suggested that the tumor deposits arose from cells which were seeded at the time of the original surgery.

PHEOCHROMOCYTOMA IN CHILDHOOD

Pheochromocytoma is a rare but curable cause of hypertension in children. In contrast to the high frequency of episodic hypertension in adults with pheochromocytoma, sustained hypertension is present in almost 90 percent of children with this tumor (Manger and Gifford). The most common symptoms, as in adults, include headache, sweating, nausea, vomiting, weight loss, and visual disturbances. In children, polydipsia and polyuria may be found in up to 25 percent of cases. In children with tumors confined to the adrenal (Stackpole et al.), 20 had bilateral tumors, while the remainder had unilateral pheochromocytomas. The remaining 31 patients in this series of 100 children had one or more extra-adrenal paragangliomas, and of these, 8 patients had one or more associated intra-adrenal tumors. In 9 patients, there was a family history of pheochromocytoma. This observation suggests that the high frequency of bilaterality, multicentricity, and association with extra-adrenal paragangliomas in children reflects a genetic predisposition to the development of neoplasia in the adrenal medulla and associated paraganglia. The vast majority of tumors in children weighed between 10 and 30 g. Microscopically, the tumors do not differ significantly from those noted in adults. The most important single cause of death during operative and immediate postoperative periods is the presence of an unsuspected pheochromocytoma in the contralateral adrenal or an extra-adrenal paraganglioma.

FAMILIAL PHEOCHROMOCYTOMA

It has been estimated that approximately 10 percent of all pheochromocytomas are familial (Neville; Manger and Gifford). In contrast to sporadic pheochromocytomas which are almost always unilateral, the familial tumors are frequently bilateral and multicentric (pl. XIII). In a review of 59 previously reported cases of pheochromocytoma associated with familial medullary thyroid carcinoma, for example, bilateral tumors were found in 66 percent of cases, while multicentric pheochromocytomas were present in 30 percent of patients with unilateral adrenal medullary abnormalities (DeLellis et al., 1976). The age of onset of tumors in patients with a positive family history is less than in patients with sporadic pheochromocytoma. Moreover, the frequency of extra-adrenal paragangliomas may be increased in some patients with familial pheochromocytoma syndromes.

The major familial pheochromocytoma syndromes are summarized in Table 8. These syndromes, which exhibit autosomal dominant patterns of inheritance, may be divided into two major groups on the basis of the frequency of pheochromocytoma. Pheochromocytomas have been reported to occur in 30 to 70 percent of patients with type II (IIA) and III (IIB) multiple endocrine neoplasia (Carney et al.; DeLellis et al., 1976; figs. 198, 199). In patients with neurocutaneous phakomatosis syndromes, including Lindau-von Hippel disease, von Recklinghausen's disease, and the Sturge-Weber syndrome, on the other hand, the frequency of pheochromocytoma has been estimated to be approximately 5 percent (Wander and Das Gupta). More recent studies indicate that the overall frequency of pheochromocytoma in patients with von Recklinghausen's disease is considerably less and ranges from 0.5 to 1.0 percent. The incidence of pheochromocytomas in some kindreds with neurocutaneous phakomatoses syndromes, however, may be considerably higher. Moreover, the adrenal medullary tumors may represent the first manifestation of the syndrome. In a recently studied kindred with Lindau-von Hippel disease reported by Atuk and associates, 7

PLATE XIII
FAMILIAL MEDULLARY CARCINOMA.

(Plate XIII-A through G from same patient.)

A. This left adrenal was resected from a patient with familial medullary thyroid carcinoma. The external surface (A) of the gland is distorted by multiple smooth-surfaced nodules. Approx. X1.5.

B. The nodules vary from pink white to tan. The intervening medulla is diffusely expanded.

C. The right adrenal, resected from the same patient, has an overall normal external configuration.

D—G. There is both diffuse and nodular expansion of the medullary region.

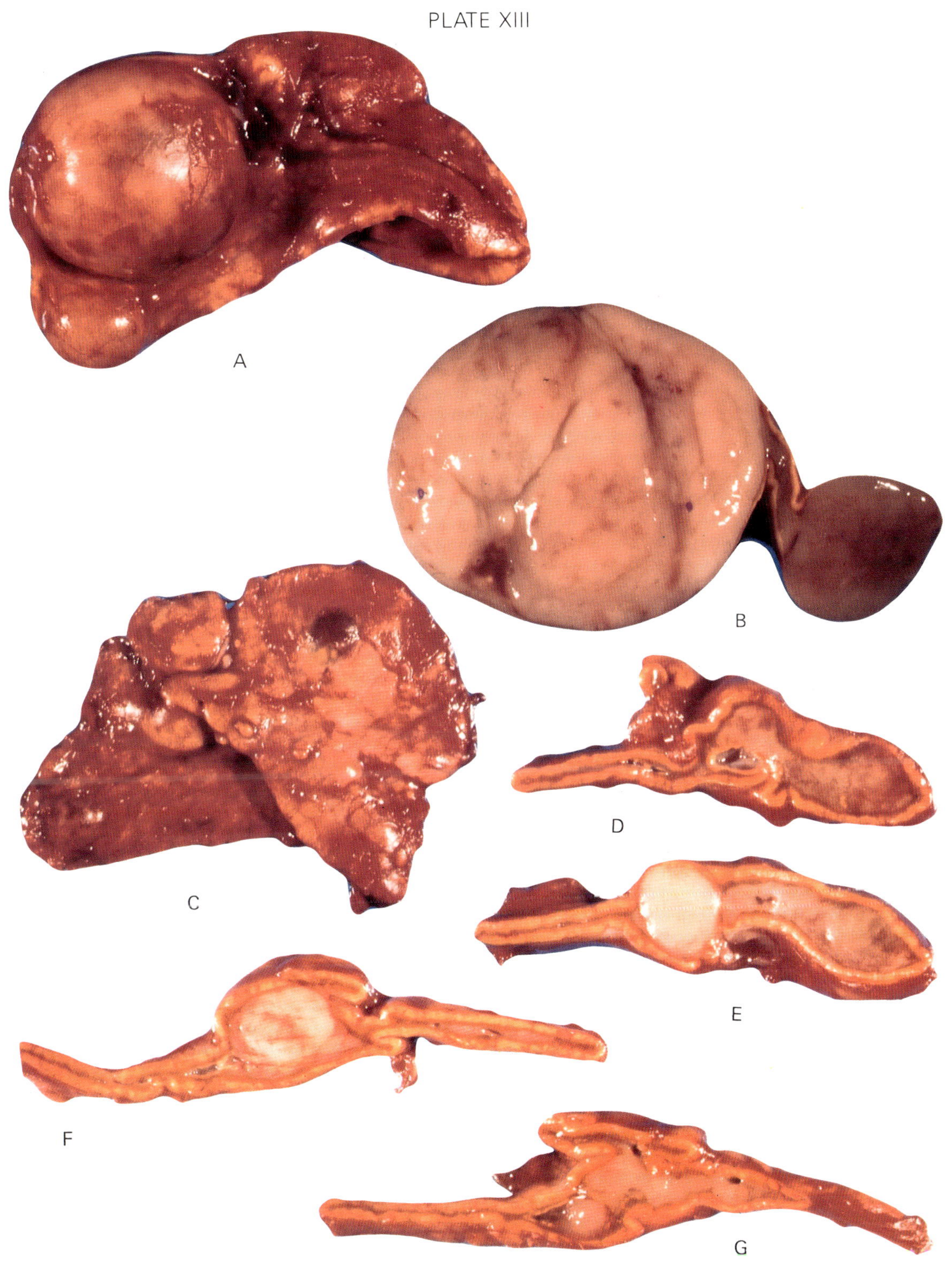

PLATE XIII
A
B
C
D
E
F
G

Table 8

FAMILIAL PHEOCHROMOCYTOMA SYNDROMES

Syndrome	Components of Syndrome
Multiple endocrine neoplasia (type II, type IIA)	C-cell hyperplasia-medullary thyroid carcinoma; adrenal medullary hyperplasia-pheochromocytoma; parathyroid hyperplasia-adenoma
Multiple endocrine neoplasia (type III, type IIB)	C-cell hyperplasia-medullary thyroid carcinoma; adrenal medullary hyperplasia-pheochromocytoma; corneal, mucocutaneous, and gastrointestinal ganglioneuromatosis; Marfanoid habitus
Lindau-von Hippel disease	Angiomatosis retinae; hemangioblastomas of central nervous system; renal, pancreatic hepatic, and epididymal cysts; renal carcinoma; pheochromocytoma
von Recklinghausen's disease	Cutaneous or visceral neurofibromas; café au lait spots; benign and malignant schwannoma; meningioma; glioma; pheochromocytoma
Sturge-Weber syndrome	Cavernous hemangiomas involving the first or all of the three divisions of the fifth cranial nerve; pheochromocytoma

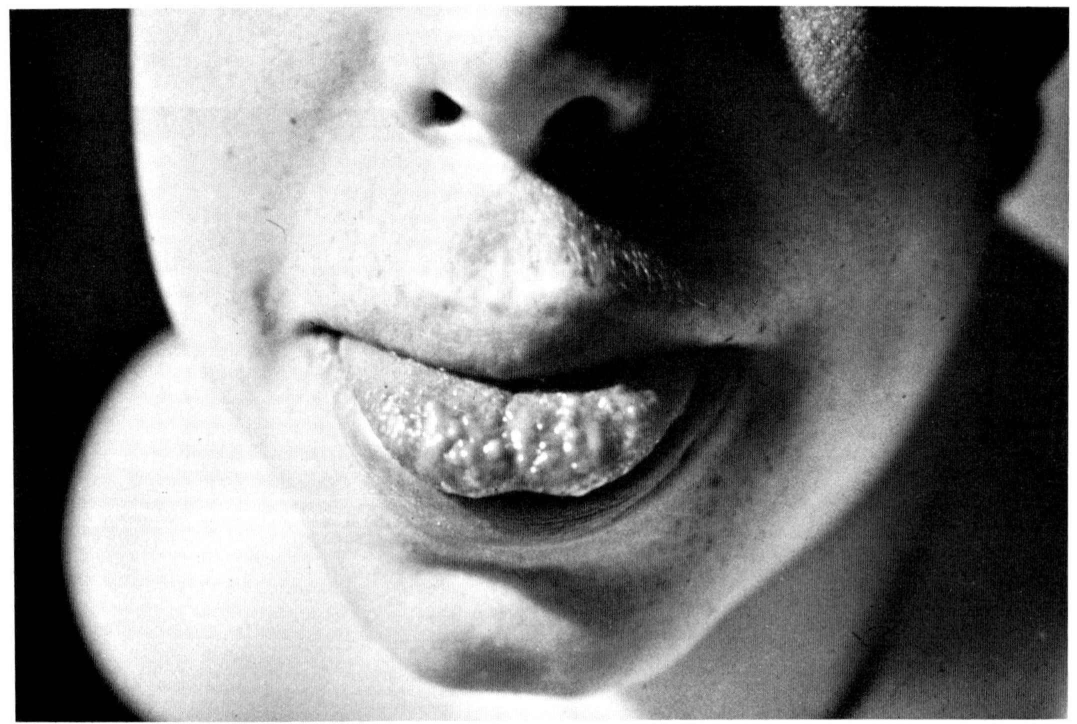

Figure 198
MULTIPLE ENDOCRINE NEOPLASIA SYNDROME
TYPE IIB (III)
This 11 year old boy has type IIB (III) multiple endocrine neoplasia. Multiple mucosal neuromas are present in the tongue, and the lips appear thickened.

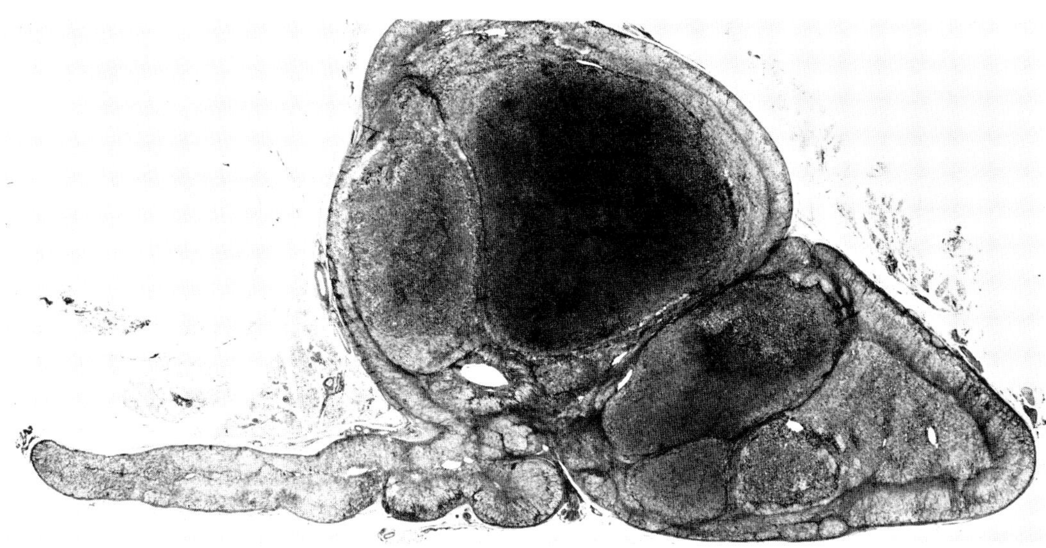

Figure 199
DIFFUSE AND NODULAR ADRENAL MEDULLARY HYPERPLASIA
The left adrenal was resected from a 27 year old man with a history of familial medullary thyroid carcinoma. Multiple medullary nodules are present in the crest and right alar regions. A narrow band of medullary tissue is present in the left alar region. X4.5. (From DeLellis, R.A., Wolfe, H.J., Gagel, R.F., Feldman, Z.T., et al. Adrenal medullary hyperplasia. Am. J. Pathol. 83:177-196, 1976.)

of 13 affected patients had pheochromocytoma alone. Of the remaining 6 patients, 1 had pheochromocytoma combined with Lindau-von Hippel disease, 4 had pheochromocytoma with retinal disease only, and a single patient had a retinal lesion alone. Although there are kindreds in which pheochromocytomas are inherited as autosomal dominant traits without other associated abnormalities, these familial occurrences may represent multiple endocrine adenomatosis or neurocutaneous phakomatosis syndrome in which only the adrenal medullary abnormalities are apparent.

Studies of DeLellis and associates (1976) in patients with familial medullary thyroid carcinoma (MTC) have shown that one of the earliest manifestations of adrenal medullary hyperfunction is an increased ratio of epinephrine to norepinephrine in the urine. Morphometric analyses of adrenal glands resected from these patients have revealed adrenal medullary hyperplasia as reflected by a two- to threefold increase in medullary volume and weight as compared to age and sex matched controls (figs. 200, 201). (See Adrenal Medullary Hyperplasia.) The increase in medullary mass resulted from diffuse and nodular proliferations of adrenal medullary cells primarily within the head and body regions of the glands (fig. 199). Similar findings have also been reported by Carney and associates in patients with familial MTC. These results support the hypothesis that the pheochromocytomas in patients with familial MTC may, in fact, represent extreme degrees of nodular hyperplasia of the medulla (fig. 202). Diffuse and nodular adrenal medullary hyperplasia similar to that seen in patients with familial MTC has also been reported in patients with Lindau-von Hippel disease.

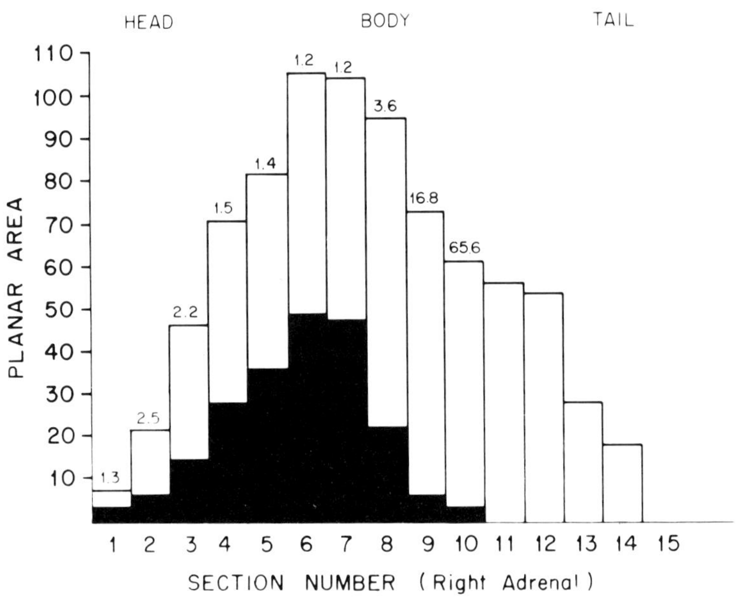

Figure 200
(Figures 200–202 from same patient)
ADRENAL MEDULLARY HYPERPLASIA
This histogram is based on a morphometric analysis of cortical and medullary areas of the right adrenal in a 68 year old man with familial medullary thyroid carcinoma. The combined corticomedullary ratio for the head and body regions of the gland was 3.7:1 (normal 10:1). The estimated medullary weight was 1.12 g (normal 0.47 ± 0.15 g). A single small nodule was present in the head of this gland, while the remaining medulla was diffusely hyperplastic. (From DeLellis, R.A., Wolfe, H.J., Gagel, R.F., Feldman, Z.T., et al. Adrenal medullary hyperplasia. Am. J. Pathol. 83:177-196, 1976.)

In contrast to the unilobular appearance of sporadic pheochromocytomas, adrenals resected from patients with one of the familial syndromes are characteristically multilobular (fig. 199; pl. XIII). On cross section, individual nodules may vary from several mm to up to 10 cm in diameter. Although the cortex overlying larger nodules is often compressed, the nodules are not truly encapsulated. The nodules, which are characteristically soft and gray tan to pink, blend imperceptibly into the adjacent medullary tissue. Larger nodules often appear to form by coalescence of multiple smaller nodules (fig. 199). Associated diffuse hyperplasia is characterized by a general expansion of the medullary zone with extension of medullary cells into both alar regions of the body and into the tail of the glands.

Individual nodules offer a wide range of cytologic characteristics. In some, the predominant cells resemble pheochromoblasts and measure 5 to 6 μ in diameter, with small, centrally placed round to ovoid hyperchromatic nuclei, scanty cytoplasm, and ill-defined cell borders. Other nodules may be composed of round to polyhedral cells with finely granular basophilic cytoplasm or with extensively vacuolated cytoplasm and slightly eccentric nuclei. Occasional nodules may be composed exclusively of spindle shaped cells. Individual nuclei within nodules may measure up to 50 μ in diameter, with frequent irregular hyperchromatic forms. The cytoplasm of the round to

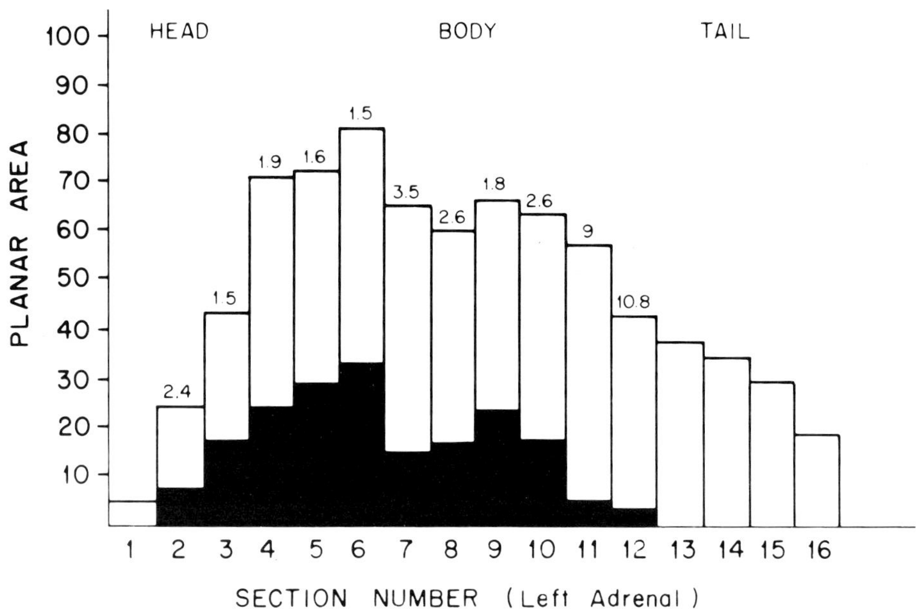

Figure 201
ADRENAL MEDULLARY HYPERPLASIA
This histogram was based on analysis of the left adrenal from the same patient presented in the previous figure. The combined corticomedullary ratio of this gland was 3.4.1 and the estimated weight was 1.07 g. This medulla was diffusely hyperplastic.

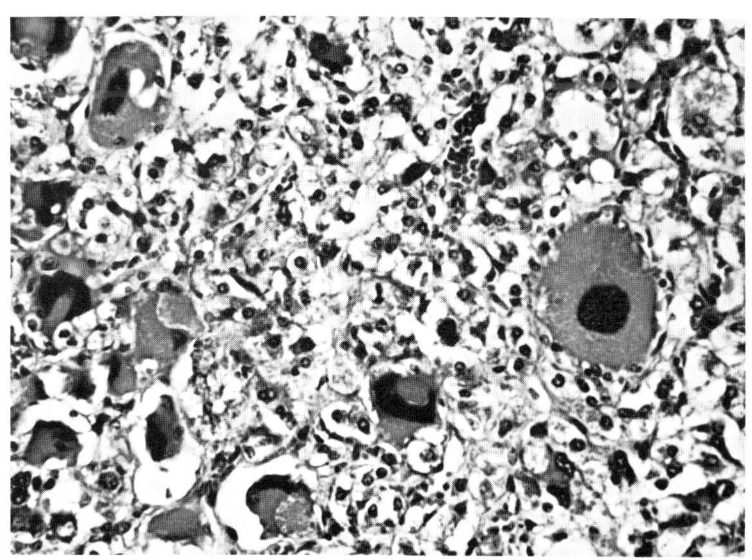

Figure 202
ADRENAL MEDULLARY HYPERPLASIA
In this area of diffuse adrenal medullary hyperplasia, there is a marked degree of nuclear hyperchromasia and pleomorphism. This photomicrograph was taken from the right adrenal of the patient in figures 200 and 201. X320.

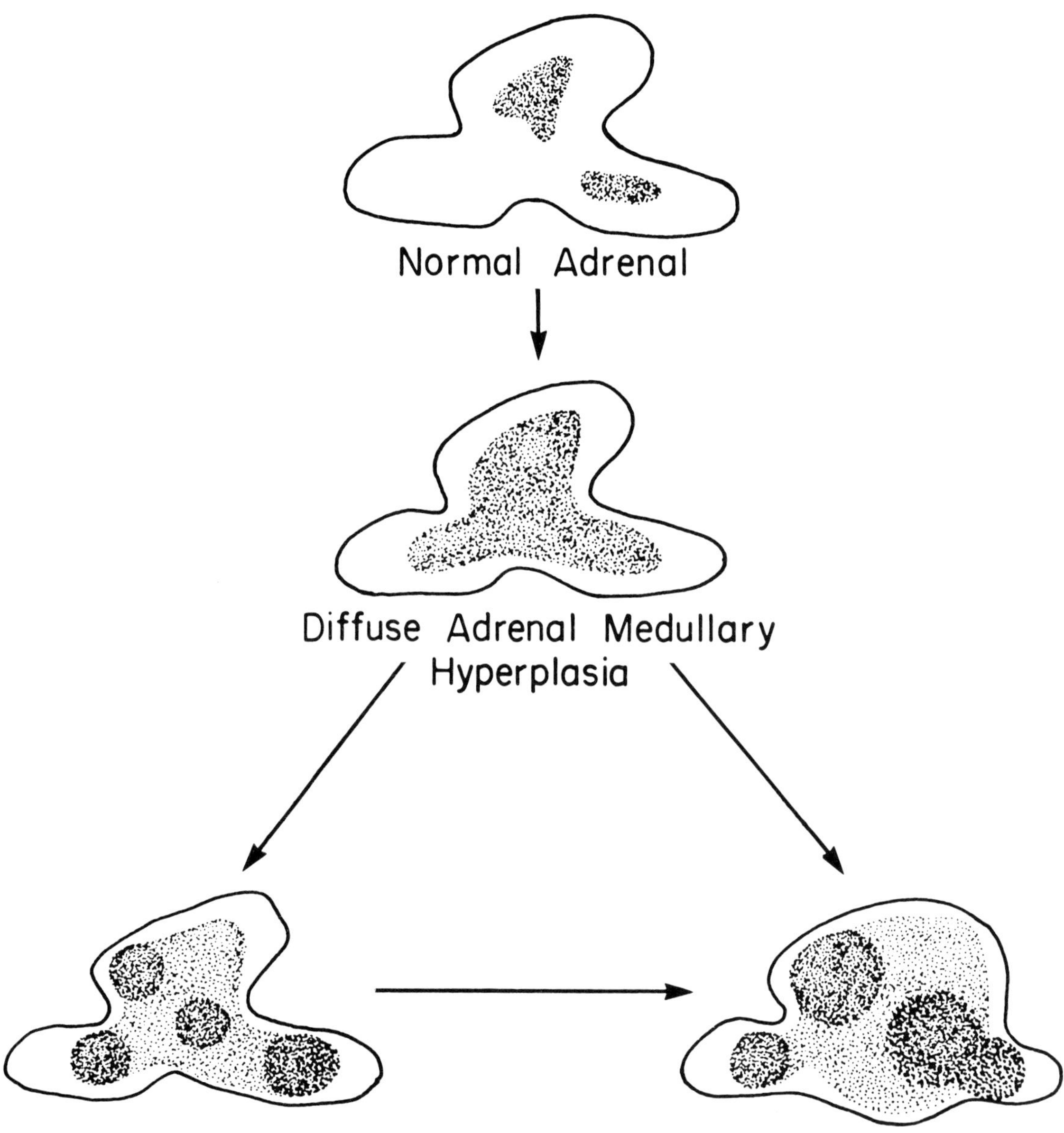

Figure 203
ADRENAL MEDULLARY HYPERPLASIA
Diagram summarizes the proposed histogenesis of adrenal medullary abnormalities seen in patients with types II and III multiple endocrine neoplasia. The diagram represents progressive abnormalities in the medulla and is based on sections through the body of the gland. (From DeLellis, R.A., Wolfe, H.J., Gagel, R.F., Feldman, Z.T., et al. Adrenal medullary hyperplasia. Am. J. Pathol. 83:177-196, 1976.)

polyhedral cells may contain large numbers of hyaline inclusions which may also be seen in some spindle shaped cells. Diffusely hyperplastic tissue between the nodules may exhibit identical characteristics, including variation in cell size and shape, bizarre giant nuclei, cytoplasmic hyaline inclusions, and occasional mitotic activity (fig. 203).

Carney and associates have recently summarized the results of a study of 19 patients with adrenal medullary disease associated with familial medullary thyroid carcinoma. In this series, nodules were classified as pheochromocytomas if they measured more than 1 cm in diameter, while nodules measuring less than 1 cm were classified as examples of nodular hyperplasia. Diffuse medullary hyperplasia was diagnosed when the corticomedullary ratio was less than 10:1 or when the medulla extended into the tail region of the gland. Carney and associates found synchronous bilateral pheochromocytomas in nine patients, while an example of asynchronous bilateral tumors was noted in one case. Unilateral pheochromocytoma with contralateral diffuse and/or nodular hyperplasia was found in four patients. Bilateral diffuse hyperplasia was found in one patient, while another patient had bilateral diffuse and nodular hyperplasia. Two patients had no apparent adrenal medullary abnormalities; however, these cases were not subjected to detailed planimetric or morphometric analysis. The decision to classify medullary nodules solely on the basis of size as pheochromocytomas or nodular hyperplasias, however, seems arbitrary. We have classified all the medullary nodules observed in these patients as examples of nodular hyperplasia, regardless of size. Additional studies, such as those reported by Baylin

and associates, utilizing isoenzymes of glucose-6-phosphate dehydrogenase as markers will be required to determine if the individual nodules represent clonal expansions or mixed cell populations.

ADRENAL MEDULLARY HYPERPLASIA

Although the pathology of pheochromocytomas has been well described, there are relatively few reports of adrenal medullary hyperplasia. Since all the medullary tissue in human adrenals is present in the head and body regions of the gland, random sectioning technics cannot be used to assess medullary volume in normal or disease states (DeLellis et al., 1976). Neville has suggested that a diagnosis of adrenal medullary hyperplasia should be made only when there is a marked diminution in the corticomedullary ratio in several areas of the head and body of the gland and when there is extension of medullary tissue into the tail region. These criteria, however, do not consider abnormalities in the corticomedullary ratios which might result from cortical atrophy. In the presence of severe cortical atrophy, the corticomedullary ratio may be spuriously decreased.

Most of the previously reported studies of human adrenal medullary hyperplasia have not employed quantitative technics, but have been based on the examination of random sections which have shown hypercellularity, nuclear and cytoplasmic pleomorphism, or increased mitotic activity. From a clinical point of view, the case reported by Montalbano and associates was most convincing since hypertension disappeared after resection of a diffusely enlarged right adrenal and biopsy of an apparently normal left gland. In a review of pheochromocytomas, Sherwin (1964) suggested that there was a close relationship between the development of pheochromocytoma and adrenal medullary hyperplasia. This hypothesis was based on the following observations: (1) transitional areas between tumor and adjacent medulla; (2) similarity of cell type of tumor and medulla; (3) large tumor veins similar to the thick-walled type of the medulla; (4) areas of tumor suggesting differentiation toward ganglion cells; and (5) cytoplasmic changes including vacuoles and droplets both in the tumor and in the medulla. These changes were most striking in patients with ganglioneuromas, neurofibromatosis, and angiomatosis.

Both Carney and associates (1975) and DeLellis and associates (1976) have described adrenal medullary hyperplasia in association with types II and III multiple endocrine neoplasia (see Familial Pheochromocytoma). According to DeLellis and associates (1976) and Visser and Axt, a definite diagnosis of adrenal medullary hyperplasia should be made only on the basis of the demonstration of increased medullary volume or weight as demonstrated morphometrically (figs. 200, 201). Other findings suggestive of adrenal medullary hyperplasia include extension of the medulla into the tail of the gland and the presence of medullary tissue in both alar regions. A diagnosis of adrenal medullary hyperplasia based solely on abnormalities in corticomedullary ratios should be interpreted with caution. Visser and Axt and Rudy and co-workers have described adrenal medullary hyperplasia unassociated with multiple endocrine neoplasia or one of the neurocutaneous phakomatosis syndromes. Naeye has described adrenal medullary hyperplasia in patients with sudden infant death syndrome and has suggested that these changes result from chronic hypoxemia.

References

Alpert, L. I., Pai, S. H., Zak, F. G., and Werthamer, S. Cardiomyopathy associated with a pheochromocytoma. Arch. Pathol. 93:544-548, 1972.

Atuk, N. O., McDonald, T., Wood, T., Carpenter, J. T., et al. Familial pheochromocytoma, hypercalcemia, and von Hippel-Lindau disease. Medicine 58:209-218, 1979.

Baylin S. B., Gann, D. S., and Hsu, S. H. Clonal origin of inherited medullary thyroid carcinoma and pheochromocytoma. Science 193:321-323, 1976.

Berenyi, M. R., Singh, G., Gloster, E. S., Davidson, M. I., and Woldenberg, D. H. ACTH-producing pheochromocytoma. Arch. Pathol. Lab. Med. 101:31-35, 1977.

Blaivas, M., Lloyd, R. V., and Wilson, B. Distribution of chromogranin and S-100 protein in normal and abnormal adrenal medullary tissue. Lab. Invest. 52:8A, 1985.

Bravo, E. L. and Gifford, R. W. Pheochromocytoma: Diagnosis, localization and management. N. Engl. J. Med. 311:1298-1303, 1984.

Brown, W. J., Barajas, L., Waisman, J., and DeQuattro, V. Ultrastructural and biochemical correlates of adrenal and extra-adrenal pheochromocytoma. Cancer 29:744-759, 1972.

Carney, J. A., Sizemore, G. W., and Sheps, S. G. Adrenal medullary disease in multiple endocrine neoplasia, type 2. Am. J. Clin. Pathol. 66:279-290, 1976.

————, Sizemore, G. W., and Tyce, G. M. Bilateral adrenal medullary hyperplasia in multiple endocrine neoplasia, type 2. Mayo Clin. Proc. 50:3-10, 1975.

Dawson, D. W. and Tapp, E. A compound tumour of the adrenal medulla. J. Pathol. 97:231-233, 1969.

Dekker, A. and Oehrle, J. S. Hyalin globules of the adrenal medulla of man. Arch. Pathol. 91:353-364, 1971.

de la Torre, J. C. and Surgeon, J. W. A methodological approach to rapid and sensitive monoamine histofluorescence using a modified glyoxylic acid technique: the SPG method. Histochem. 49:81-93, 1976.

DeLellis, R. A. Formaldehyde-induced fluorescence technique for the demonstration of biogenic amines in diagnostic histopathology. Cancer 28:1704-1710, 1971.

————, Suchow, E., and Wolfe, H. J. Ultrastructure of nuclear "inclusions" in pheochromocytoma and paraganlioma. Hum. Pathol. 11:205-207, 1980.

————, Tischler, A. S., Lee, A. K., Blount, M., and Wolfe, H. H. Leu-enkephalin-like immunoreactivity in proliferative lesions of the human adrenal medulla and extra-adrenal paraganglia. Am. J. Surg. Pathol. 7:29-37, 1983.

————, Wolfe, H. J., Gagel, R. F., Feldman, Z. T., et al. Adrenal medullary hyperplasia. Am. J. Pathol. 83:177-196, 1976.

Falck, B. and Owman, C. A detailed methodological description of the fluorescence method for the cellular demonstration of biogenic monoamines. Acta Univ. Lund. Section 2, No. 7:5-23, 1965.

Feldman, J. M., Blalock, J. A., Zern, R. T., Shelburne, J. D., et al. Deficiency of dopamine-B-hydroxlase. Am. J. Clin. Pathol. 72:175-185, 1979.

Garcia, R. and Jennings, J. M. Pheochromocytoma masquerading as a cardiomyopathy. Am. J. Cardiol. 29:568-571, 1972.

Glenner, G. G. and Grimley, P. M. Tumors of the Extra-adrenal Paraganglion System (Including Chemoreceptors). Atlas of Tumor Pathology, Fascicle 9, Second Series. Washington: Armed Forces Institute of Pathology, 1974.

Hamilton, B. P., Landsberg, L., and Levine, R. J. Measurement of urinary epinephrine in screening for pheochromocytoma in multiple endocrine neoplasia type II. Am. J. Med. 65:1027-1032, 1978.

Harrison, T. S., Freier, D. T., and Cohen, E. L. Recurrent pheochromocytoma. Arch. Sug. 108:1027-1032, 1978.

Hassoun, J., Monges, G., Giraud, P., Henry, J. F., Charpin, C., Payan, H., and Toga, M. Immunohistochemical study of pheochromocytomas. Am. J. Pathol. 114:56-63, 1984.

Heath, H. III and Edis, A. J. Pheochromocytoma associated with hypercalcemia and ectopic secretion of calcitonin. Ann. Int. Med. 91:208-210, 1979.

Karsner, H. T. Tumors of the Adrenal. Atlas of Tumor Pathology, Fascicle 29, First Series. Washington: Armed Forces Institute of Pathology, 1950.

Kennedy, J. S., Symington, T., and Woodger, B. A. Chemical and histochemical observations in benign and malignant phaeochromocytoma. J. Pathol. Bacteriol. 81:409-418, 1961.

Lattes, R. Nonchromaffin paraganglioma of ganglion nodosum, carotid body, and aortic-arch bodies. Cancer 3:667-694, 1950.

Lauper, N. T., Tyce, G. M., Sheps, S. G., and Carney, J. A. Pheochromocytoma. Am. J. Cardiol. 30:197-204, 1972.

Lewis, P. D. A cytophotometric study of benign and malignant phaeochromocytomas. Virchows Arch. [Zellpathol.] 9:371-376, 1971.

Linnoila, R. I., Diaugustine, R. P., Hervonen, A., and Miller, R. J. Distribution of (met[5])- and (leu[5])-enkephalin-, vasoactive intestinal polypeptide- and substance P-like immunoreactivities in human adrenal glands. Neuroscience 5:2247-2259, 1980.

Lloyd, R. V. and Warner, T. F. Immunohistochemistry of Neuron Specific Enolase. In: Advances in Immunohistochemistry. DeLellis, R. A. (Ed.). New York: Masson Publishing USA, Inc., 1984.

———— and Wilson, B. S. Specific endocrine tissue marker defined by a monoclonal antibody. Science 222:628-630, 1983.

Lundberg, J. M., Hamberger, B., Schultzberg, M., et al. Enkephalin and somatostatin-like immunoreactivity in human adrenal medulla and pheochromocytoma. Proc. Natl. Acad. Sci. USA 76:4079-4083, 1979.

Manger, W. M. and Gifford, R. W., Jr. Pheochromocytoma. New York: Springer-Verlag, 1977.

Medeiros, L. J., Wolf, B. C., Balogh, K., and Federman, M. Adrenal pheochromocytoma. A clinicopathologic review of 60 cases. Hum. Pathol. 16:580-589, 1985.

Melicow, M. M. One hundred cases of pheochromocytoma (107 tumors) at the Columbia Presbyterian Medical Center, 1926-1976. Cancer 40:1987-2004, 1977.

Meloni, C. R., Tucci, J., Canary, J. J., and Kyle, L. H. Cushing's syndrome due to bilateral adrenocortical hyperplasia caused by a benign adrenal medullary tumor. J. Clin. Endocrinol. Metab. 26:1192-1200, 1966.

Miettinen, M., Lehto, V-P., and Virtanin, I. Immunofluorescence microscopic evaluation of the intermediate filament expression of the adrenal cortex and medulla and their tumors. Am. J. Pathol. 118:360-366, 1985.

Montalbano, F. P., Baronofsky, I. D., and Ball, H. Hyperplasia of the adrenal medulla. J.A.M.A. 182:264-267, 1962.

Naeye, R. L. Brain-stem and adrenal abnormalities in the sudden-infant-death syndrome. Am. J. Clin. Pathol. 66:526-530, 1976.

Neville, A. M. The Adrenal Medulla, pp. 217-324. In: Functional Pathology of the Human Adrenal Gland. Symington, T. (Ed.). Baltimore: The Williams & Wilkins Company, 1969.

O'Connor, D. T., Burton, D., and Deftos, L. J. Chromogranin A: Immunohistology reveals its universal occurrence in normal polypeptide hormone producing endocrine glands. Life Sci. 33:1657-1663, 1983.

Pick, L. Das ganglioma embryonale sympathicium (sympathoma embryonale). Berl. Klin. Wochenschr. 49:16-22, 1912.

Remine, W. H., Chong, G. C., vanHeerden, J. A., Sheps, S. G., and Harrison, E. G., Jr. Current management of pheochromocytoma. Ann. Surg. 179:740-748, 1974.

Robinson, R., Smith, P., and Whittaker, S. R. F. Secretion of catecholamines in malignant phaeochromocytoma. Br. Med. J. 1:1422-1424, 1964.

Rudy, F. R., Bates, R. D., Cimorelli, A. J., Hill, G. S., and Engelman, K. Adrenal medullary hyperplasia: a clinicopathologic study of four cases. Hum. Pathol. 11:650-657, 1980.

Schmechel, D., Marangos, P. J., and Brightman, M. Neurone-specific enolase is a molecular marker for peripheral and central neuroendocrine cells. Nature 276:834-836, 1978.

Sellwood, R. A., Wapnick, S., Breckenridge, A., Williams, E. D., and Welbourn, R. B. Recurrent phaeochromocytoma. Br. J. Surg. 57:309-312, 1970.

Sherwin, R. P. Present status of the pathology of the adrenal gland in hypertension. Am. J. Surg. 107:136-143, 1964.

————. The Adrenal Medulla, Paraganglia and Related Tissues, pp. 256-315. In: Endocrin Pathology. Bloodworth, J. M. B. (Ed.). Baltimore: The Williams & Wilkins Company, 1968.

Shin, W-Y., Groman, C. S., and Berkman, J. I. Pheochromocytoma with angiomatous features. Cancer 40:275-283, 1977.

Sisson, J. C., Kalff, V., Thompson, N. W., and Beierwaltes, W. A. Pheochromocytomas and intraabdominal paragangliomas: A histologic and immunohistochemical study. Lab. Invest. 48:52A, 1983.

Solcia, E., Vasallo, G., Capella, C. Selective staining of endocrine cells by basic dyes after acid hydrolysis. Stain Techn. 43:257-263, 1968.

Spark, R. F., Connolly, P. B., Gluckin, D. S., et al. ACTH secretion from a functioning pheochromocytoma. N. Engl. J. Med. 301:416-418, 1979.

Stackpole, R. H., Melicow, M. M., and Uson, A. C. Pheochromocytoma in children. J. Pediatr. 63:315-330, 1963.

Tannenbaum, M. Ultrastructural pathology of adrenal medullary tumors. Pathol. Ann. 5:145-171, 1970.

Tapia, F. J., Polak, J. M., Barbosa, A. J. A., Bloom, S. R., et al. Neurone-specific enolase is produced by neuroendocrine tumours. Lancet 1:808-811, 1981.

Tischler, A. S. and Greene, L. A. Phenotypic Plasticity of Pheochromocytoma and Normal Adrenal Medullary Cells, pp. 61-63. In: Histochemistry and Cell Biology of Autonomic Neurons, SIF Cells and Paraneurons. Eranko, O., Soinila, S., and Paivarinta, H. (Eds.). New York: Raven Press, 1980.

Tramezzani, J. H., Chiocchio, S., and Wassermann, G. F. A technique for light and electron microscopic identification of adrenalin- and noradrenalin-storing cells. J. Histochem. Cytochem. 12:890-899, 1964.

VanWay, C. W. III, Scott, H. W., Jr., Page, D. L., and Rhamy, R. K. Pheochromocytoma. Curr. Prob. in Surg. 1-59, 1974.

Verhofstad, A. A. J., Stewbusch, H. W. M., Joosten, H. W. J., Penke, B., et al. Immunocytochemical Localization of Noradrenaline, Adrenaline and Serotonin, pp. 143-168. In: Immunocytochemistry. Practical Applications in Pathology and Biology. Polak, J. M. and VanNoorden, S. (Eds.). London: Wright PSG, 1983.

Visser, J. W. and Axt, R. Bilateral adrenal medullary hyperplasia: A clinicopathological entity. J. Clin. Pathol. 28:298-304, 1975.

Wander, J. V. and Das Gupta, T. K. Neurofibromatosis. Curr. Probl. Surg. 14:1-81, 1977.

Wantanabe, H., Burnstock, G., Jarrott, B., and Louis, W. J. Mitochondrial abnormalities in human phaeochromocytoma. Cell Tissue Res. 172:281-288, 1976.

Weinstein, R. S. and Ide, L. F. Immunoreactive calcitonin in pheochromocytomas. Proc. Soc. Exp. Biol. Med. 165:215-217, 1980.

Yokoyama, M. and Takayasu, H. An electron microscopic study of the human adrenal medulla and pheochromocytoma. Urol. Int. 24:79-95, 1969.

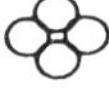

NEUROBLASTOMA

Definition and Terminology. The neuroblastomas represent a group of highly malignant neoplasms that arise most commonly from the adrenal medulla and sympathetic ganglia and occur predominantly during infancy and early childhood. The most poorly differentiated neoplasms in this group have been referred to as sympathicogoniomas on the basis of their resemblance to sympathogonia, the most primitive precursors of sympathetic neurons. Those tumors composed of cells resembling the more differentiated sympathicoblasts, on the other hand, have been referred to as sympathicoblastomas (Karsner). Admixtures of sympathicogoniomas and sympathicoblastoma are found in most tumors of this group and, for this reason, we will use the term neuroblastoma to include both cytologic patterns. Those tumors showing unequivocal evidence of mature ganglion cell differentiation are classified as ganglioneuroblastomas.

Incidence. Neuroblastoma represents the most common solid extracranial tumor of infancy and childhood. According to the Third National Cancer Survey, the incidence of neuroblastoma has been reported at approximately 9.6 cases per million children (Young and Miller). In autopsy studies of infants less than three months of age, however, the incidence of so-called in situ neuroblastoma has been reported to range from 1:39 to 1:259 cases (Beckwith and Perrin; Bolande). The marked discrepancy between the incidence of this tumor in neonates and in older children has been explained on the basis of spontaneous tumor regression in the neonatal group.

Age, Sex, Site. Approximately 70 percent of neuroblastomas become clinically apparent before the age of four years. In a series of 212 cases reported by deLorimer and associates, 32 percent of the patients were less than 1 year old; 14 percent were between 1 and 2 years; 37 percent were between 2 and 7 years; and 17 percent were from 7 to 19 years of age. Pooled data on age distribution reported by Jaffe revealed that 60 percent of the patients were under 1 year; 26 percent between 1 and 2 years; and 13 percent above 2 years. Occasional tumors may be diagnosed at birth. In most series, males appear to be affected slightly more often than females.

The most common sites of origin include the adrenal gland and sympathetic chains of the retroperitoneum, posterior mediastinum, and neck. Rarely, these tumors may arise within the cerebrum (Horten and Rubinstein). The primary sites of involvement are summarized in Table 9. Mackay

Table 9

PRIMARY SITES OF NEUROBLASTOMA*

Site	Incidence (%)
Abdomen	54
Adrenal	(36)
Extra-adrenal	(18)
Mediastinum	14
Neck	5
Pelvis	5
Head	2
Other	10
Unknown	10

*Adapted from Jaffe, N. Neuroblastoma: review of the literature and an examination of factors contributing to its enigmatic character. Cancer Treat. Rev. 3:61-82, 1976.

and associates have reported a series of tumors in adults with ultrastructural features of neuroblastomas. In contrast to the high frequency of abdominal and mediastinal involvement reported in children, the tumors in adults tended to occur more often in peripheral sites, including the leg, buttock, head, and neck. In two patients, the primary tumor was located in the nasal cavity and one contained areas of olfactory differentiation. Hashimoto and coworkers have reported 15 additional cases of peripheral neuroblastoma (malignant neuro-epithelioma), in which the patients were primarily young adults with a median age of 21 years. Tumors of similar morphology have also been reported as primary neoplasms of the chest wall, possibly arising from intercostal nerves (Askin et al.; Triche and Askin). Primary neuroblastomas of the sciatic nerve have also been described (Nesbitt and Vidone). At least some of the reported neuroblastomas in adults may represent metastatic small cell undifferentiated carcinoma or Merkel cell tumors (Warner et al.).

Clinical. The most common presenting signs and symptoms in children with neuroblastoma are summarized in Table 10. Particularly in those children less than two years of age, the presence of an abdominal mass is the most common sign. Signs and symptoms in other groups are dependent upon both the initial site of tumor involvement and the extent of disease at the time of diagnosis. Fever, bone pain, and weight loss are common presenting symptoms. Various staging systems have been suggested for children with neuroblastoma (Gerson and Koop). In general, these staging schemes are based on clinical patterns of disease known to affect the prognosis.

Table 10

PRESENTING SIGNS AND SYMPTOMS IN NEUROBLASTOMA*

Signs and Symptoms	Percentage of Patients
Mass	54
Fever	37
Pain	37
Irritability/malaise	25
Proptosis/orbital ecchymosis	23
Paraplegia	19
Lymphadenopathy	14
Anorexia	12
Weight loss	9
Pallor	5
Urinary problems	5
Vomiting	2

*Adapted from Evans, A. E., D'Angio, G. J., and Koop, C. E. Diagnosis and treatment of neuroblastoma. Pediatr. Clin. North Am. 23:161-170, 1976.

The staging system devised by Evans is the most commonly employed and is summarized in Table 11.

Intravenous pyelography is of particular value in determining the origin of intra-abdominal neuroblastomas (fig. 204). With adrenal primaries, the kidneys are typically depressed and the calyces appear displaced rather than distorted. Retroperitoneal tumors arising in the para-aortic sympathetic ganglia are usually associated with lateral displacement of the kidneys (fig. 205). Recent studies comparing intravenous pyelography with computerized axial tomography have stressed the superiority of the latter technic in the workup of abdominal masses in infancy and childhood (Leonidas et al.; fig. 205). In three cases of neuroblastoma, CT scanning gave superior

Table 11
STAGING OF NEUROBLASTOMA
(Evans, A. E. et al.)

Stage I	Tumor confined to the structure or organ of origin
Stage II	Tumor extending in continuity beyond the organ or structure of origin but not crossing the midline, with or without ipsilateral lymph node involvement[*]
Stage III	Tumors extending in continuity beyond the midline, with or without bilateral lymph node involvement
Stage IV	Remote disease involving skeleton, viscera, soft tissue, or distant lymph node groups
Stage IVs	Patients who would otherwise be Stage I or Stage II, but who have remote disease confined to one or more of the following sites: liver, skin, or bone marrow (without radiographic evidence of bone involvement)

*Tumors with extension into extradural space are considered in Stage II unless the paravertebral portion crosses the midline. It then becomes Stage III.

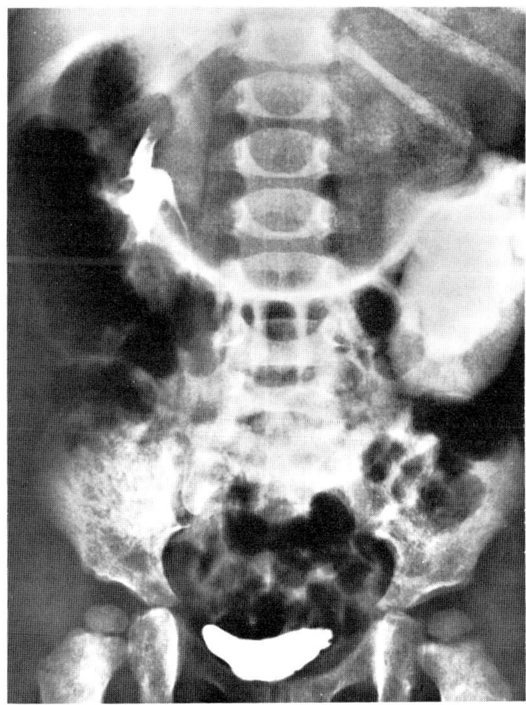

Figure 204
(Figures 204 and 205 from same patient)
NEUROBLASTOMA
Intravenous pyelogram was obtained from a child with a large retroperitoneal neuroblastoma. The kidneys are displaced laterally, and there is also evidence of metastatic disease in the pelvis.

information, including better definition of intraspinal tumor extension, calcification enhancement, and correct localization of tumor in the presacral space (Leonidas et al.). Skeletal surveys including films of the chest should be made in all patients. As noted by Evans and associates, even for abdominal tumors, the chest x-rays may show signs of disease extending through the diaphragm posteriorly into the mediastinum. Radionuclide scans of bone and liver may be of considerable value for the detection of metastatic disease (Evans et al., 1976a).

Biochemical Abnormalities. Abnormally high levels of catecholamines and/or their metabolites are found in the urine of the majority of children with neuroblastoma (Gitlow et al., 1970). Measurements of these substances are useful not only in establishing the diagnosis of neuroblastoma, but also in following the course of the disease after therapy. A number of studies have revealed that there is a great deal of

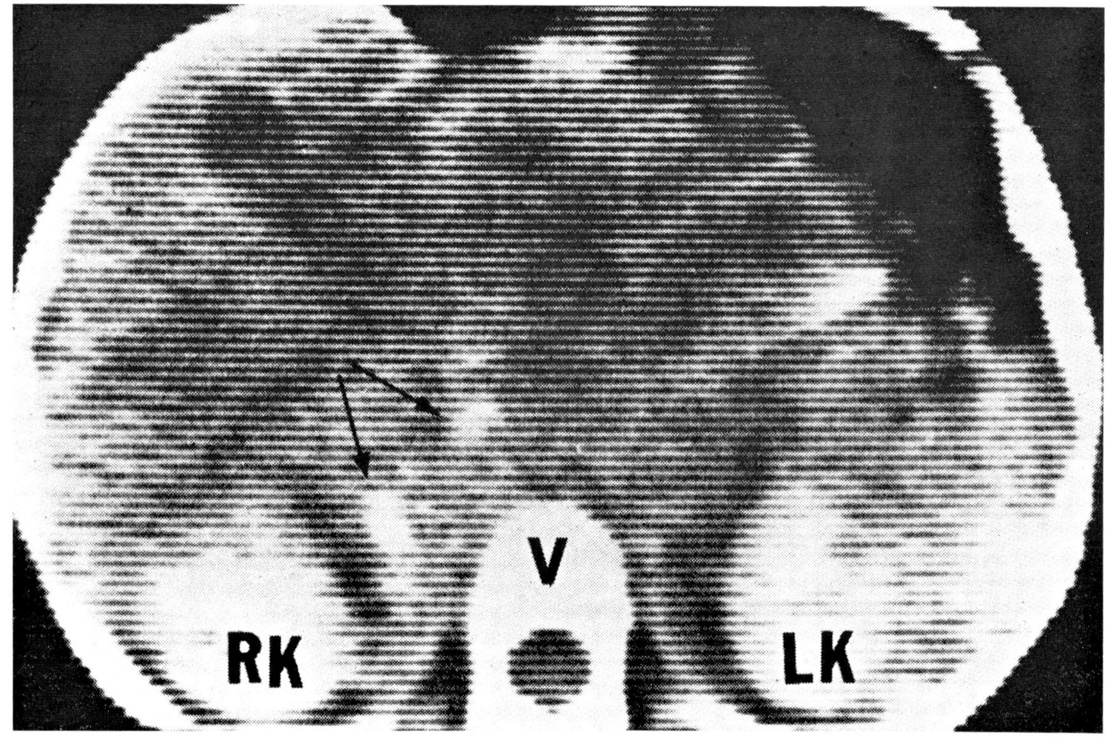

Figure 205
NEUROBLASTOMA
A computerized axial tomography scan in the same patient illustrated in figure 204 shows lateral displacement of both the right (RK) and left kidneys (LK) by a large mass anterior to the vertebrae (V). The arrows indicate areas of calcification within the tumor mass.

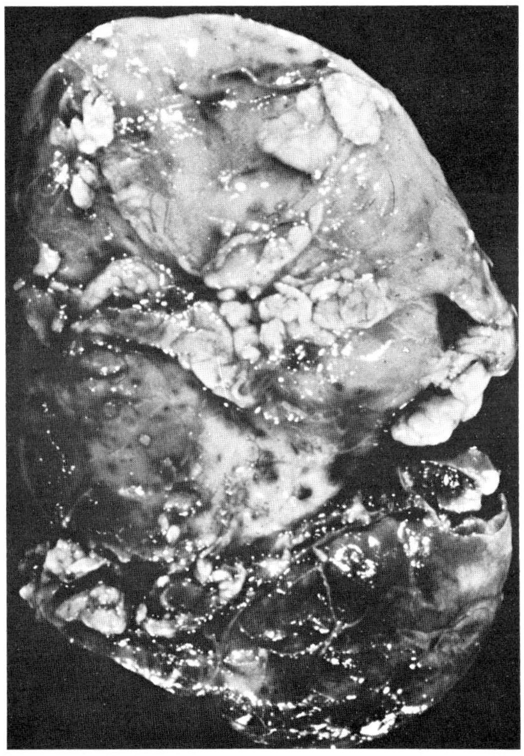

Figure 210
(Figures 210 and 211 from same patient)
NEUROBLASTOMA
This neuroblastoma was discovered in the left adrenal of
a one month old boy. The capsular surface illustrated in this
figure contains a few small lobules of adherent fibroadipose
tissue. X1.6.

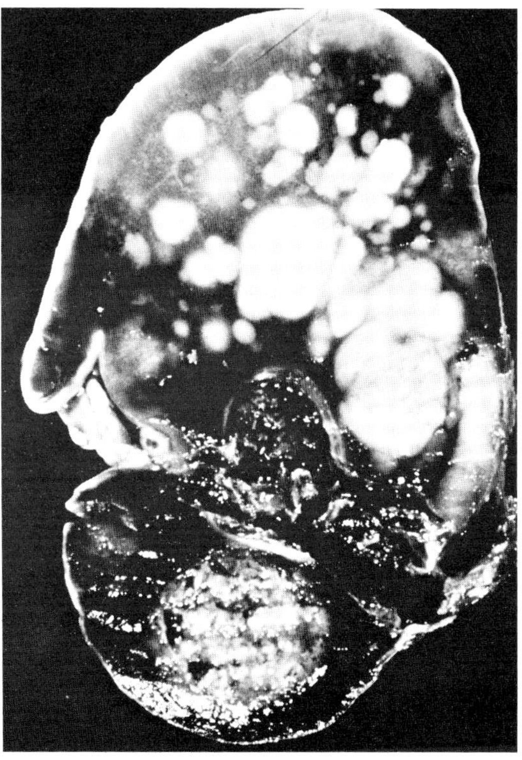

Figure 211
NEUROBLASTOMA
The figure represents the cut surface of the tumor illustrated in figure 210. A rim of intact cortical tissue is
apparent in the upper portion of the illustration. The tumor
shows extensive areas of hemorrhagic necrosis. Viable
tumor is apparent in the form of multiple soft white nodules.
X1.6.

from the retroperitoneal sympathetic chains
may show evidence of invasion of the vertebral bodies. Those tumors arising adjacent to the spine may assume a dumbbell
configuration, due to their passage through
the vertebral foramina. Mediastinal neuroblastomas may invade thoracic vertebrae
and ribs, but rarely involve the pulmonary
parenchyma.

Microscopic. The neuroblastomas show
a wide range of histologic characteristics
(figs. 215–221). The most primitive tumors
are composed of sheets of cells with round

to ovoid hyperchromatic "lymphocyte"-like
nuclei measuring 7 to 10 μm in diameter
(figs. 215, 217). The chromatin often has a
blocklike configuration. Occasional cells
with triangular or carrot shaped nuclei may
be evident. Nucleoli are generally incon-
spicuous. In tissue sections, the tumor
cells appear loosely cohesive and have
some tendency to grow in a "streaming"
fashion (fig. 217). The cytoplasm is usually
scanty and cell borders are difficult to
resolve in routine histologic preparations.
Mitotic activity is quite variable, but may be
most prominent in very young individuals.

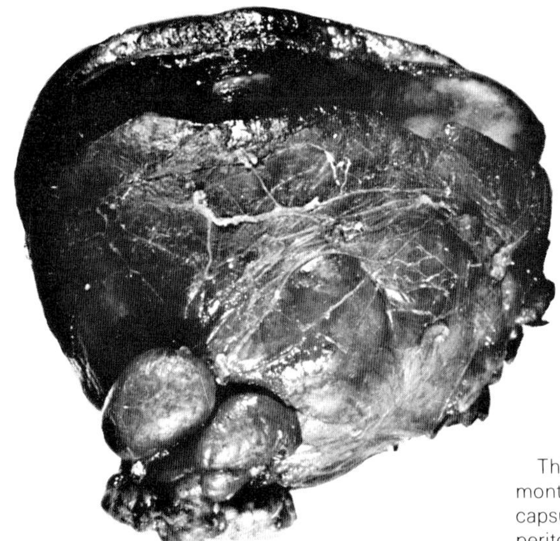

Figure 212
(Figures 212 and 213 from same patient)
NEUROBLASTOMA
This retroperitoneal neuroblastoma was resected from an eight month old boy. Multiple tumor nodules have extended beyond the capsule of the tumor and metastases were found in multiple retroperitoneal lymph nodes. X1.1.

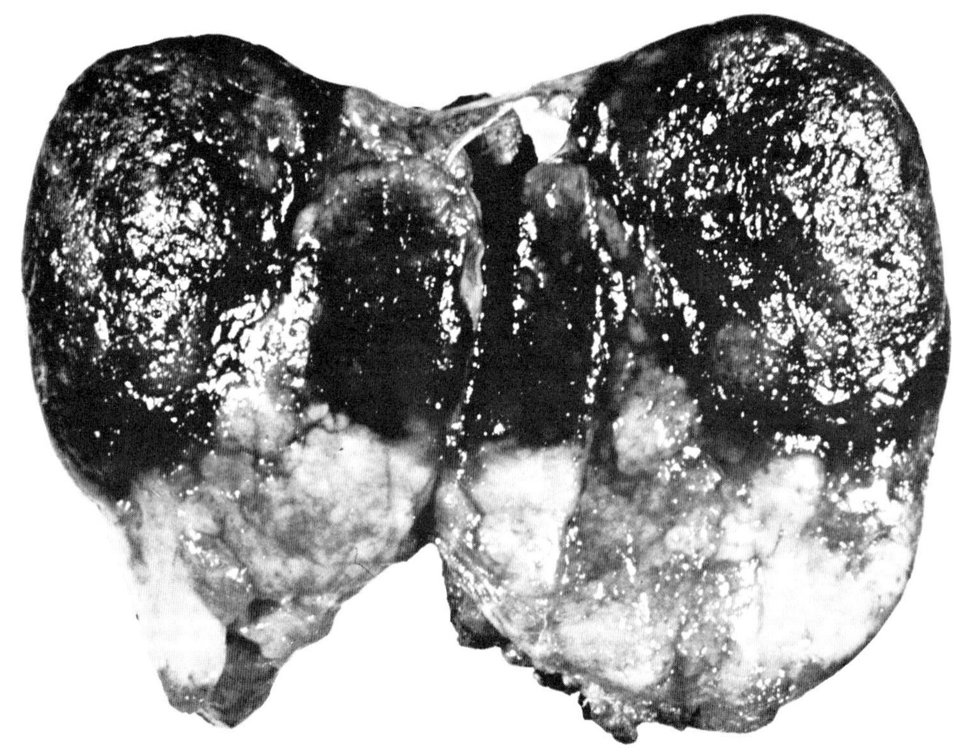

Figure 213
NEUROBLASTOMA
Most of the tumor exhibits hemorrhagic necrosis. The viable portions of the tumor appear white. X2.1.

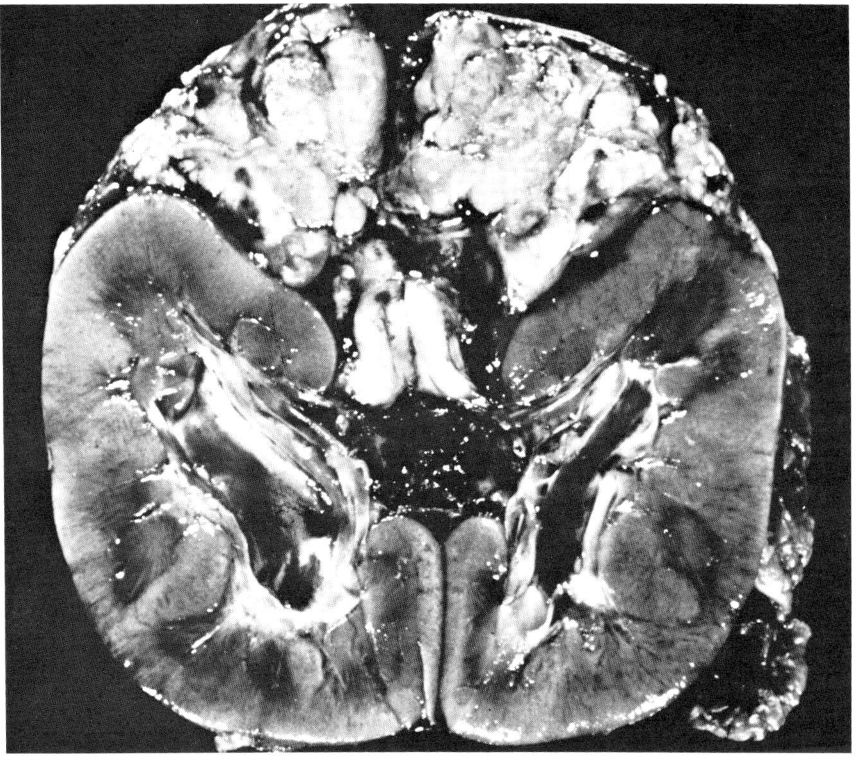

Figure 214
NEUROBLASTOMA
This right adrenal neuroblastoma was found in a four year old boy. The tumor has extended beyond the confines of the adrenal into the surrounding adipose tissue. Although the tumor has compressed the underlying kidney, there is no evidence of invasion of the renal parenchyma. X1.2.

In some cases, the cells may form small clusters, particularly at the edges of the tumor. These clusters of cells are thought to represent the earliest stages in the development of rosettes. Thin fibrovascular bands may impart a distinct lobular appearance to the tumor (fig. 215). These connective tissue septa are often infiltrated by lymphocytes and other mononuclear cells. Invasion of both lymphatic and vascular channels is seen frequently, even in tumors of small size. Similarly, necrosis, hemorrhage, and calcification are frequent microscopic findings.

A notable feature of neuroblastomas is the presence of a finely fibrillar eosinophilic matrix in which the tumor cells are embedded. Special stains as well as ultrastructural studies have revealed that these eosinophilic areas represent tangles of predominantly unmyelinated nerve fibrils (figs. 218–221). Occasional lobules of some tumors may be composed of nerve fibrils exclusively. Although the presence of Homer-Wright rosettes (pseudorosettes) has been stressed in the differential diagnosis of neuroblastomas, they are seen in only approximately one-third of cases (figs.

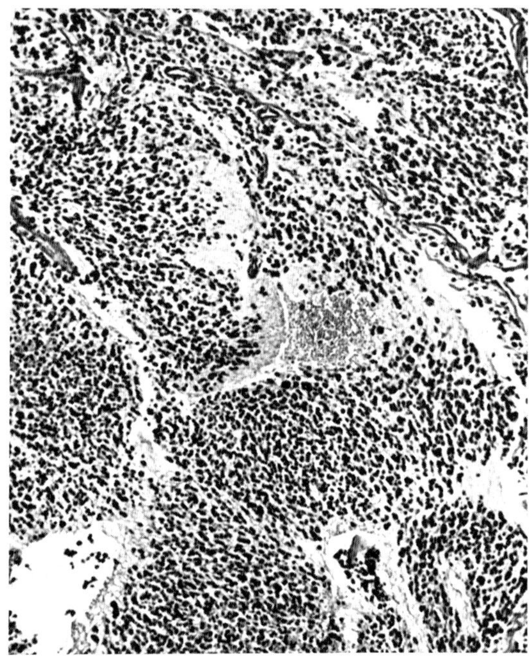

Figure 215
NEUROBLASTOMA
The neuroblastoma shows an indistinct lobular pattern
with a few thin fibrous septa between groups of tumor cells.
X125.

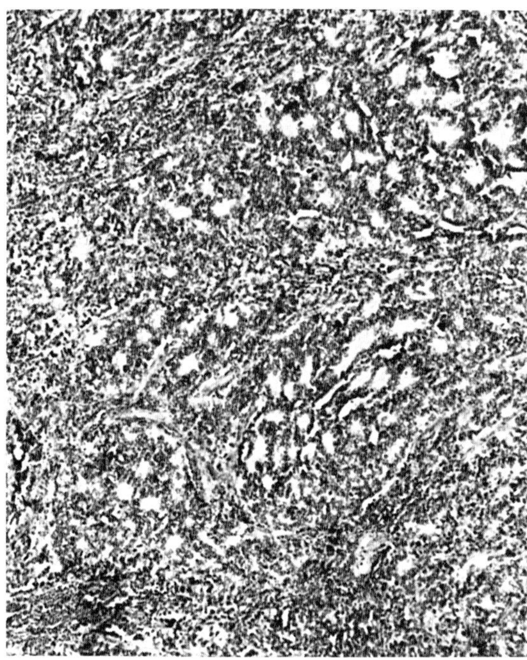

Figure 216
NEUROBLASTOMA
Neuroblastoma shows extensive areas of pseudorosette
and tubule formations. X125.

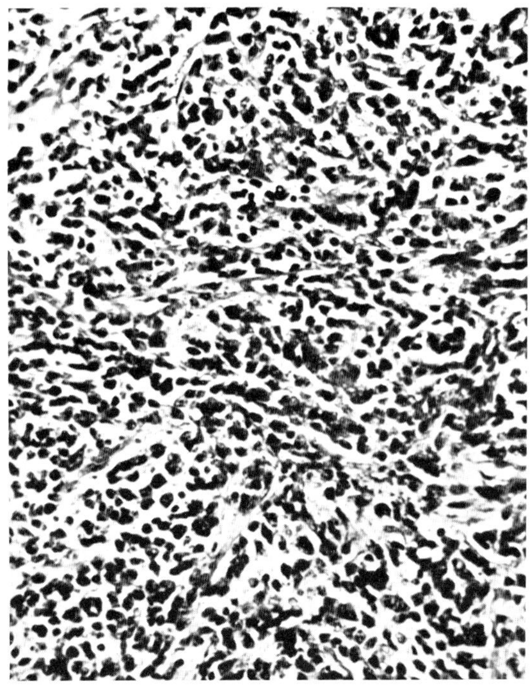

Figure 217
NEUROBLASTOMA
The tumor cells in this neuroblastoma appear somewhat
elongated and show a streaming pattern. X320.

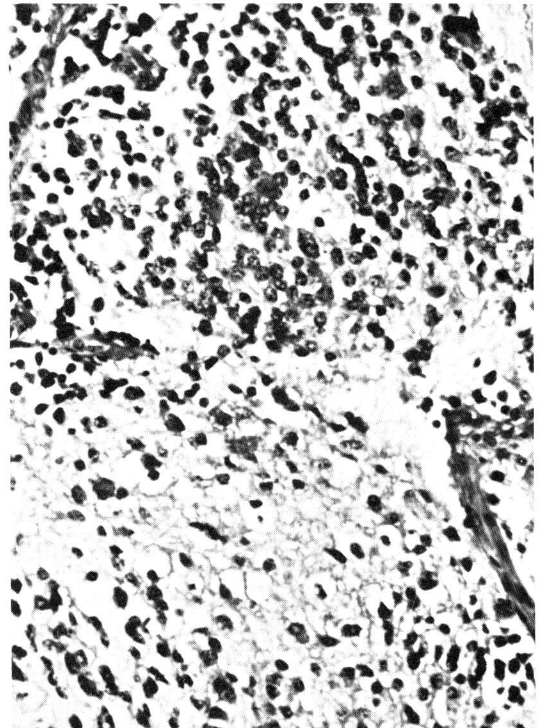

Figure 218
NEUROBLASTOMA
The tumor in the lower portion of this field shows the typical fibrillary matrix characteristic of neuroblastoma. The tumor cells in this region show slight nuclear enlargement and other features suggestive of early maturation. X320.

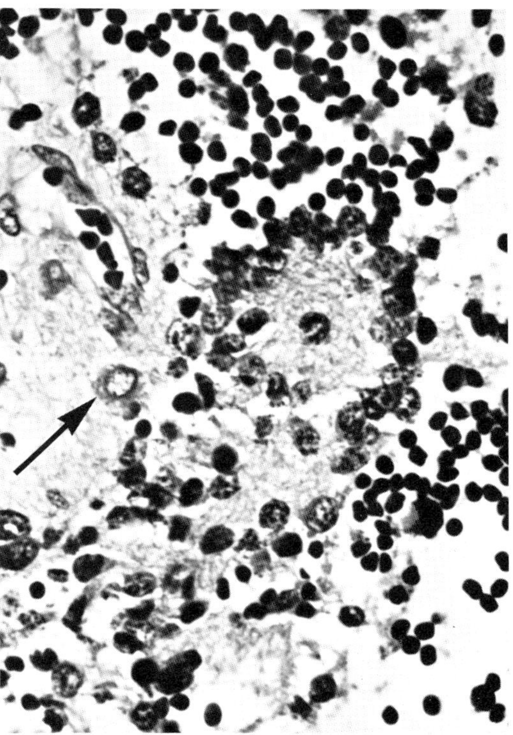

Figure 219
NEUROBLASTOMA
This field shows the histologic features of a Homer-Wright rosette. The central portion of this structure is composed of a tangle of neurofibrillary processes. A portion of a nucleus is also noted in this rosette. Occasional cells (arrow) show evidence of early maturation. X800.

216, 219, 220). Pseudorosettes may be present in only small areas of the tumors or may form the predominant histologic element of the neoplasm. The pseudorosettes are composed of one or two layers of neuroblasts which surround a central zone of nerve fibrils. In suitable histologic preparations, the fibrils may be traced to the apices of the tumor cells and may show a radial pattern. Occasional tumors may contain short tubule-like structures which, on cross section, may resemble rosettes (fig. 216).

Maturing neuroblastoma cells are characterized by large vesicular nuclei with coarsely clumped chromatin and a single

prominent nucleolus (Beckwith and Martin; fig. 221). The cytoplasm is more abundant than in the primitive tumor cell forms and cytoplasmic processes may be seen to emanate from some of these cells. Maturing neuroblastoma cells may measure up to 30 μm in diameter. These cells may be present singly or in small clusters in the midst of largely undifferentiated elements or may form the bulk of the tumor. Cells which may measure up to 60 μm in diameter and which resemble developing ganglion type cells may also be present. As summarized by Makinen, histologic criteria of advancing maturation in a neuroblastoma include: (1) enlargement of individual

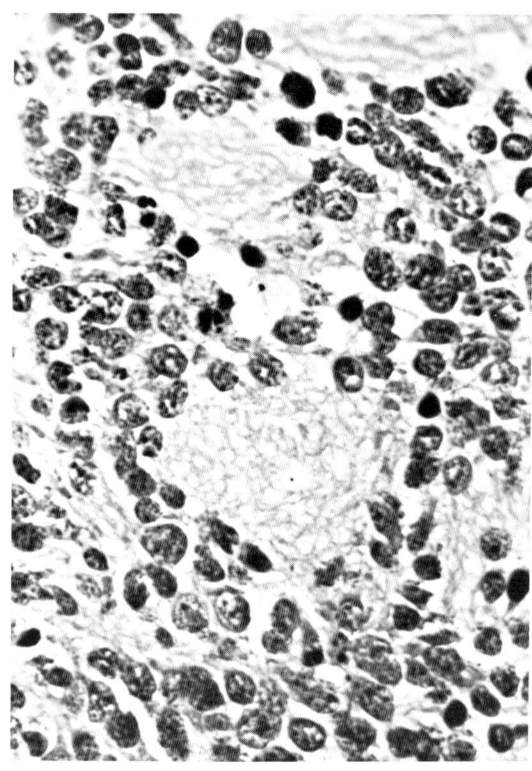

Figure 220
NEUROBLASTOMA
Two Homer-Wright pseudorosettes are seen in this area of tumor. As compared to the previous illustration, the tumor cells in this case have larger nuclei and more prominent nucleoli. X800.

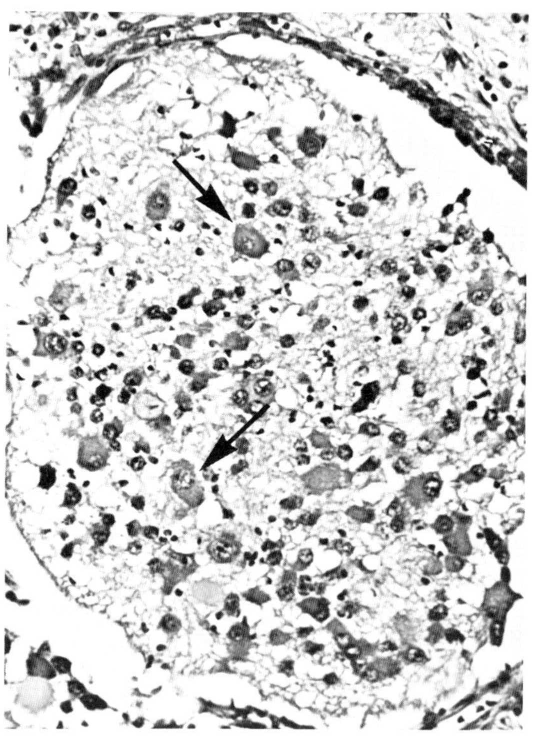

Figure 221
NEUROBLASTOMA
The maturing neuroblasts (arrows) in this field have large vesicular nucleoli and abundant eosinophilic cytoplasm. The cells are surrounded by an eosinophilic neurofibrillary matrix. There were no mature ganglion cells in this case. X320.

nuclei with the emergence of large vesicular forms; (2) development of prominent nucleoli; (3) development of increasing amounts of cytoplasm; (4) development of cell processes; (5) formation of rosettes; (6) development of a fibrous stroma; and (7) development of ganglion cells.

Although most reports indicate that neuroblastoma cells are PAS negative, recent studies have called attention to the presence of occasional glycogen containing tumors (Triche and Ross; fig. 222). Attempts to demonstrate the catecholamine content of these tumors by standard histochemical methods have been almost in-

variably unsuccessful. The chromaffin reaction, with rare exception, has been reported to be negative. Catecholamines, however, may be demonstrated with the formaldehyde or glyoxylic acid induced fluorescence technics (DeLellis; Helson and Biedler; pl. XIV-A, B). These methods may be particularly valuable in the differential diagnosis of small cell tumor infiltrates in bone marrow or other metastatic sites. In addition to catecholamines, recent studies have demonstrated that the presence of neuron specific enolase might be useful to classify small cell undifferentiated malignancies. This neuron specific protein has

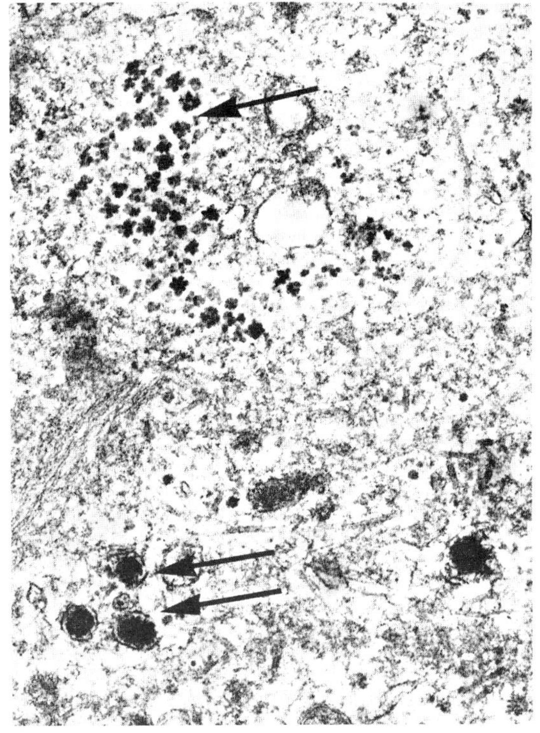

Figure 222
NEUROBLASTOMA
This neuroblastoma contains both neurosecretory gran-
ules (double arrows) and glycogen deposits (single arrow).
X34,000. (Courtesy of Dr. T. Triche, National Cancer Insti-
tute, Bethesda, MD.)

been demonstrated not only in neuroblastomas and pheochromocytomas, but also
in a variety of normal and neoplastic neuroendocrine cells of the APUD series (Tapia
et al.; Lloyd and Warner).

Ultrastructure. Characteristic features of
neuroblastomas at the ultrastructural level
include the presence of membrane-bound,
dense core, secretory granules, as well as
variable numbers of cytoplasmic processes
(Misugi et al.; Yokoyama et al.; Triche,
1982a; figs. 222, 223). The least differentiated tumors are composed of loosely
cohesive cells with only occasional desmosome-like structures between adjacent

cells. The nuclei are round to ovoid, with
moderately condensed to coarsely clumped
heterochromatin. The cytoplasm contains
scattered ribosomes, small numbers of
mitochondria, a few clear vesicles, and
generally small amounts of granular endoplasmic reticulum. The Golgi regions tend
to be poorly developed. With increasing
differentiation, the cytoplasm becomes
more abundant, with the appearance of
increased amounts of granular and smooth
endoplasmic reticulum, mitochondria, Golgi
saccules and vesicles, and round membrane-
bound neurosecretory type granules which
measure between 80 to 150 μm in diameter.
Heterogeneous membrane bound osmiophilic granules, which measure from 250 to
550 μm in diameter, are also present. The
intercellular spaces contain variable numbers of dendritic type processes which contain microtubules, microfilaments, neurosecretory type granules, and clear vesicles.
Often, the processes show areas of bulbous
expansion which are particularly rich in
dense core granules and vesicles (fig. 223).
In approximately 10 percent of cases,
deposits of glycogen may be present within
the cytoplasm of the tumor cells (Triche
and Ross; fig. 222).

Schwann cells, which may not be apparent by light microscopy, may be noted
by electron microscopic analysis of some
neuroblastomas and it has been suggested
that the presence of these cells may reflect
an early phase of tumor maturation (Taxy).
The identification of these cells may be
facilitated at the light microscopic level by
immunohistochemical technics for the
demonstration of S-100 protein (Nakajima
et al.; Shimada et al.).

Metastases. Neuroblastomas often metastasize widely via the lymphatic system
and blood stream (Ashley; Karsner; Russell

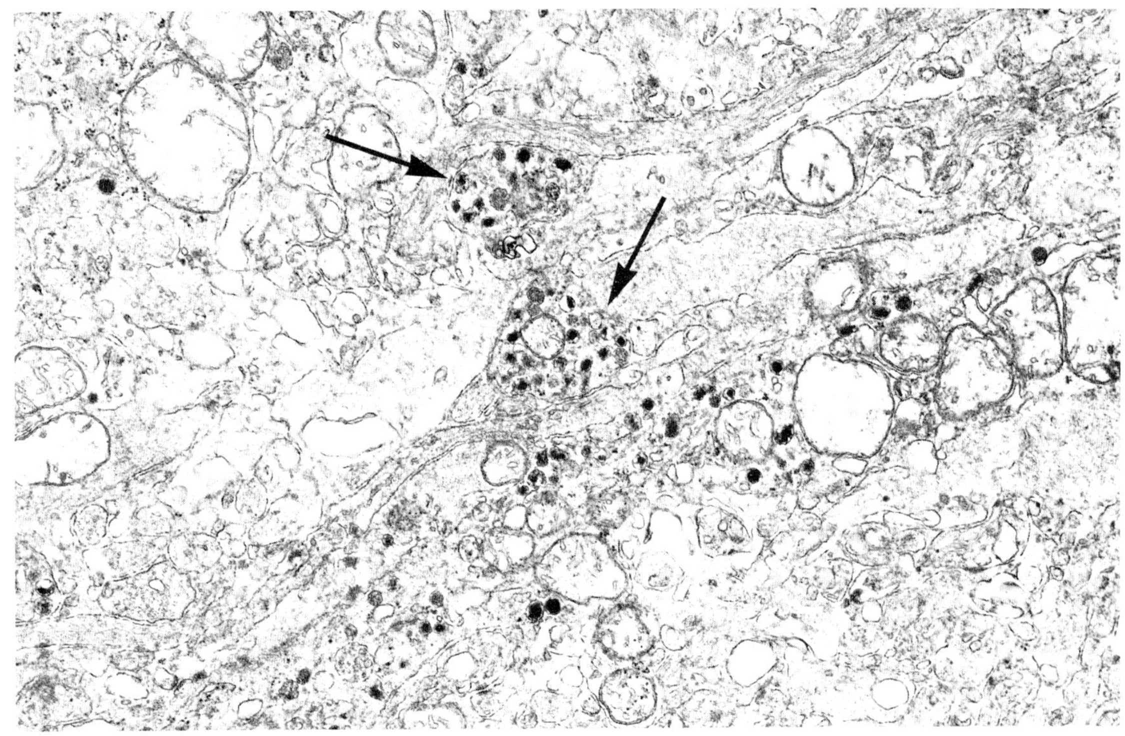

Figure 223
NEUROBLASTOMA
The neuritic processes in this neuroblastoma exhibit focal bulbous expansions. Collections of dense core neurosecretory granules are present within these expanded regions (arrows). X18,000.

and Rubinstein). The most frequent sites of secondary spread include bone, regional nodes, liver, skull, and cervical lymph nodes. Early tumor deposits in bones appear as soft white nodules within the medullary cavity. As the tumors enlarge, they become more diffuse with further extension into marrow spaces and haversian canals. In affected bones, the tumor deposits often elicit subperiosteal new bone formation, producing a characteristic sunburst or onionskin pattern. Metastatic neuroblastomas characteristically form fusiform swellings about the ribs and long bones or plaquelike lesions in flat bones. In the skull and rib, a sunburst periosteal reaction is common, while long bones often show concentric onionskin periosteal new bone formation. The development of extensive skeletal metastases, particularly involving the skull, has been referred to as Hutchinson's syndrome.

Involvement of the liver may occur as a result of direct invasion in the case of right-sided adrenal primary tumors (fig. 224) or by extensive hematogenous metastases. Pepper's syndrome refers to massive hepatomegaly secondary to metastatic neuroblastoma. Striking degrees of hepatomegaly may be apparent at birth in patients with congenital neuroblastoma. Although it had

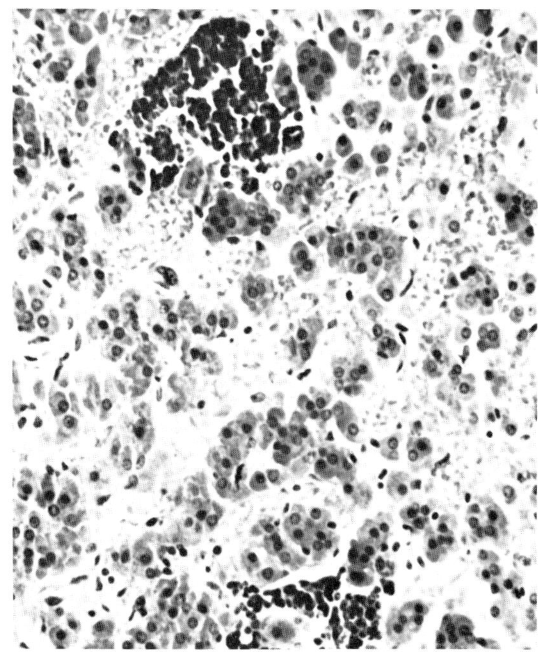

Figure 224
NEUROBLASTOMA
Clusters of metastatic neuroblastoma cells are present in the sinusoids of this liver biopsy from a four year old boy with a primary right adrenal neuroblastoma. X320.

been thought that left- and right-sided adrenal primary tumors gave rise to different patterns of metastasis, more recent studies have failed to confirm any distinctive patterns of spread based on the laterality of the primary tumors. In addition to regional nodes, liver, and bone, other common sites of metastasis include lungs, subcutaneous tissue, kidneys, spleen, pancreas, ovaries, and pituitary. Cerebral metastases are rare.

Differential Diagnosis. The differential diagnosis of neuroblastoma includes Ewing's sarcoma and other sarcomas of bone, Wilms' tumor (nephroblastoma), rhabdomyosarcoma, and malignant lymphoma. Occasional intrarenal neuroblastomas may be extremely difficult to differentiate from Wilms' tumors, since pseudorosettes may resemble the im-

mature tubules found in nephroblastomas. In general, the tubules of Wilms' tumors contain a central lumen around which a single layer of epithelial cells is aligned; moreover, a basement membrane is present. Pseudorosettes lack a lumen and are surrounded by a multilayered epithelium without a basement membrane. Since ganglion cells may be found in some Wilms' tumors, the presence of this cell type should not lead to an immediate diagnosis of neuroblastoma or one of its mature congeners (Beckwith). Moreover, the stroma of neuroblastic tumors consists only of fibrovascular and neurofibrillary tissue, while the stroma of Wilms' tumors is usually fibromyxoid and often contains other mesenchymal cell types. The major light microscopic and ultrastructural features of these tumors are summarized in Table 12.

Table 12

DIFFERENTIAL DIAGNOSIS OF SMALL ROUND CELL TUMORS
OF INFANCY AND CHILDHOOD

TUMOR TYPE (and Incidence per 10^6 Children*)	LIGHT MICROSCOPY	ELECTRON MICROSCOPY
Neuroblastoma (9.6)	Tumor shows a solid and sometimes lobular pattern of growth with frequent areas of hemorrhage, necrosis, and calcification. The nuclei are round to ovoid and are hyperchromatic with inconspicuous nucleoli. Cytoplasm is scanty and cell borders are poorly defined. The tumor cells are embedded in a fibrillar eosinophilic matrix. Homer-Wright type pseudorosettes may be present. (See text for further description.)	Nuclear chromatin is moderately condensed to dispersed, nucleoli are small and inconspicuous except in cases showing maturation, where they may be prominent and nuclear blebs are inconspicuous. Cells often show prominent process formation. Cytoplasm contains large numbers of mono- and polyribosomes, small amounts of granular endoplasmic reticulum, few mitochrondria, and inconspicuous Golgi regions. Small numbers of desmosome-like junctions, which in some cases resemble synapses, may be seen. Membrane-bound dense core secretory granules measuring 50-200 nm in diameter are present in perinuclear cytoplasm and processes. Large granules measuring up to 900 nm in diameter (lysosomes) may be present. Processes contain 10 nm in width intermediate filaments and 25-30 nm in width microtubules. Glycogen may be present in considerable quantities in up to 10 percent of cases. Basal lamina is absent except around Schwann cells, which may be present within the tumor. (Ghadially; Henderson and Papadimitriou; Misugi et al.; Triche; Yokoyama et al.)
Wilms' Tumor (7.8)	The tumor frequently shows a trabecular pattern of growth with epithelial, blastematous, and sarcomatous areas. Those tumors composed of blastematous elements are most difficult to differentiate from other small cell malignancies of infancy and childhood. Blastematous foci are characterized by cells with round to ovoid hyperchromatic nuclei and prominent nucleoli. Cytoplasm is usually scanty and cell borders are ill defined.	In the undifferentiated monomorphic nephroblastoma, chromatin is dispersed and nucleoli tend to be prominent and marginated. Nuclear blebs are inconspicuous. Cells show some process formation. Cytoplasm contains prominent mono- and polyribosomes, moderate numbers of mitochondria, and occasional cisternae of granular endoplasmic reticulum. Cells in blastematous areas may be surrounded by an electron dense flocculent material and basal lamina. Tubular areas show luminal polarity and are surrounded by a basal lamina. Both desmosomes and junctional complexes may be evident in tubular areas. These cells may have microvilli and cilia. (Ghadially; Ito and Johnson; Balsaver et al.; Tannenbaum)
Non-Hodgkin's Lymphoma (7.4)	The tumor most often shows a diffuse pattern of growth. Nuclear size varies from that of a small nonactivated lymphocyte to that of a large transformed lymphocyte. Nuclei may be round, cleaved, or convoluted. Chromatin may be dispersed or condensed, depending on lymphoma subtype. Cytoplasm is generally scanty. Small amounts of glycogen may be present. In Burkitt's lymphoma, the cells often contain neutral lipid-filled vacuoles.	Chromatin pattern and number and size of nucleoli may show considerable variation, depending on subtype. Nuclear blebs are prominent in all subtypes. Process formation may be prominent, but is not as striking as in neuroblastoma. Cytoplasm contains large numbers of mono- and polyribosomes and few mitochondria. Granular endoplasmic reticulum and Golgi regions may be especially prominent in immunoblastic subtypes. Intercellular junctions are absent between individual lymphoma cells, but desmosomes may be present between interdigitating reticulum cells of follicular center cell tumors. Ten nm intermediate type filaments may be present. Basal lamina is absent. (Ghadially; Henderson and Papadimitriou; Rice et al.)

Table 12 (Continued)

TUMOR TYPE (and Incidence per 10^6 Children*)	LIGHT MICROSCOPY	ELECTRON MICROSCOPY
Rhabdomyosarcoma (5.3)	Embryonal type shows considerable variation in cellularity, with hypercellular areas alternating with hypocellular areas in a loose myxoid background. The least differentiated cells have round to ovoid hyperchromatic nuclei with prominent nucleoli. The cytoplasm is often indistinct. The more differentiated cells may have a racquet or tadpole shape, with densely eosinophilic cytoplasm containing cross striations. Moderate to large amounts of glycogen may be present. The alveolar type of tumor is composed of groups of round to ovoid cells which show loss of cohesion centrally with the formation of irregular alveolar spaces. (Enzinger and Weiss)	Chromatin tends to be condensed and is often marginated, nucleoli are prominent, and nuclear blebs are inconspicuous. Process formation is inapparent. Cytoplasm contains large numbers of mono- and polyribosomes, occasional cisternae of granular endoplasmic reticulum, and moderate numbers of mitochondria. Golgi regions may be prominent. Intracellular glycogen is present and may be extensive in some cases. Occasional lysosomes may be evident. A few desmosome-like junctions may be present, particularly in the alveolar type. Occasional basal lamina may be present. The cytoplasm contains thin (actin, 6-8 nm) and thick (myosin, 12-15 nm) filaments. Well differentiated tumor cells may contain a 6-1 (actin-myosin) hexagonal array of myofilaments as well as Z-band-like material. Ten nm in width intermediate type filaments are also evident. At the ultrastructural level, the primitive mesenchymal cells are identical to immature fibroblasts. (Ghadially; Henderson and Papadimitriou)
Ewing's Sarcoma (1.7)	Tumor shows a solid and occasionally lobular pattern of growth, both in extraskeletal and skeletal variants. Nuclei are round to ovoid with finely dispersed chromatin and small but distinct nucleoli. Cytoplasm is scanty and occasionally vacuolated. Cytoplasmic borders are indistinct. Cells contain abundant glycogen, which may also be evident in extracellular spaces. Tumor cells tend to aggregate around blood vessels and create a rosette-like pattern.	Nuclear chromatin is generally dispersed, nucleoli are small and may be filamentous, and nuclear blebs are inconspicuous. Process formation is generally absent. Cytoplasm contains abundant mono- and polyribosomes and few mitochrondria. Large amounts of glycogen are present in aggregates within the cytoplasm and may also be apparent in intercellular spaces (matrix glycogen). Occasional pinocytotic vesicles may be apparent. Desmosome-like junctions and some tight junctions may be seen. Ten nm in width intermediate filaments may be present. (Ghadially; Henderson and Papadimitriou; Hou Jensen et al.; Llombart-Busch et al.)

*Incidence figures based on Third National Cancer Survey (Young and Miller).

In addition to electron microscopy, immunohistochemical technics employing both poly- and monoclonal antisera for the localization of a battery of markers have proven to be extremely useful in the differential diagnosis of small cell malignant tumors of infancy and childhood. Neuron specific enolase, for example, has been reported to be present in neuroblastomas, but is not demonstrable in cases of rhabdomyosarcoma, Ewing's sarcoma, or malignant lymphoma (Tapia et al.; Lloyd and Warner; Triche, 1982b). This isoenzyme is expressed in malignant small cell tumors of the thoracopulmonary region (Askin et al.; Triche and Askin) and has also been reported in small cell carcinomas (oat cell carcinomas) (Tapia et al.) and in some Merkel cell tumors. Myoglobin, on the other hand, has been reported to be present in a high proportion of rhabdomyosarcomas and in some Wilms' tumors with skeletal muscle differentiation, but is absent from other small cell undifferentiated malignancies (Brooks). Other markers that have been reported to be present in rhabdomyosarcomas include skeletal muscle myosin and creatine phosphokinase (MM and BB isoenzymes) (Tsokos et al.). Using monoclonal antibodies, Andres and Kadin have reported that hematopoietic neoplasms of all types react with antibody T29/33, which detects a glycoprotein antigen (T200), while other small cell malignant tumors are T200-negative. Similarly, the HLA-DR antigen has been reported to be present only in lymphomas (Andres and Kadin).

An additional approach to the differential diagnosis of the small round cell tumors of infancy and childhood is an analysis of their intermediate filament profiles. These filaments, which measure 10 nm in diameter, are present in most normal and neoplastic cells (Gabbiani et al.). The five major intermediate filament types and their cells of origin are vimentin (mesenchymal cells), desmin (muscle cells), cytokeratins (epithelial cells), glial fibrillary acidic protein (glial cells), and neurofilaments (neuronal cells). These various cell products exhibit a high degree of tissue specificity and have been used as specific markers both in embryologic studies and for the analysis of different tumor types (Osborn and Weber). Neurofilament proteins, for example, are suitable as differentiation markers, since they are present in neural crest and neuroectodermal derivatives. Studies of bronchogenic carcinomas, for example, have revealed that neurofilament proteins are present in oat cell carcinomas, but are not detectable in other tumor types (Lehto et al.). In the adrenal medulla, neurofilament proteins have been identified in pheochromocytomas and ganglioneuroblastomas; moreover, neuroblastomas have also been shown to exhibit neurofilament positivity (Osborn and Weber). In contrast, other small round cell tumors of infancy are neurofilament protein negative, but exhibit varying degrees of positivity for cytokeratins, desmin, and vimentin (Kahn et al.; Table 13).

Table 13

INTERMEDIATE FILAMENT PROFILE OF SMALL ROUND CELL TUMORS OF INFANCY AND CHILDHOOD

Tumor Type	Cytokeratins	Desmin	Vimentin	Neurofilaments
Neuroblastoma	−	−	−	+
Lymphoma	−	−	+	−
Rhabdomyosarcoma	−	+	+	−
Wilms' tumor	+*	−	+*	−
Ewing's sarcoma	−	−	+	−

*In Wilms' tumors, the tubular elements are cytokeratin positive, while the spindle cell elements are vimentin positive. Those Wilms' tumors that contain skeletal muscle elements may also be positive for desmin.

Maturation of Neuroblastoma. Maturation of primitive neuroblastic tumors into mature ganglioneuromas, although extensively discussed in the literature, is an infrequent occurrence (Gerson and Koop). In the case reported by Cushing and Wolbach in 1927, an 18 month old boy presented with a paravertebral mass associated with progressive weakness of the legs and arms, inability to coordinate eye movements, ptosis, and loss of sphincter control. A biopsy of the mass revealed a sympathetic neuroblastoma. Following treatment with Coley's toxin, the patient's symptoms improved. At the age of 12 years, he was noted to have marked spasticity with sustained clonus of the ankles and knees. Laminectomy revealed an extradural mass that proved to be a benign ganglioneuroma. Follow-up study 46 years after the initial diagnosis showed that he was free of residual or recurrent tumor (Fox et al.). A second patient reported by Fox and associates was noted to have extensive subcutaneous deposits of metastatic neuroblastoma at the age of seven months. This patient was treated with Coley's toxin and local radiation to the skin, with resolution of the tumor deposits. He was well until the age of 19 years, when he was hospitalized because of severe headaches. Abdominal x-rays revealed a calcified mass in the right suprarenal region. No tumor was palpable at the sites of previous irradiation; however, two subcutaneous nodules were palpated in the right flank. These nodules were biopsied and showed mature ganglioneuromas. Excision of the suprarenal mass revealed a ganglioneuroblastoma. The patient died five years after operation, with evidence of widely metastatic neuroblastoma. These cases, together with several additional cases reported in the literature, indicate that maturation of neuroblastomas into mature ganglion cell tumors may occur.

In Vitro Studies. The classical experiments of Murray and Stout demonstrated that neuroblastoma cells in vitro exhibit spontaneous outgrowth of processses and these authors suggested the possibility of using this characteristic as a diagnostic tool. In addition to the spontaneous outgrowth of processes, there is abundant evidence based on in vitro studies that this phenomenon can be augmented by the addition of a variety of agents to cultured cells (Prasad and Kumar). Some of the agents used to induce this type of differentiation include nerve growth factor (NGF), cyclic AMP, prostaglandins, and vitamin B12. It has been shown recently that some neuroblastomas may exhibit a marked dependency on NGF for survival in primary cultures. These findings suggest that tumors that require NGF for survival might constitute a biologically distinctive subset of neuroblastomas or that NGF might function as a survival factor for some human neuroblastomas only in suboptimal or deleterious environments (Tischler et al.). The C1300 murine neuroblastoma has been studied extensively with regard to differentiation (Blume et al.). Cessation of cell division in these cultures has been characterized by an increase in cholinesterase and protein content, process formation, formation of electrically active membranes, and synthesis of acetylcholine receptors. The PC12 rat pheochromocytoma line has been shown to respond to the addition of NGF with a series of similar changes (Tischler and Greene). The factors that are responsible for neuronal differentiation in humans with these neural crest neoplasms, however, remain to be determined.

Spontaneous Regression. Neuroblastomas have been reported to undergo spontaneous regression or maturation by a number of authors. In a review of 1276 cases of spontaneous regression of various tumors, 17 percent were in patients with neuroblastoma (Everson and Cole). Cases of spontaneous regression include patients who have recovered after no therapy, after therapy that was directed at only part of the disease, or after systemic therapy that by most standards would be considered insufficient. In an analysis of 57 patients with neuroblastoma showing spontaneous regression, Evans and associates (1976b) showed that most patients were infants with stages II or IVs disease. Spontaneous regression consisted of complete disappearance of the disease or maturation to ganglioneuroma. Evans and associates (1976b) reported that approximately two-thirds of patients exhibiting spontaneous

regression were less than six months of age. The sites of metastasis may also influence the phenomenon of spontaneous regression. Of 37 patients who had spontaneous regression with disseminated disease, 28 had metastases in liver and/or skin, and only 9 had bone metastases. It has been suggested that tumor deposits in the subcutaneous tissue are capable of stimulating a particularly effective immune response in draining lymph nodes. A number of studies have shown that lymphocytes from neuroblastoma patients inhibit the growth of the tumor cells in vitro (Jaffe). In addition, serum of neuroblastoma patients and their family members has been shown to contain complement dependent cytotoxic antibodies against tumor cells. The exact relationships of these immunologic events to the phenomenon of spontaneous regression, however, remain to be determined.

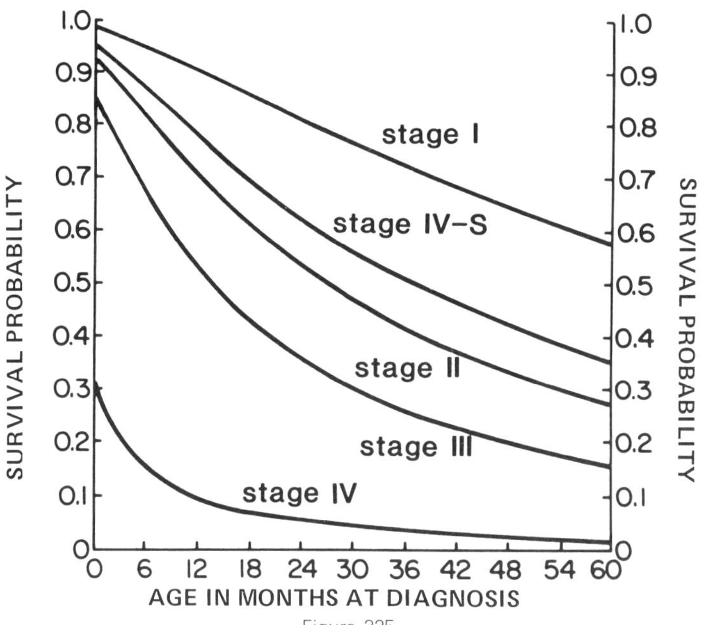

Figure 225
NEUROBLASTOMA / SURVIVAL PATTERNS
(From Evans, A.E., D'Angio, G.J., and Koop, C.E. Diagnosis and treatment of neuroblastoma. Pediatr. Clin. North Am. 23:161-170, 1976.)

Prognosis. The prognosis of neuroblastoma is dependent upon a number of variables, including age at diagnosis, stage, site of primary involvement, histologic grade, and sex (Jaffe; Hassenbusch et al.; Wilson and Draper). The results of most recent series have indicated that age at diagnosis is the single most important prognostic parameter. In a review of 246 patients with neuroblastoma, Breslow and McCann showed that the two-year survival rate by age at diagnosis was 74 percent for ages 0 to 11 months, 26 percent for 12 to 23 months, and 12 percent for children older than 24 months. The probability of survival for two years free of disease by stage and age in months at diagnosis is summarized in figure 225. Results of a number of series have indicated that the prognosis for children with mediastinal tumors is considerably better than for those with primary subdiaphragmatic involvement. In the series reported by Jaffe, two-year survivals after diagnosis were 61 percent for patients with thoracic tumors and 20 percent for those with primary subdiaphragmatic disease. In the latter group, those patients with extraadrenal tumors had a considerably better prognosis than those with a primary tumor within the adrenal (32 percent vs. 9 percent). There is some evidence that the better prognosis of patients with thoracic tumors results from the fact that the disease is detected at a less advanced stage than those with intra-abdominal primary tumors. Other studies indicate that stage for stage, the prognosis is better for tumors arising above the diaphragm. Data from several series indicate that prognosis is better for females than males.

Prognosis has also been related to the degree of histologic differentiation in neuroblastomas. Beckwith and Martin have divided neuroblastomas into four major grades on the basis of the extent of differentiating elements within the tumor (Table 14). In this study, a cell was identified as differentiating when nuclear enlargement,

Table 14

HISTOLOGIC GRADE AND PROGNOSIS *

Grade	% Differentiating Elements	Total Cases	Survival
I	>50%	5	100%
II	5 to 50%	4	75%
III	<5%	13	32%
IV	0	28	4%

*Adapted from Beckwith, J. B. and Martin, R. F. Observations on the histopathology of neuroblastomas. J. Pediatr. Surg. 3:106-110, 1968.

cytoplasmic enlargement with clear cell borders and increased affinity for eosin, as well as nerve processes were clearly evident in routinely stained sections. Other studies, however, have not supported as clear-cut a relationship between the extent of histologic differentiation and survival. Factors that do not appear to have an adverse effect on prognosis include high numbers of mitoses and the extent of hemorrhage or necrosis (Gitlow et al., 1973). Other factors that do appear to affect prognosis include the absolute numbers of circulating lymphocytes at diagnosis, as well as the percentage of bone marrow lymphoblasts and the immune competence of the patient at diagnosis and during therapy (Jaffe).

PLATE XIV

A. NEUROBLASTOMA
External (left) and cut surface (right) of a left adrenal neuroblastoma from a one year old boy. A thin rim of yellow cortical tissue is apparent along one pole of the tumor. A few small calcific flecks are apparent on the cut surface of the tumor. X1.8.

B. NEUROBLASTOMA
This bone marrow smear is from a patient with neuroblastoma and suspected bone metastases. The dried bone marrow smear was reacted with formaldehyde vapor for one hour. The intense yellow green cytoplasmic fluorescence is indicative of intracellular catecholamine stores. X400.

C. GANGLIONEUROBLASTOMA
This ganglioneuroblastoma shows a typically variegated pattern with focally hemorrhagic, raised cellular nodules admixed with a glistening fibrous stroma. Focal areas of calcification are present in the lower left portion of the tumor mass. X0.75.

PLATE XIV

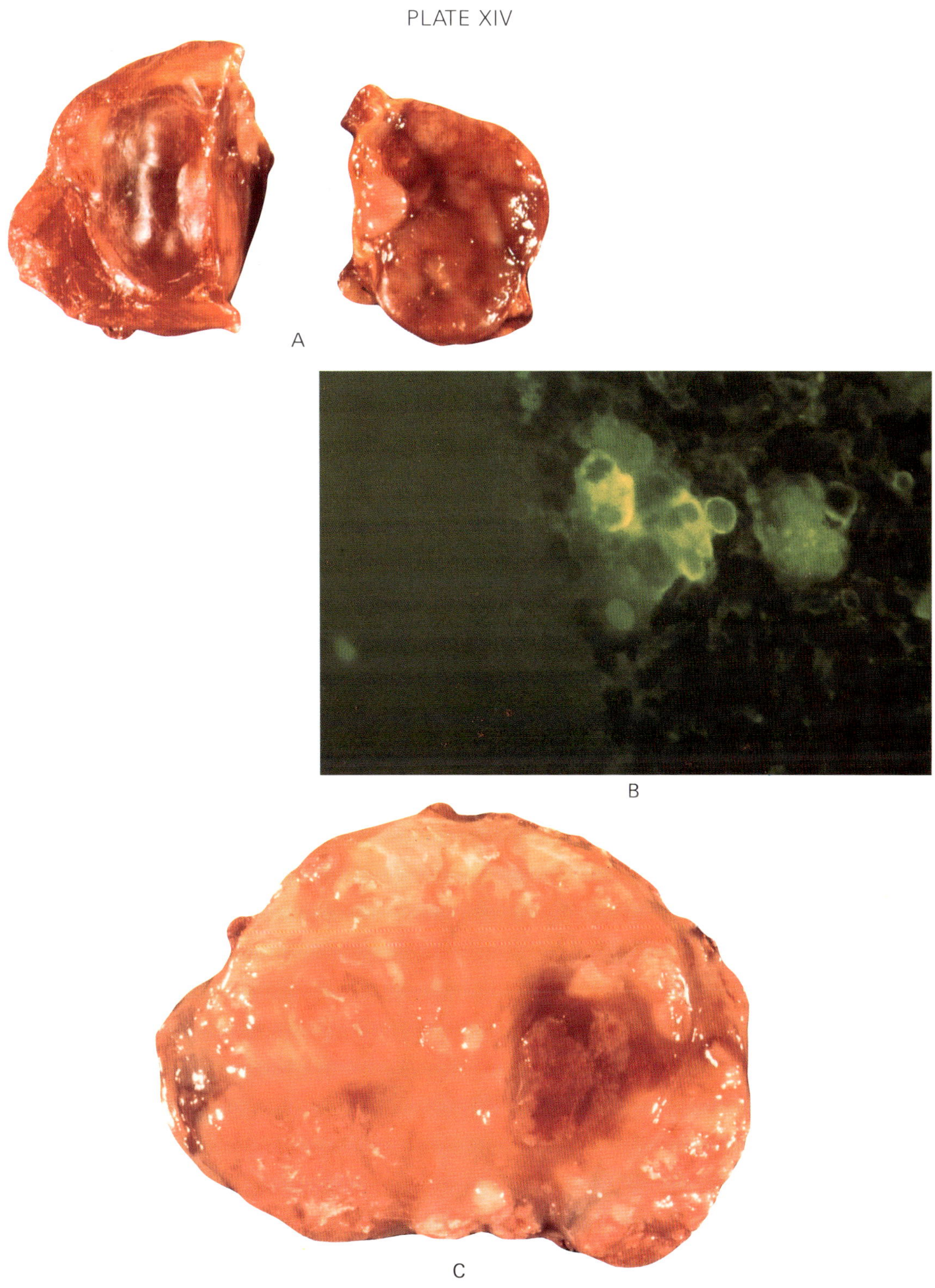

A

B

C

References

Andres, T. L. and Kadin, M. E. Immunologic markers in the differential diagnosis of small round cell tumors from lymphocytic leukemia. Am. J. Clin. Pathol. 79:546-552, 1983.

Ashley, D. J. B. Evans' Histological Appearances of Tumours. Edinburgh: Churchill Livingstone, 1978.

Askin, F. B., Rosai, J., Sibley, R. K., Dehner, L. P., and McAlister, W. W. Malignant small cell tumor of the thoracopulmonary region in childhood. Cancer 43:2438-2451, 1979.

Balsaver, A. M., Gibley, C. W., Jr., and Tessmer, C. F. Ultrastructural studies in Wilms's tumor. Cancer 22:417-427, 1968.

Beckwith, J. B. Wilms' tumor and other renal tumors of childhood: A selective review from the National Wilms' Tumor Study Pathology Center. Hum. Pathol. 14:481-492, 1983.

——— and Martin, R. F. Observations on the histopathology of neuroblastomas. J. Pediatr. Surg. 3:106-110, 1968.

——— and Perrin, E. V. In situ neuroblastomas: A contribution to the natural history of neural crest tumors. Am. J. Pathol. 43:1089-1104, 1963.

Blume, A., Gilbert, F., Wilson, S., Farber, J., Rosenberg, R., and Nirenberg, M. Regulation of acetylocholinesterase in neuroblastoma cells. Proc. Natl. Acad. Sci. 67:786-792, 1970.

Bolande, R. P. Developmental pathology. Am. J. Pathol. 94:627-684, 1979.

——— and Towler, W. F. A possible relationship of neuroblastoma to von Recklinghausen's disease. Cancer 26:162-175, 1970.

Breslow, N. and McCann, B. Statistical estimation of prognosis for children with neuroblastoma. Cancer Res. 31:2098-2103, 1971.

Brooks, J. J. Immunohistochemistry of Myoglobin, pp. 343-348. In: Advances in Immunohistochemistry. DeLellis, R. A. (Ed.) New York: Masson Publishing USA, Inc. 1984.

Cushing, H. and Wolbach, S. B. The transformation of a malignant paravertebral sympathicoblastoma into a benign ganglioneuroma. Am. J. Pathol. 3:203-216, 1927.

DeLellis, R. A. Formaldehyde-induced fluorescence technique for the demonstration of biogenic amines in diagnostic histopathology. Cancer 28:1704-1710, 1971.

deLorimier, A. A., Bragg, K. U., and Linden, G. Neuroblastoma in childhood. Am. J. Dis. Child. 118:441-450, 1969.

Emery, L. G., Shields, M., Shah, N. R., and Garbes, A. Neuroblastoma associated with Beckwith-Wiedemann syndrome. Cancer 52:176-179, 1983.

Enzinger, F. M. and Weiss, S. W. Soft Tissue Tumors. St. Louis: The C. V. Mosby Company, 1983.

Evans, A. E., D'Angio, G. J., and Koop, C. E. Diagnosis and treatment of neuroblastoma. Pediatr. Clin. North Am. 23:161-170, 1976a.

———, Gerson, J., and Schnaufer, L. Spontaneous regression of neuroblastoma. Natl. Cancer Inst. Monogr. 44:49-54, 1976b.

Everson, T. C. and Cole, W. H. Spontaneous Regression of Cancer. Philadelphia: W. B. Saunders Company, 1966.

Fox, F., Davidson, J., and Thomas, L. B. Maturation of sympathicoblastoma into ganglioneuroma. Cancer 12:108-116, 1959.

Gabbiani, G., Kapanci, Y., Barazzone, P., and Franke, W. W. Immunochemical identification of intermediate-sized filaments in human neoplastic cells. A diagnostic aid for the surgical pathologist. Am. J. Pathol. 104:206-216, 1981.

Gerson, J. M. and Koop, C. E. Neuroblastoma. Semin. Oncol. 1:35-46, 1974.

Ghadially, F. N. Diagnostic Electron Microscopy of Tumours. London: Butterworth, 1980.

Gitlow, S. E., Bertani, L. M., Rausen, A., Gribetz, D., and Dziedzic, S. W. Diagnosis of neuroblastoma by qualitative and quantitative determination of catecholamine metabolites in urine. Cancer 25:1377-1383, 1970.

———, Dziedzic, L. B. Strauss, L., Greenwood, S. M., and Dziedzic, S. W. Biochemical and histologic determinants in the prognosis of neuroblastoma. Cancer 32:898-905, 1973.

Goldstein, M., Freedman, L. S., Bohuon, A. C., and Guerinot, F. Serum dopamine-B-hydroxylase activity in neuroblastoma. N. Engl. J. Med. 286:1123-1125, 1972.

Hashimoto, H., Enjoji, M., Nakajima, T., Kiryu, H., and Daimaru, Y. Malignant neuroepithelioma (peripheral neuroblastoma). Am. J. Surg. Pathol. 7:309-318, 1983.

Hassenbusch, S., Kaizer, H., and White, J. J. Prognostic factors in neuroblastic tumors. J. Pediatr. Surg. 11:287-297, 1976.

Helson, L. and Biedler, J. L. Catecholamines in neuroblastoma cells from human bone marrow, tissue culture and murine C-1300 tumor. Cancer 31:1087-1091, 1973.

Henderson, D. W. and Papadimitriou, J. M. Ultrastructural Appearances of Tumours. A Diagnostic Atlas. Edinburgh: Churchill Livingstone, 1982.

Horten, B. C. and Rubinstein, L. J. Primary cerebral neuroblastoma. Brain 99:735-756, 1976.

Hou-Jensen, K., Priori, E., and Dmochowski, L. Studies on ultrastructure of Ewing's sarcoma of bone. Cancer 29:280-286, 1972.

Ito, J. and Johnson, W. W. Ultrastructure of Wilms' tumor. 1. Epithelial cell. J. Natl. Cancer Inst. 42:77-99, 1969.

Jaffe, N. Neuroblastoma: review of the literature and an examination of factors contributing to its enigmatic character. Cancer Treat. Rev. 3:61-82, 1976.

Kahn, H. J., Yeger, H., Baumal, R., Thom, H., and Phillips, J. M. Categorization of pediatric neoplasms by immunostaining with antiprekeratin and antivimentin antisera. Cancer 51:645-653, 1983.

Karsner, H. T. Tumors of the Adrenal. Atlas of Tumor Pathology, Fascicle 29, First Series. Washington: Armed Forces Institute of Pathology, 1950.

Knudson, A. G. and Meadows, A. T. Developmental genetics of neuroblastoma. J. Natl. Cancer Inst. 57:675-682, 1976.

Laug, W. E., Siegel, S. E., Shaw, K. N. F., Landing, B., et al. Initial urinary catecholamine metabolite concentrations and prognosis in neuroblastoma. Pediatrics 62:77-83, 1978.

Lehto, V-P., Stenman, S., Miettinen, M., Dahl, D., and Virtanen, I. Expression of a neural type of intermediate filament as a distinguishing feature between oat cell carcinoma and other lung cancers. Am. J. Pathol. 110:113-118, 1983.

Leonidas, J. C., Carter, B. L., Leape, L. L., Ramenofsky, M. L., and Schwartz, A. M. Computed tomography in diagnosis of abdominal masses in infancy and childhood. Arch. Dis. Child. 53:120-125, 1978.

Li, F. P., Cassady, J. R., and Jaffe, N. Risk of second tumors in survivors of childhood cancer. Cancer 35:1230-1235, 1975.

Llombart-Bosch, A., Blache, R., and Peydro-Olaya, A. Ultrastructural study of 28 cases of Ewing's sarcoma: typical and atypical forms. Cancer 41:1362-1373, 1978.

Lloyd, R. V. and Warner, T. F. C. S. Immunohistochemistry of Neuron Specific Enolase, pp. 127-140. In: Advances in Immunohistochemistry. DeLellis, R. A. (Ed.). New York: Masson Publishing USA, Inc., 1984.

Lynch, H. T. Cancer Genetics. Springfield, IL: C. C. Thomas Pub., 1976.

Mackay, B., Luna, M. A., and Butler, J. J. Adult neuroblastoma. Cancer 37:1334-1351, 1976.

Mäkinen, J. Microscopic patterns as a guide to prognosis of neuroblastoma in childhood. Cancer 29:1637-1646, 1972.

Misugi, K., Misugi, N., and Newton, W. A., Jr. Fine structural study of neuroblastoma, ganglioneuroblastoma, and pheochromocytoma. Arch. Pathol. 86:160-170, 1968.

Murray, M. R. and Stout, A. P. Distinctive characteristics of the sympathicoblastoma cultivated in vitro. A method for prompt diagnosis. Am. J. Pathol. 23:429-441, 1946.

Nakajima, T., Kameya, T., Watanabe, S., Hirota, T., et al. S-100 Protein Distribution in Normal and Neoplastic Tissues, pp. 141-158. In: Advances in Immunohistochemistry. DeLellis, R. A. (Ed.). New York: Masson Publishing USA, Inc., 1984.

Nesbitt, K. A. and Vidone, R. A. Primitive neuroectodermal tumor (neuroblastoma) arising in sciatic nerve of a child. Cancer 37:1562-1570, 1976.

Osborn, M. and Weber, K. Biology of disease. Tumor diagnosis by intermediate filament typing. A novel tool for surgical pathology. Lab. Invest. 48:372-394, 1983.

Prasad, K. N. and Kumar, S. Role of cyclic AMP in differentiation of human neuroblastoma cells in culture. Cancer 36:1338-1343, 1975.

Rice, R. W., Cabot, A., and Johnston, A. D. The application of electron microscopy to the diagnostic differentiation of Ewing's sarcoma and reticulum cell sarcoma of bone. Clin. Orthop. 91:174-185, 1973.

Russell, D. S. and Rubinstein, L. J. Pathology of Tumors of the Nervous System. Baltimore: The Williams & Wilkins Company, 1971.

Shimada, H., Aoyama, C., Chiba, T., and Newton, W. Prognostic subgroups for undifferentiated neoblastoma: Immunohistochemical study with anti-S100 protein antibody. Hum. Pathol. 16:471-476, 1985.

Sy, W. M. and Edmonson, J. H. The developmental defects associated with neuroblastoma — etiologic implications. Cancer 22:234-238, 1968.

Tannenbaum, M. Renal Tumors. In: Electron Microscopy in Human Medicine, Vol. 9, Urogenital System and Breast. Johannessen, V. (Ed.). New York: McGraw-Hill International Book Company, 1979.

————. Ultrastructural Pathology of Human Renal Cell Tumors. In: Kidney Pathology Decennial (1966-1975). Sommers, S. C. (Ed.). New York: Appleton-Century-Crofts, 1975.

Tapia, F. J. Barbosa, A. J. A., Marangos, P. J., Polak, J. M., et al. Neurone-specific enolase in produced by neuroendocrine tumours. Lancet 1:808-811, 1981.

Taxy, J. B. Electron microscopy in the diagnosis of neuroblastoma. Arch. Pathol. Lab. Med. 104:355-360, 1980.

Tischler, A. S. and Greene, L. A. Morphologic and cytochemical properties of a clonal line of rat adrenal pheochromocytoma cells which respond to nerve growth factor. Lab. Invest. 39:77-89, 1978.

————, Slayton, V. W., Costopoulos, D., Leape, L. L., DeLellis, R. A., and Wolfe, H. J. Nerve growth factor as a survival factor in human neuroblastoma. Cancer 54:1344-1347, 1984.

Triche, T. Pathology of Cancer in the Young. In: Cancer in the Young. Levine, A. S. (Ed.). New York: Masson Publishing USA, Inc., 1982a.

————. Round Cell Tumors in Childhood: The Application of Newer Techniques to the Differential

Diagnosis. In: Perspectives in Pediatric Pathology, Vol. 7. Rosenberg, H. S. and Berstein, J. (Eds.). New York: Masson Publishing USA, Inc., 1982b.

Triche, T. and Askin, F. B. Neuroblastoma and the differential diagnosis of small-, round-, blue cell tumors. Hum. Pathol. 14:568-595, 1983.

———— and Ross, W. E. Glycogen-containing neuroblastoma with clinical histopathologic features of Ewing's sarcoma. Cancer 41:1425-1432, 1978.

Tsokos, M., Howard, R., and Costa, J. Immunohistochemical study of alveolar and embryonal rhabdomyosarcoma. Lab. Invest. 48:148-155, 1982.

Turkel, S. B. and Itabashi, H. H. The natural history of neuroblastic cells in the fetal adrenal gland. Am. J. Pathol. 76:225-244, 1974.

Wang, J. J., Sinks, L. F., and Chu, T. M. Carcinoembryonic antigen in patients with neuroblastoma. J. Surg. Oncol. 6:211-217, 1974.

Warner, T. F. C. S., Uno, H., Hafez, R., Burgess, J., et al. Merkel cells and Merkel cell tumors. Cancer 52:238-245, 1983.

Wick, M. R., Scheithauer, B. W., and Kovacs, K. Neuron-specific enolase in neuroendocrine tumors of the thymus, bronchus, and skin. Am. J. Clin. Pathol. 79:703-707, 1983.

Wilson, L. M. K. and Draper, G. J. Neuroblastoma, its natural history and prognosis. Br. Med. J. 3:301-307, 1974.

Witzleben, C. L. and Landy, R. A. Disseminated neuroblastoma in a child with von Recklinghausen's disease. Cancer 34:786-790, 1974.

Yokoyama, M., Okada, K., Tokue, A., Takayasu, H., and Yamada, R. Ultrastructural and biochemical study of neuroblastoma and ganglioneuroblastoma. Invest. Urol. 9:156-164, 1971.

Young, J. L. and Miller, R. W. Incidence of malignant tumors in children. J. Pediatrics 86:254-260, 1975.

GANGLIONEUROBLASTOMA

Definition. The ganglioneuroblastoma is a composite tumor containing both mature ganglion cells and primitive neuroblastic elements together with cells of intermediate differentiation and Schwann cells. This term was introduced by Robertson in 1915 to describe a transitional tumor of sympathetic cell origin, which was composed of malignant neuroblastic elements and benign ganglioneuromatous areas (Adam and Hochholzer). While some authors regard these neoplasms as a distinct tumor type (Russell and Rubinstein), others consider them to represent a neuroblastoma showing evidence of ganglionic differentiation or maturation (Ashley).

Age, Sex, Site. Ganglioneuroblastomas occur most commonly in children less than 10 years of age, with an approximately equal male to female ratio. In the series reported by Stowens, approximately 65 percent of tumors were located in the retroperitoneum, while the remaining cases were equally distributed in the mediastinum, neck, and adrenal. Kilton and associates have reviewed 19 ganglioneuroblastomas in adults. These tumors occurred most commonly in the retroperitoneum, mediastinum, and neck.

Clinical. The symptoms of ganglioneuroblastoma are most often referable to the local effects of the neoplasm and do not separate ganglioneuroblastomas from other malignant tumors. Although these tumors are capable of synthesizing, storing, and secreting catecholamines, hypertension occurs rarely (Staley et al.). Occasional cases of intractable watery diarrhea have been found in some patients with ganglioneuroblastomas (Jansen-Goemans and Engelhardt; Mitchell et al.). In these cases, vasoactive intestinal polypeptide (VIP), the presumed diarrheogenic agent, has been localized immunohistochemically to the mature ganglion cells within the tumor (Mendelsohn et al.).

Gross. Ganglioneuroblastomas show considerable variation in size, but, in general, the adrenal primary tumors tend to be smaller than the mediastinal or retroperitoneal tumors. Those tumors that show spinal extension often assume a dumbbell configuration. Both intra- and extra-adrenal primary tumors often appear encapsulated grossly. On cut section, they show considerable variation, depending in part upon the extent of differentiated elements within the neoplasm (pl. XIV-C). The best differentiated tumors may resemble ganglioneuromas with a glistening, pink tan, fibrous cut surface (fig. 226). In these cases, careful sectioning may reveal small soft and focally hemorrhagic areas which represent primitive neuroblastic foci. Some tumors may show multifocal nodular areas with more obvious areas of necrosis and hemorrhage (pl. XIV-C). Other tumors may grossly resemble neuroblastomas. Areas of calcification are found frequently.

Microscopic. Ganglioneuroblastomas are characterized cytologically by the presence of cells showing varying degrees of differentiation ranging from neuroblasts to sympathetic ganglion cells. The ganglion cells are often indistinguishable from normal sympathetic ganglion cells. They are characterized by abundant cytoplasm containing Nissl's substance and neuromelanin, a large vesicular nucleus, and a prominent nucleolus. Capsular or satellite cells frequently surround the ganglion cells (figs. 227–231). In the so-called imperfect type of ganglioneuroblastoma, tumor cells showing all degrees of differentiation are scattered throughout the tumor (figs. 227, 228). In some series, this type of tumor has also been classified as a maturing neuroblastoma. The so-called immature or composite ganglioneuroblastomas resemble mature ganglioneuromas which contain discrete

nodular collections of immature neuroblastic elements, together with mature ganglion cells and areas of proliferation of Schwann cells (figs. 229–231). The Schwann cells in these tumors may be demonstrated selectively with immunoperoxidase technics for S-100 protein (Nakajima et al.). Both neuroblastic and ganglionic cells are unreactive for this protein, but are positive for neuron specific enolase. The number of S-100 protein positive cells in these tumors has been shown to correlate with prognosis (Misugi et al.; Nakajima et al.). In both diffuse and immature variants

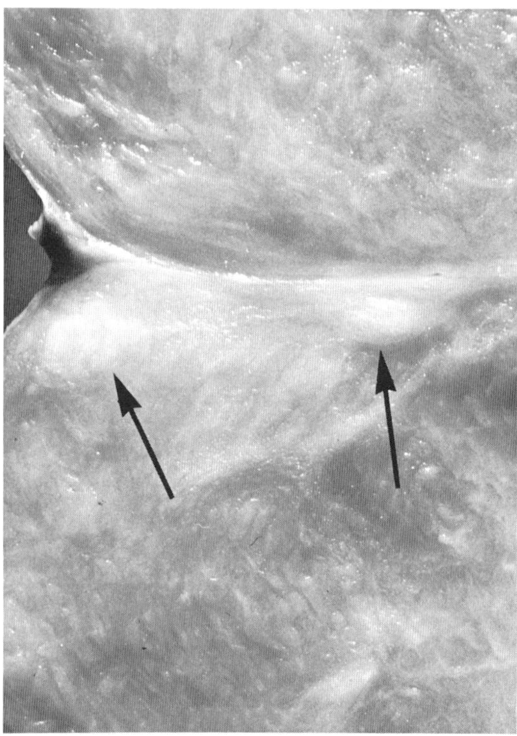

Figure 226
GANGLIONEUROBLASTOMA
On cross section, this tumor shows a predominant fibrous pattern, which is consistent with a diagnosis of ganglioneuroma. Two slightly raised white nodules (arrows), however, were composed of primitive neuroblastic elements on microscopic examination. X2.

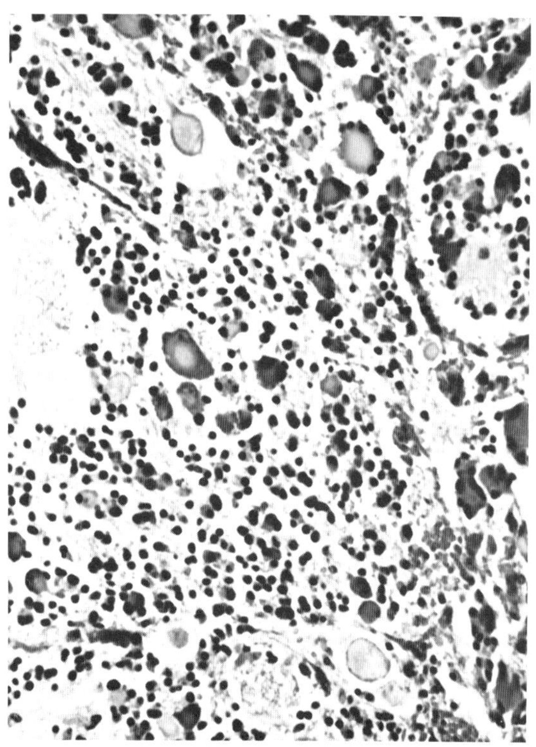

Figure 227
GANGLIONEUROBLASTOMA
This adrenal ganglioneuroblastoma contains an admixture of cell types ranging from small hyperchromatic neuroblasts to larger mono- and multinucleate ganglion type cells. Other areas of this tumor contained mature ganglion cells. X320.

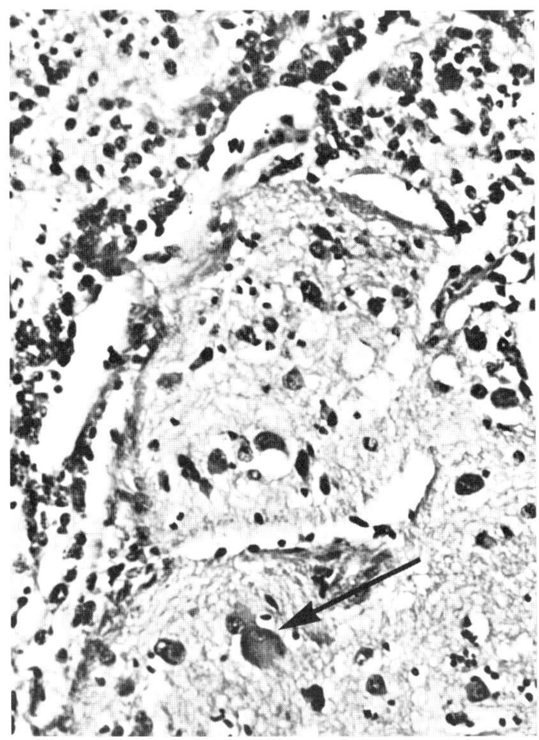

Figure 228
GANGLIONEUROBLASTOMA
In this ganglioneuroblastoma, occasional mature appearing ganglion type cells (arrow) are present in a neurofibrillary rich eosinophilic matrix. X320.

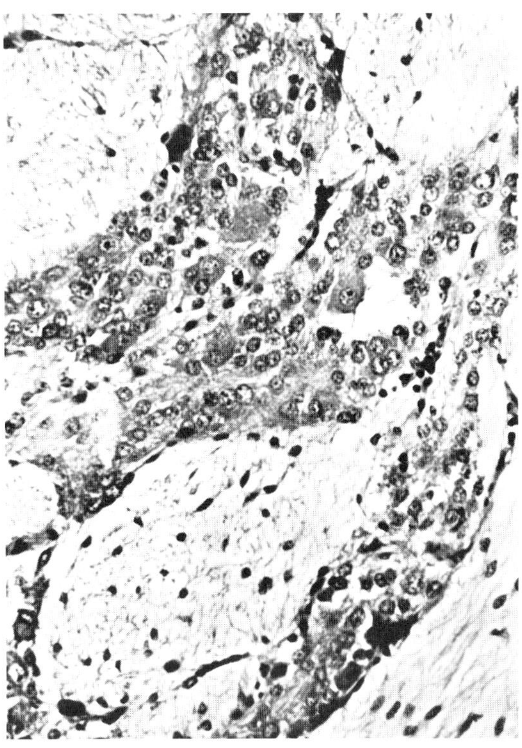

Figure 229
(Figures 229–231 from same patient)
GANGLIONEUROBLASTOMA
Ganglioneuroblastoma shows bandlike collections of neuroblastoma cells exhibiting varying degrees of maturation. The neuroblastic cells are surrounded by lobules of neurofibrillary matrix that contain elongated Schwann cells. X320.

of this tumor, some ganglion cells may be multinucleate and may appear immature (figs. 227, 228). Lymphocytic infiltration, hemorrhage, and necrosis are seen commonly. Despite the frequently apparent gross encapsulation, microscopic evidence of infiltration of tumor beyond the capsule is often noted. Rarely, the tumors may contain melanin, which is present within Schwann cells (Hahn et al.).

Ultrastructure. Reflecting the composite nature of the tumor, ultrastructural studies have revealed areas indistinguishable from ganglioneuroma as well as areas that are identical to neuroblastoma (Beltran et al.; Gonzalez-Angulo et al.). The ganglioneuromatous foci consist predominantly of abundant neuritic processes which are enclosed by Schwann cells (fig. 232). Myelin may or may not be present. Ganglion cells in these areas appear mature. The zones of immature cells are composed of neuroblasts and immature ganglionic elements (fig. 232). Powers and colleagues have reported the ultrastructure of a ganglioneuroblastoma that contained Hirano, zebra, membranous cytoplasmic bodies, and Pick bodies in the same population of neoplastic ganglion cells.

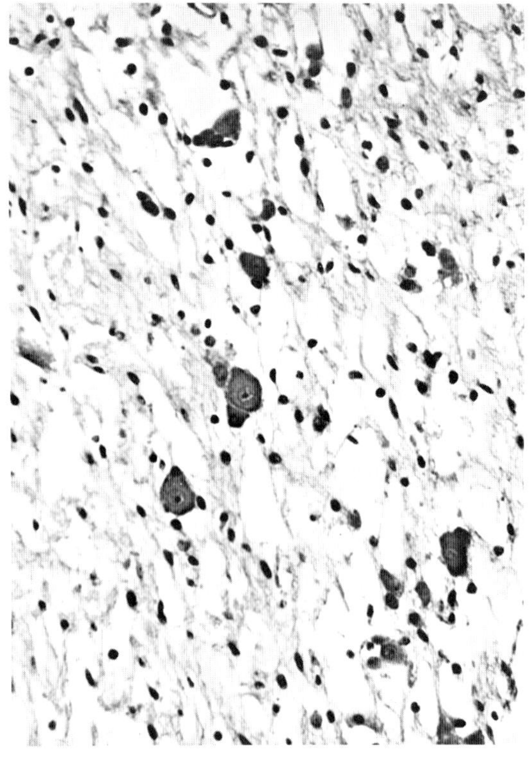

Figure 230
GANGLIONEUROBLASTOMA
This portion of the tumor contains a predominance of
mature ganglion cells with well developed Nissl's substance
and satellite type cells. The small cells in this field represent
Schwann cells. X320.

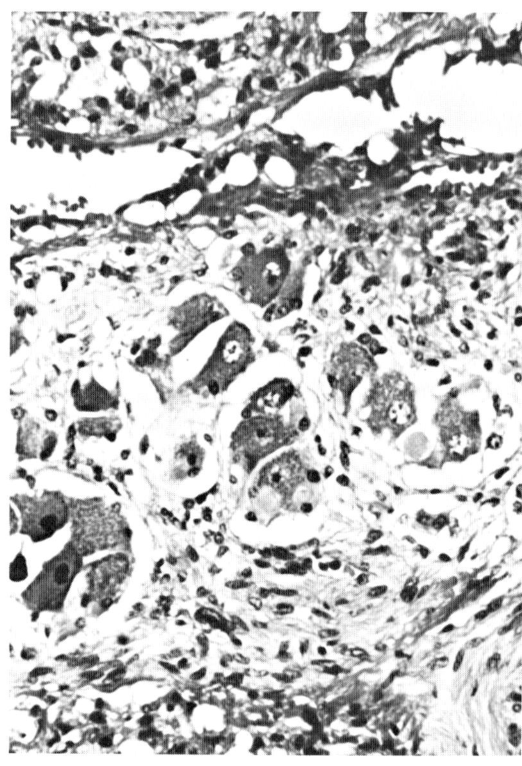

Figure 231
GANGLIONEUROBLASTOMA
This field of the case illustrated in figures 229 and 230 is
indistinguishable from a benign ganglioneuroma. X320.

Natural History. The natural history of ganglioneuroblastoma is unpredictable. In general, however, the well encapsulated neoplasms do not recur following complete surgical excision. Alternatively, the tumors may show extensive local invasion, regional node metastasis, and, finally, distant metastases similar to the neuroblastomas.

Adam and Hochholzer have devised a staging system for ganglioneuroblastomas that is similar to that employed for neuroblastomas. Stage I refers to a circumscribed noninvasive tumor, while stage II indicates a tumor which invades adjacent tissues but does not extend across the midline. Stage III refers to a tumor which extends in continuity across the midline, while stage IV patients have evidence of metastatic disease. As with neuroblastomas, the best prognosis is seen in patients with stage I disease. Stout has indicated that metastatic disease is more likely to occur in those tumors that show the immature or composite pattern (65 percent), as compared to the imperfect or diffuse pattern (18 percent). Other authors, however, have failed to confirm the better prognosis of those tumors with an immature or diffuse pattern (Kilton et al.). In the series of mediastinal tumors reported by Adam and

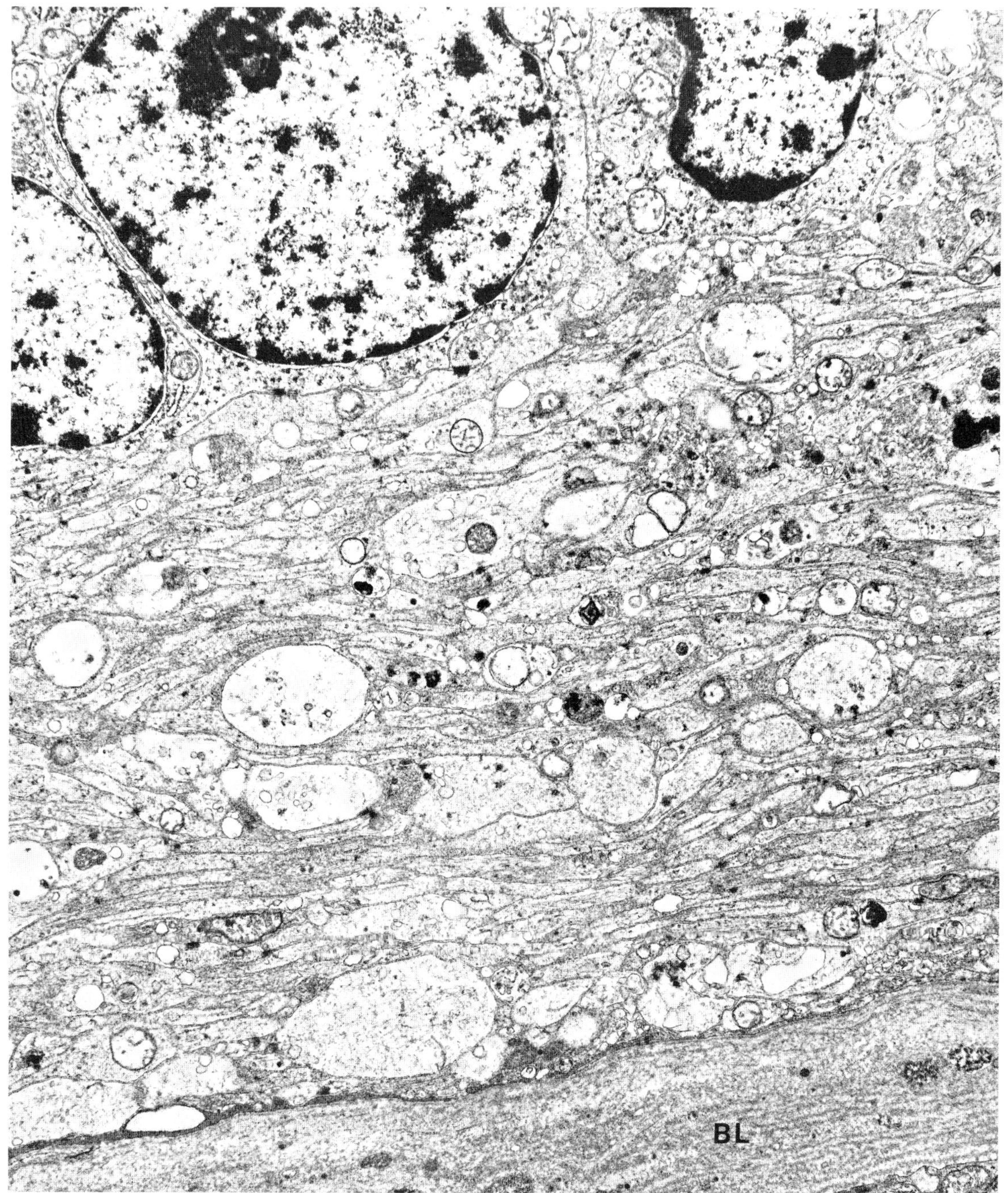

Figure 232
GANGLIONEUROBLASTOMA
Three neuroblastoma cells are present in the upper portion of the field. Just beneath these cells, there is an area showing multiple neuritic processes, some of which contain dense core neurosecretory granules. Adherens type junctions are present between the processes. A portion of a Schwann cell is present in this field. The basal lamina (BL) is extensively reduplicated. X9,800.

Hochholzer, 75 percent of the composite tumors, but only 4 percent of the diffuse ganglioneuroblastomas metastasized. These authors have concluded that the best prognosis is associated with age under three years, stage I disease, and a diffuse or imperfect pattern. Microscopic calcification, necrosis hemorrhage, and lymphocytic infiltration, however, did not correlate with prognosis.

References

Adam, A. and Hochholzer, L. Ganglioneuroblastoma of the posterior mediastinum. Cancer 47:373-381, 1981.

Ashley, D. J. B. Evans' Histological Appearances of Tumours. Edinburgh: Churchill Livingstone, 1978.

Beltran, G., Leiderman, E., Stuckey, W. J., Jr., Ferrans, V. J., and Mogabgab, W. J. Metastatic ganglioneuroblastoma. Cancer 24:552-559, 1969.

Gonzalez-Angulo, A., Reyes, H., and Reyna, A. N. The ultrastructure of ganglioneuroblastoma. Neurology 15:242-252, 1965.

Hahn, J. F., Netsky, M. G., Butler, A. B., and Sperber, E. E. Pigmented ganglioneuroblastoma: relation of melanin and lipofuscin to Schwannomas and other tumors of neural crest origin. J. Neuropathol. Exp. Neurol. 35:393-403, 1976.

Jansen-Goemans, A. and Engelhardt, J. Intractable diarrhea in a boy with vasoactive intestinal peptide-producing ganglioneuroblastoma. Pediatrics 59:710-716, 1977.

Kilton, L. J., Aschenbrener, C., and Burns, C. P. Ganglioneuroblastoma in adults. Cancer 37:974-983, 1976.

Mendelsohn, G., Eggleston, J. C., Olson, J. L., Said, S. I., and Baylin, S. B. Vasoactive intestinal peptide and its relationship to ganglion cell differentiation in neuroblastic tumors. Lab. Invest. 41:144-149, 1979.

Misugi, K., Aoki, I., Shimada, H., Kikyo, S., Sasaki, Y., Tsumoda, A., and Nakajima, T. S-100 protein distribution in neuroblastoma group tumors. Yokohama Med. Bull. 33:127-131, 1982.

Mitchell, C. H., Sinatra, F. R., Crast, F. W., Griffin, R., and Sunshine, P. Intractable watery diarrhea, ganglioneuroblastoma, and vasoactive intestinal peptide. J. Pediatr. 89:593-595, 1976.

Nakajima, T., Kameya, T., Watanabe, S., Hirota, T., Shimosato, Y., and Isobe, T. S-100 Protein Distribution in Normal and Neoplastic Tissues. In: Advances in Immunohistochemistry. DeLellis, R. A. (Ed.). New York: Masson Publishing USA, Inc., 1984.

Powers, J. M., Balentine, J. D., Wisniewski, H. M., and Terry, R. D. Retroperitoneal ganglioneuroblastoma: a kaleidoscope of neuronal degeneration. J. Neuropathol. Exp. Neurol. 35:14-25, 1976.

Robertson, H. E. Das ganglioneuroblastom, ein besonderer Typus im System der Neurome. Virchows Arch. [Pathol. Anat.] 220:147-168, 1915.

Russell, D. S. and Rubinstein, L. J. Pathology of Tumors of the Nervous System. Baltimore: The Williams & Wilkins Company, 1971.

Staley, N. A., Polesky, H. F., and Bensch, K. G. Fine structural and biochemical studies on the malignant ganglioneuroma. J. Neuropathol. Exp. Neurol. 26:634-653, 1967.

Stout, A. P. Ganglioneuroma of the sympathetic nervous system. Surg. Gynecol. Obstet. 84:101-110, 1947.

Stowens, D. Neuroblastoma and related tumors. Arch. Pathol. 63:451-459, 1957.

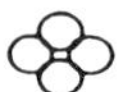

GANGLIONEUROMA

Definition. The mature ganglioneuroma is a benign neoplasm composed of sympathetic ganglion cells and sheathed neurites, with or without myelin, and with variable numbers of Schwann cells and collagen.

Age, Sex, Site. Ganglioneuromas most commonly develop from the great sympathetic chains that extend from the base of the skull to the neck, posterior mediastinum, and retroperitoneal regions, including the adrenal glands (Stout). These tumors have also been reported in a variety of other sites, including the gastrointestinal tract, uterus, ovary, and skin. In the series reported by Stowens, 56 percent of the tumors developed in the mediastinum or retroperitoneum, while 30 percent originated in the adrenals. Fourteen percent of the tumors developed in a variety of other sites. In Stout's series, only 13 percent of the tumors had an adrenal origin. The tumors have been reported to occur at all ages. Adrenal primary tumors, however, have a tendency to occur in older age groups, with a predominance of cases in the third to fifth decades (Stout). The greater frequency of adrenal ganglioneuromas in older age groups may be explained in part by their frequent discovery as incidental autopsy findings.

Clinical. Ganglioneuromas of the adrenal are most commonly asymptomatic (Russell and Rubinstein). On rare occasions, patients may present with abdominal or flank pain. Because of the high frequency of calcification, ganglioneuromas may be apparent on plain films of the abdomen. Ganglioneuromas are rarely associated with hypertension (Rosenthal et al.). Urinary levels of catecholamines and their metabolites, however, may be increased in patients with these tumors. Rarely, ganglioneuromas may be associated with a syndrome of severe watery diarrhea, hypochlorhydria, and alkalosis (Verner-Morrison syndrome). In these cases, both serum and tumor tissue levels of vasoactive intestinal polypeptide (VIP) may be increased. This hormone has been localized immunocytochemically to the ganglion cells of the tumors (Mendelsohn et al.).

Gross. The ganglioneuromas show considerable variation in size. In general, however, the adrenal primary tumors rarely weigh more than 50 g. The larger extra-adrenal tumors are spherical to ovoid in shape and are completely encapsulated. The smaller tumors that develop within the adrenal are sharply demarcated from the adjacent medulla, but are not definitely encapsulated (figs. 233–235). In some cases, finger-like projections of the tumor may extend into the adjacent medulla and may resemble thickened nerve bundles (Ashley; fig. 234). On cross section, the tumors are typically gray white and firm, with a distinct resemblance to leiomyomas. Occasionally, the tumors may be bilateral.

Microscopic. The tumors are composed of variable numbers of ganglion cells and sheathed neurites, with or without myelin, Schwann cells, and variable amounts of collagen. The ganglion cells may be distributed diffusely throughout the tumor, but are present more commonly in clusters (fig. 236). Individual cells have generally round and somewhat eccentric vesicular

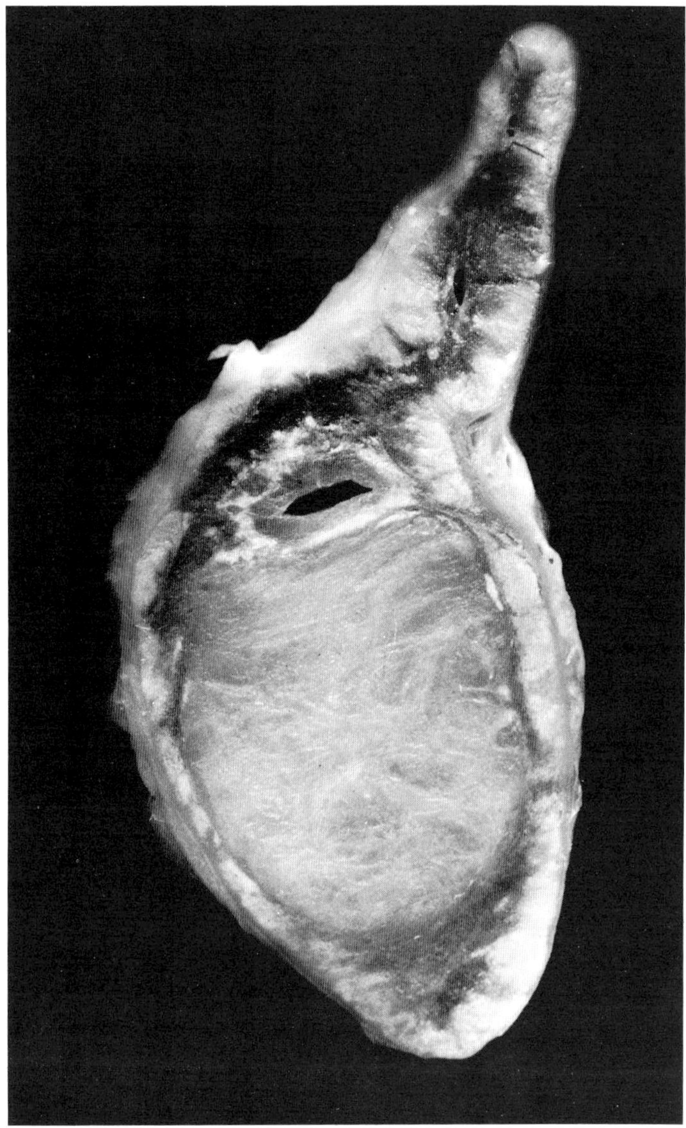

Figure 233
(Figures 233 and 234 from same patient)
GANGLIONEUROMA
Bilateral adrenal ganglioneuromas were incidental autopsy findings in this 70 year old man who died of an acute myocardial infarction. The tumor has a dense fibrous appearance and is sharply demarcated from the adjacent medulla. Approx. X2.1.

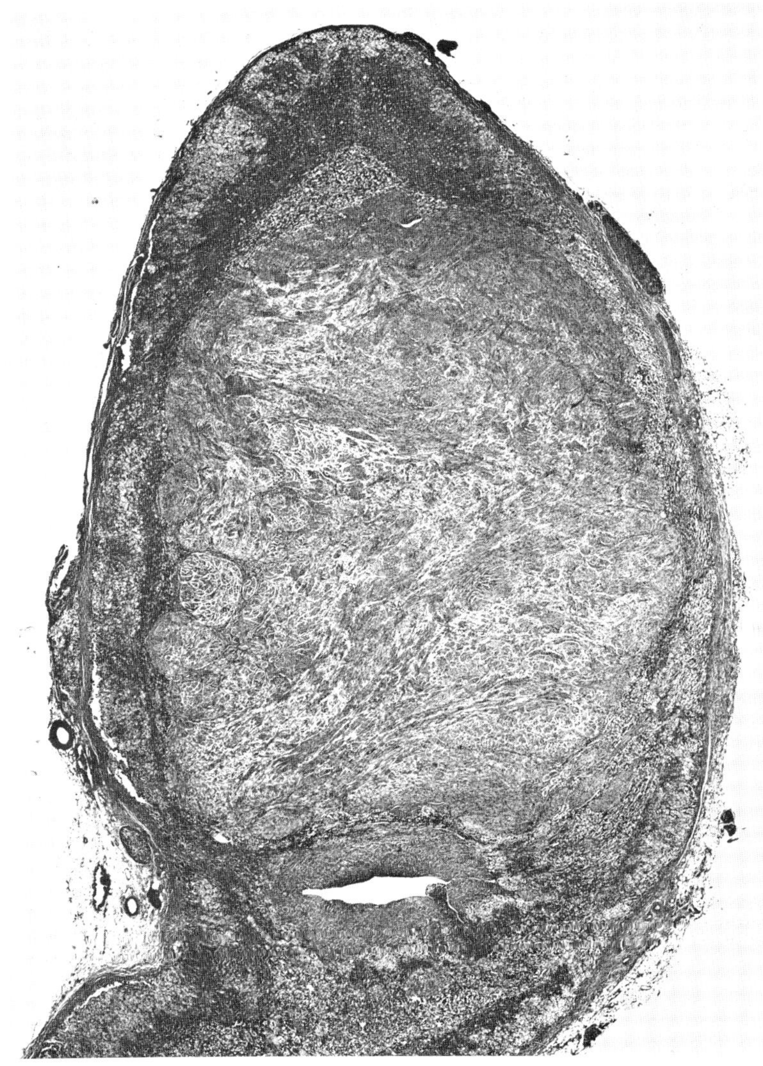

Figure 234
GANGLIONEUROMA
On low power microscopic examination, the tumor appears to be composed of thickened nerve bundles. This appearance is most striking in the lower portion of the field. X4.

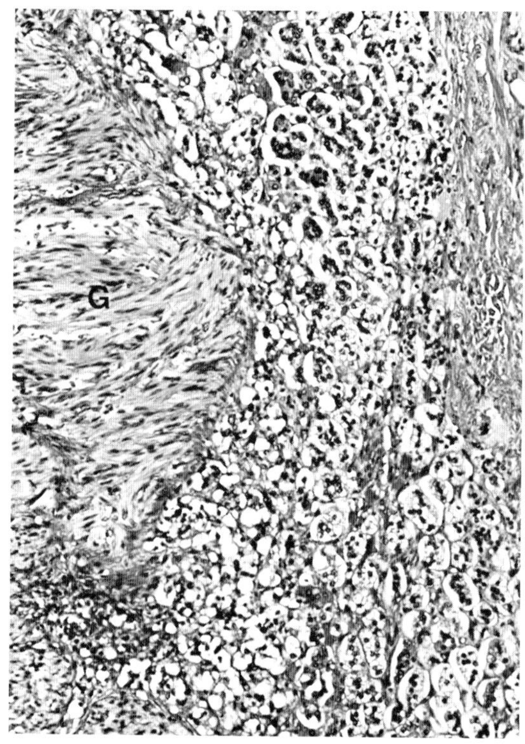

Figure 235
GANGLIONEUROMA
There is no definite capsule between the ganglioneuroma
(G) and the adjacent medullary tissue. X125.

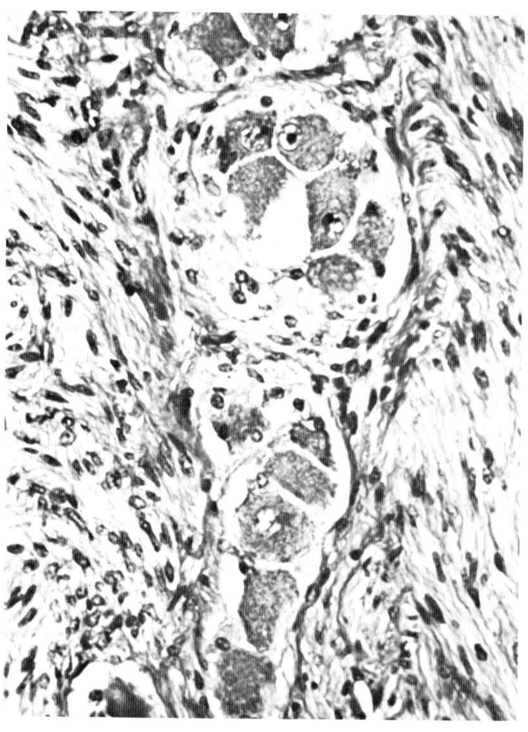

Figure 236
GANGLIONEUROMA
Ganglion cells in ganglioneuromas may be dispersed
throughout the tumor. More often, however, they are aggre-
gated into small groups, as they are in this case. X320.

nuclei with a single prominent nucleolus. Binucleate or multinucleate forms may be found and the ganglion cells may be surrounded by satellite or capsular cells. The cytoplasm of the ganglion cells in ganglioneuromas often contains well developed Nissl's substance as well as neuromelanin granules. Occasionally, the differential diagnosis may lie between ganglioneuroma and neurofibroma with entrapped ganglion cells. In the latter instance, the ganglion cells are always surrounded by satellite cells, while satellite cells are less commonly encountered in ganglioneuromas. Occasional ganglion cells may contain cytoplasmic inclusions that resemble Pick's bodies (Bender and Ghatak). Scully and Cohen

have described a ganglioneuroma that contained cells morphologically identical to ovarian hilus cells, including the presence of crystalloids of Reinke. More recently, Aguirre and Scully have reported a case of a 58 year old woman with virilization associated with a testosterone-secreting adrenal ganglioneuroma containing Leydig cells with crystalloids of Reinke.

Variable numbers of mature lymphocytes may be scattered throughout the tumor. These cells should not be mistaken for immature neuroblasts.

The stroma of ganglioneuromas may appear edematous or compact. The predominant cell is a spindle shaped Schwann cell (figs. 237, 238). Variable amounts of

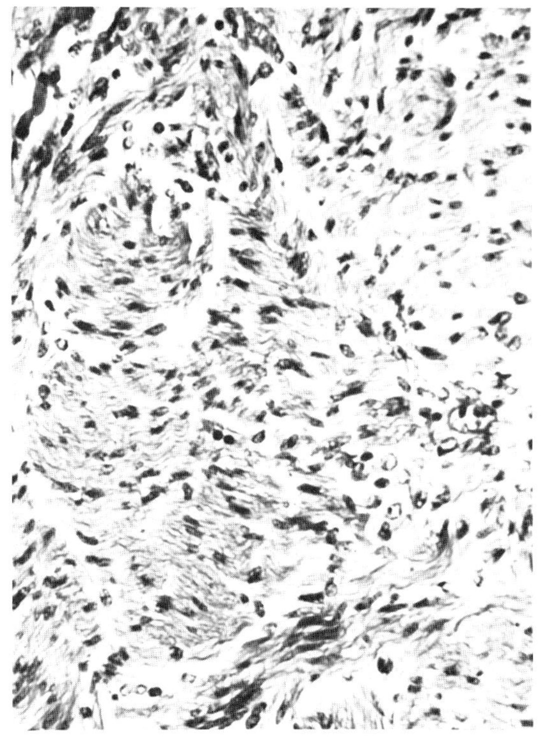

Figure 237
GANGLIONEUROMA
This field demonstrates the characteristic bundles of Schwann cells which comprise the bulk of ganglioneuromas. X320.

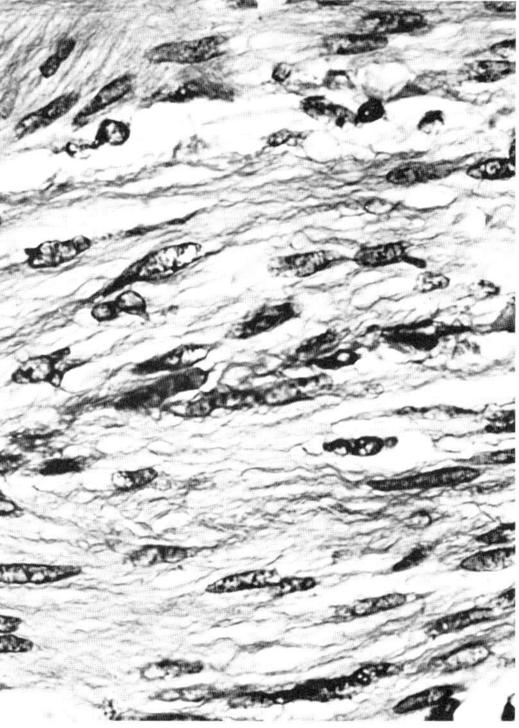

Figure 238
GANGLIONEUROMA
The Schwann cells in this field have elongated nuclei and a fibrillary eosinophilic cytoplasm. X800.

collagen separate individual stromal cells. The schwannian cells are often arranged in interlacing bundles (fig. 237). Numerous stainable neurofibrils are characteristically present within the tumor. Variable amounts of myelin may be present. Occasional tumors may show extensive areas of cystic degeneration. Particularly in mediastinal and retroperitoneal ganglioneuromas, mature adipose tissue and lymph nodes may be entrapped within the substance of the tumor.

Ultrastructure. The ganglioneuromas most closely resemble sympathetic ganglia (Razzuk et al.; Yokoyama et al.). The most impressive features of the tumors at the ultrastructural level include the presence of masses of unmyelinated nerve bundles together with large numbers of mature Schwann cells (figs. 239, 240). The latter cell type is recognized by the presence of a well formed basal lamina completely surrounding the cell (fig. 240). One Schwann cell usually ensheaths several axons. The nerve processes show considerable variation in diameter and contain typical neurofilaments and neurotubules, as well as both clear and cored vesicles. The intervening stroma contains variable amounts of collagen, which shows a normal pattern of spacing.

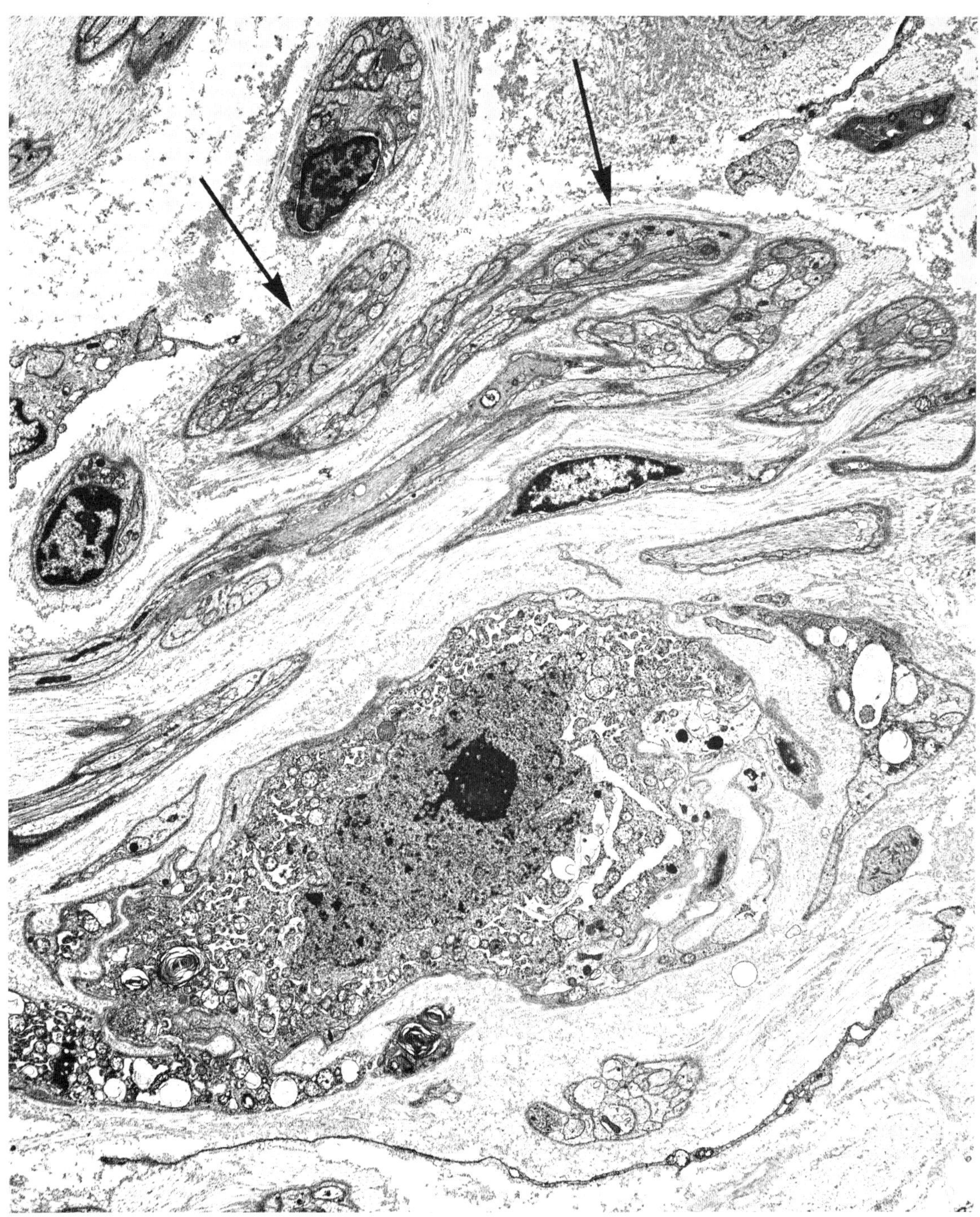

Figure 239
GANGLIONEUROMA

The mature ganglion cell in the center of the field is surrounded by collagen and processes of Schwann cells (arrows). The latter contain bundles of neurites. X4400.

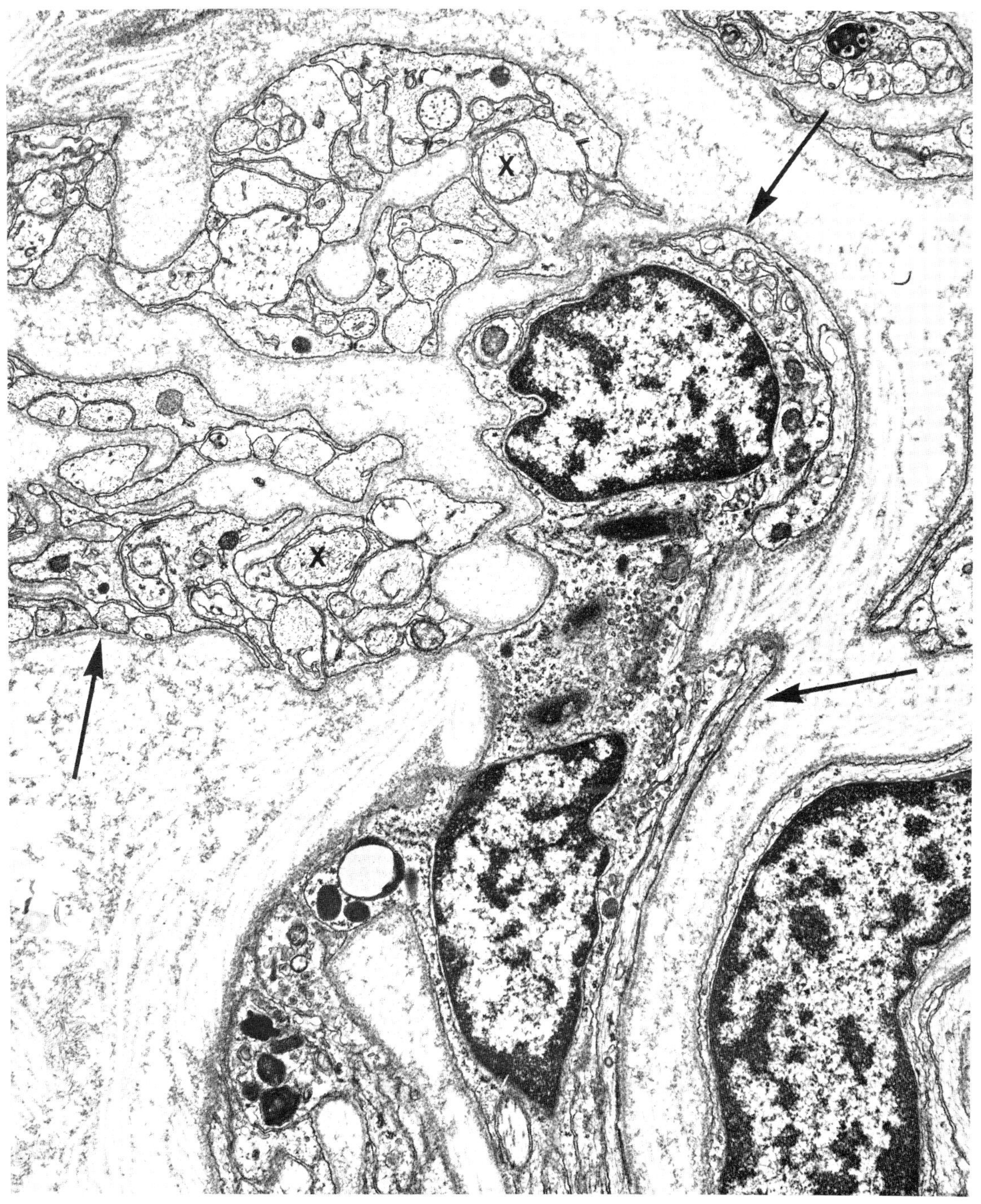

Figure 240
GANGLIONEUROMA
The Schwann cells in this field have prominent heterochromatin which is closely applied to the nuclear membranes. The Schwann cells are surrounded by a continuous basal lamina (arrows). The enclosed neurites (X) contain microfilaments and microtubules. X14,100.

Natural History. The tumors grow slowly by progressive expansion and symptoms are most frequently associated with compression of adjacent structures. The progressive growth of these lesions is undoubtedly due to proliferation of the Schwann cell compartments of the tumors. Surgical excision is usually curative.

References

Aguirre, P. and Scully, R. E. Testosterone-secreting adrenal ganglioneuroma containing Leydig cells. Am. J. Surg. Pathol. 7:699-705, 1983.

Ashley, D. J. B. Evans' Histological Appearances of Tumours. Edinburgh: Churchill Livingston, 1978.

Bender, B. L. and Ghatak, N. R. Light and electron microscopic observations on a ganglioneuroma. Acta Neuropathol. (Berl.) 42:7-10, 1978.

Mendelsohn, G., Eggleston, J. C., Olson, J. L., Said, S. I., and Baylin, S. B. Vasoactive intestinal peptide and its relationship to ganglion cell differentiation in neuroblastic tumors. Lab. Invest. 41:144-149, 1979.

Razzuk, M. A., Urschel, H. C., Jr., Martin, J. A., Kingsley, W. B., and Paulson, D. L. Electron microscopical observations on mediastinal neurolemmoma, neurofibroma and ganglioneuroma. Ann. Thorac. Surg. 15:73-83, 1973.

Rosenthal, I. M., Greenberg, R., Kathan, R., Falk, G. S., and Wong. R. Catecholamine metabolism of a ganglioneuroma. Pediatr. Res. 3:413-424, 1969.

Russell, D. S. and Rubinstein, L. J. Pathology of Tumors of the Nervous System. Baltimore: The Williams & Wilkins Company, 1971.

Scully, R. E. and Cohen, R. B. Ganglioneuroma of adrenal medulla containing cells morphologically identical to hilus cells (extraparenchymal Leydig cells). Cancer 14:421-425, 1961.

Stout, A. P. Ganglioneuroma of the sympathetic nervous sytem. Surg. Gynecol. Obstet. 84:101-110, 1947.

Stowens, D. Neuroblastoma and related tumors. Arch. Pathol. 63:451-459, 1957.

Yokoyama, M., Okada, K., Tokue, A., Takayasu, H. Ultrastructural and biochemical study of benign ganglioneuroma. Virchows Arch. [Pathol. Anat.] 361:195-209, 1973.

MISCELLANEOUS TUMORS

MALIGNANT MELANOMA

Malignant melanomas rarely have been reported to arise within the adrenal, but some authors have expressed considerable doubt as to the existence of this entity. DasGupta and associates have suggested that most of these cases may represent metastases to the adrenals rather than true primary neoplasms. In a detailed autopsy study of the distribution of metastases from cutaneous and ocular melanomas, DasGupta and Brasfield found secondary deposits within the adrenals in 50 percent of cases. Since melanomas of the skin or eye may undergo spontaneous regression, those cases classified as primary melanomas of the adrenal may represent metastases from occult or regressed primary tumors (Das Gupta et al.).

Fu and colleagues have reported three cases of primary melanocytic tumors of sympathetic ganglia. Ultrastructural studies of one case revealed evidence of true melanogenesis. Clinically, two of the tumors behaved as malignant melanomas. These results support the concept that primary malignant melanomas may arise within sympathetic ganglia and, presumably, within the adrenal medulla (fig. 241). Other melanocytic tumors arising in various derivatives of neural crest have been reported rarely. These include melanotic neurofibroma, melanotic schwannoma, melanotic meningioma, and melanotic medullary thyroid carcinoma. Pigmented ganglioneuroblastomas have also been reported (Hahn).

OTHER TUMORS

Both neurilemomas and neurofibromas have been reported to occur within the adrenal medulla. Some of these tumors may represent ganglioneuromas, with small numbers of ganglion type cells. Lipomas, leiomyomas, osteomas, and angiomas have also been reported to arise within the adrenal. These lesions are discussed in the section on Adrenal Cortex.

References

DasGupta, T. and Brasfield, R. Metastatic melanoma. Cancer 17:1323-1339, 1964.

————, Brasfield, R. D., and Paglia, M. A. Primary melanomas in unusual sites. Surg. Gynecol. Obstet. 128:841-848, 1969.

Fu, Y-S., Kay, G. I., and Lattes, R. Primary malignant melanocytic tumors of the sympathetic ganglia, with ultrastructural study of one. Cancer 36:2029-2041, 1975.

Hahn, J. F., Netsky, M. G., Butler, A. B., and Sperber, E. E. Pigmented ganglioneuroblastoma: relation of melanin and lipofuscin to Schwannomas and other tumors of neural crest origin. J. Neuropathol. Exp. Neurol. 35:393-403, 1976.

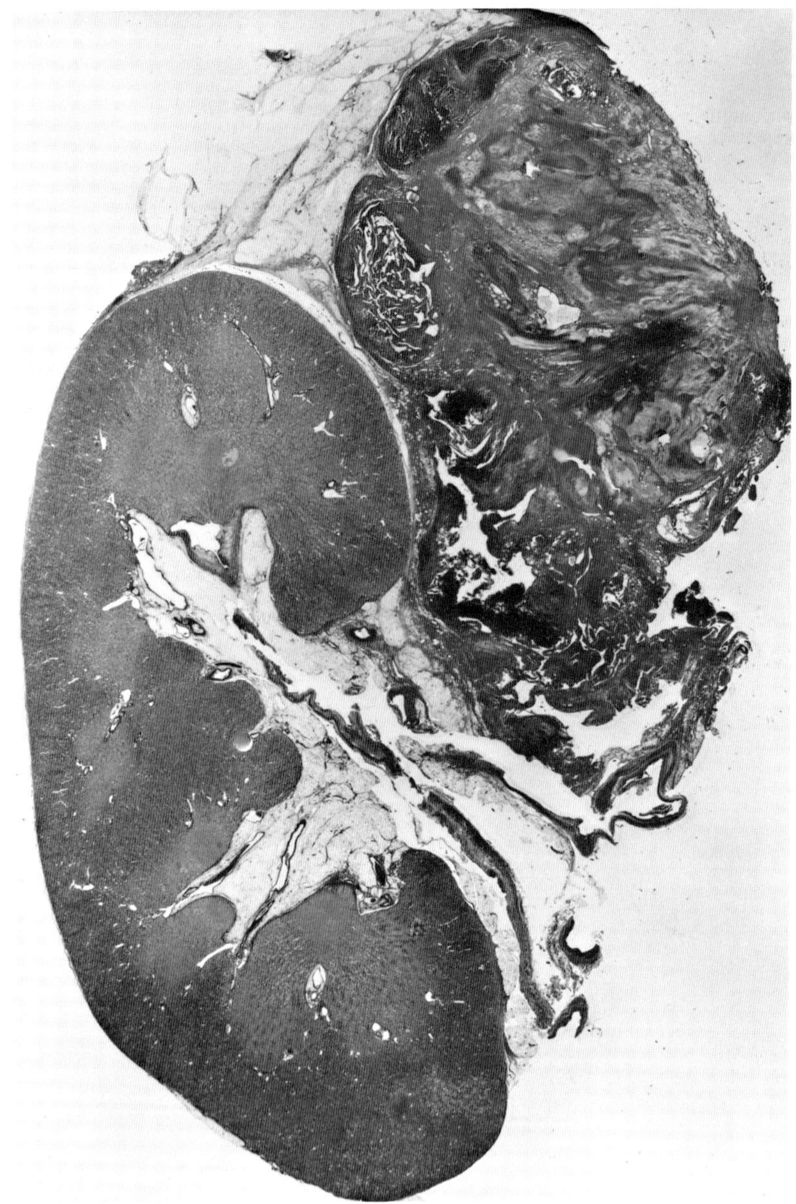

Figure 241
ADRENAL MEDULLA
A large adrenal melanoma was present in a 48 year old man who presented with left lower cervical lymph node metastases. There was no primary cutaneous or mucosal melanoma present nor was there a history of that. The patient expired shortly after operation. This case is probably an example of melanoma primary in the adrenal medulla. X1.2.

INDEX

Note: See Adrenal, Adrenal cortex, or Adrenal medulla for many subjects.